Human Cytogenetics: malignancy and acquired abnormalities

Third Edition

A Practical Approach

Edited by

D. E. Rooney

NE London Regional Cytogenetics Laboratory,
Great Ormond Street Hospital for Children
NHS Trust, Queen Square House,
London WC1N 3BG

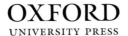

OXFORD
UNIVERSITY PRESS

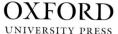

UNIVERSITY PRESS

Great Clarendon Street, Oxford OX2 6DP

Oxford University Press is a department of the University of Oxford.
It furthers the University's objective of excellence in research, scholarship,
and education by publishing worldwide in

Oxford New York

Athens Auckland Bangkok Bogotá Buenos Aires Kolkata Cape Town
Chennai Dar es Salaam Delhi Florence Hong Kong Istanbul Karachi
Kuala Lumpur Madrid Melbourne Mexico City Mumbai Nairobi Paris
São Paulo Shanghai Singapore Taipei Tokyo Toronto Warsaw

with associated companies in Berlin Ibadan

Oxford is a registered trade mark of Oxford University Press in the UK and
in certain other countries

Published in the United States by Oxford University Press Inc., New York

First edition published 1986
Reprinted 1987
Second edition published 1992
Third edition published 2001

A catalogue record for this title is available from
the British Library

Library of Congress Cataloguing in Publication Data
(Data available)

1 3 5 7 9 10 8 6 4 2

ISBN 0 19 963842 X (Hbk.)
ISBN 0 19 963841 1 (Pbk.)

Typeset in Swift by Footnote Graphics, Warminster, Wilts
Printed in Great Britain on acid-free paper
by Bookcraft (Bath) Ltd,
Midsomer Norton, Avon.

Preface

Some of you may still possess a copy or two of the first edition of *Human Cytogenetics: A Practical Approach*. Published in 1986, it included a chapter entitled 'Specialist Techniques in Research and Diagnostic Clinical Cytogenetics' which covered three technologies which, at that time, were considered to be research tools with the potential to impact on diagnostic cytogenetic analysis. Five pages of that chapter were devoted to *in situ* hybridization. By the time the second edition appeared in 1992, *in situ* hybridization occupied a whole chapter comprising 33 pages and part of the meiosis chapter as well as providing a blaze of colour, both inside the volume and on the cover. It is now the year 2000, and FISH as we now call fluorescence *in situ* hybridization is referred to in the majority of the following chapters, occupies two full chapters (one in each volume) and is even more colourful. FISH technology has now been integrated into most cytogenetic laboratories by virtue of commercially prepared kits and the availability of affordable computerized imaging systems.

This pretty much says it all regarding the evolution of cytogenetics over the last 14 years or so, and this new edition of *Human Cytogenetics* has been extensively revised to include the up-to-date technologies and applications of FISH both to diagnostic and research cytogenetics. However, despite these exciting advances, the new millennium sees us still sitting at the microscope analysing G-banded chromosomes, having grown our cells and stained our chromosomes by hand. Automated cell harvesters are with us, but have not replaced us entirely, and the gardening, cookery and 'jiggery-pokery' aspects of practical cytogenetics remain. Chapters dealing with these traditional cytogenetic methodologies have been updated, and 'freshened up' where necessary, with an emphasis on safety issues in the protocols.

I have greatly appreciated all comments, reviews and general feedback over the years. However, the greatest satisfaction is always the sight of faded, dog-eared and generally well-used copies of the previous editions lying around on desks in laboratories I have visited. I can only say that if in a year's time or so I start to see this new edition in the same state, I shall be well pleased.

13 April 2000   DER

Contents

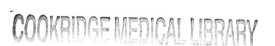

Protocol list

Abbreviations

aCML	atypical CML
AILD	angioimmunoblastic T-cell lymphoma
ALCL	anaplastic large cell lymphoma
ALL	acute lymphoblastic leukaemia
AMCA	aminomethylcoumarin acetic acid
AML	acute myeloid leukaemia
AP	acid phosphatase
APES	3'aminopropyl trieth oxysilane
APAAP	alkaline phosphatase anti-alkaline phosphatase
APML	acute promyelocytic leukaemia
A-T	Ataxia telangiectasia
ATL/L	adult T-cell lymphoma/leukaemia
ATRA	all-*trans* retinoic acid
BAC	bacterial artificial chromosome
B-CLL	B-cell chronic lymphocytic leukaemia
Bio	biotin
BMT	bone marrow transplant
BrdU	5-bromo-2'-deoxyuridine
BS	Bloom Syndrome
BSA	bovine serum albumin
CALLA	common acute lymphoblastic leukaemia antigen
CCD	charged coupled device
cDNA	complementary DNA
CGH	comparative genomic hybridization
CGL	chronic granulocytic leukaemia
cIgμ	cytoplasmic immunoglobulin μ-chain
CLL	chronic lymphocytic leukaemia
CLL/PL	CLL, mixed type
CML	chronic myeloid leukaemia
CMML	chronic myelomonocytic leukaemia
CNS	central nervous system
CR	complete remission
Cyt B	cytochalasin B

DAPI   4′,6-diamidino-2-phenylindole
DEB   diepoxybutane = 1,3 butadiene diepoxide
D-FISH   double-fusion FISH
Dig   digoxigenin
DLBCL   diffuse large B-cell lymphoma
dmin   double minute
DMSO   dimethyl sulphoxide
DNA   deoxyribonucleic acid
DOP-PCR   degenerate oligonucleotide primer-polymerase chain reaction
DTT   dithiothreitol
EBV   Epstein–Barr virus
ET   essential thrombocythaemia
FA   Fanconi anaemia
FAB   French–American–British
FBS   fetal bovine serum
FCS   fetal calf serum
FdU   fluorodeoxyuridine
FISH   fluorescence *in situ* hybridization
FITC   fluorescein isothiocyanate
FPG   fluorescence plus Giemsa
HBSS   Hanks' balanced salt solution
HN2   mustine hydrochloride = nitrogen mustard
hsr   homogeneously staining region
IRS   interspersed repetitive sequences
ISCN   International Standing Committee on Human Cytogenetic Nomenclature
kb   kilobase
LGL   large cell granular lymphocyte leukaemia
LOH   loss of heterozygosity
LPL   lympho-plasmacytoid lymphoma
LRF   Leukaemia Research Fund
MALT   mucosal associated lymphoid tissues
Mb   megabase
MDS   myelodysplastic syndrome
MF   myelofibrosis
M-FISH   multiplex fluorescence *in situ* hybridization
MI   mitotic index
MIC   Morphology–Immunology–Cytogenetics
MIC-M   Morphology, Immunophenotyping, Cytogenetics, Molecular genetic analysis
MMC   mitomycin C
MPD   myeloproliferative disease
MPO   myeloperoxidase
mRNA   messenger RNA
MTX   methotrexate
NHL   non-Hodgkin's lymphomas
NK   natural killer

NSE	non-specific esterase
PAC	P1 artificial chromosome
PAS	periodic acid–Schiff reaction
PBS	phosphate buffered saline
PCD	premature centromere division
PCL	plasma cell leukaemia
PCR	polymerase chain reaction
Ph	Philadelphia chromosome
PHA	phytohaemagglutinin
PI	propidium iodide
PLL	prolymphocytic leukaemia
PMA	4-phorbol-12-myristate-13-acetate
PPE	personal protective equipment
PRV	polycythaemia rubra vera
PWM	pokeweed mitogen
RA	refractory anaemia
RAEB	refractory anaemia with excess blasts
RAEBt	RAEB in transformation
RARS	refractory anaemia with ringed sideroblasts
RBC	red blood cells
REAL	revised European–American Classification of Lymphoid Neoplasms
RFLP	restriction fragment length polymorphism
RMD	region of minimal deletion
RNA	ribonucleic acid
RT-PCR	reverse transcriptase PCR
SBB	Sudan black B
SCE	sister chromatid exchange/s
SDS	sodium dodecyl sulphate
S-FISH	single-fusion FISH
SKY	spectral karyotyping
SLVL	splenic lymphoma with villous lymphocytes
SmIg	surface membrane immunoglobulin
SSC	standard saline citrate
TAM	transient abnormal myelopoiesis
TPA	12-0 tetradecanocylphorbol-13-acetate
T-PLL	T-cell prolymphocytic leukaemia
UKCCG	UK Cancer Cytogenetics Group
WHO	World Health Organization
YAC	yeast artificial chromosome

Chapter 1

Basic techniques for the preparation and analysis of chromosomes from bone marrow and leukaemic blood

B. Czepulkowski

King's College Hospital Cytogenetics Department, The Rayne Institute, 123, Coldharbour Lane, London SE5 9NU, UK

1 Introduction

This chapter is the first of five covering all aspects of the cytogenetic study of the leukaemias and related disorders. It serves to provide basic and general information on the culture, staining and analysis of the tissues normally used for such studies, namely bone marrow and peripheral blood. Protocols for the use of other sample types such as lymph node and solid tumour tissue, and further techniques specific to particular disease types are provided in subsequent chapters.

DNA technology plays a major role in the detection of chromosomal alterations which occur in malignant cells, particularly subtle rearrangements that cannot be detected by non-molecular techniques, or changes which occur at a molecular level. This technology is a necessary part of the arsenal for the haematological cytogeneticist, and a brief summary of how it is used to complement existing non-molecular techniques is therefore included.

Throughout this volume, a basic understanding and expertise of sterile technique, tissue culture, and general karyotype analysis is assumed. The inexperienced should refer to Human Cytogenetics: constitutional analysis, where these topics are dealt with in greater detail.

Some cytogeneticists may be unfamiliar with some of the haematological terms used throughout this book, so the reader is referred to a helpful glossary of terms commonly encountered when dealing with oncological material (Appendix 4). It is recommended that the novice haematological cytogeneticist be acquainted with at least some of the principles of haematology and oncology. Such knowledge is essential for the application of appropriate culture regimes to a sample according to the suspected disease type, for the interpretation of results and for effective liaison with the clinician dealing with the patient's management (1–4).

1.1 Safety considerations

Appendix 2 provides a brief overview of basic safety considerations for the cytogeneticist. General safety regulations, such as forbiddance of eating, drinking and smoking in the laboratory, as well as accident procedure and record keeping, are assumed to be in place (5,6). *Croner's Laboratory Manager* (7) is a useful source of information.

2 Cell culture techniques

2.1 Culture of bone marrow aspirates

Bone marrow is the tissue of choice for the cytogenetic study of most haematological conditions. Exceptions to this are CGL (see Chapter 2) and CLL, where a blood sample is more appropriate because of the high white cell count, since chronic disorders are extremely hypercellular, and even the most dilute sample can overgrow and subsequently fail. In the case of lymphomas, a lymph node biopsy would be more informative than a bone marrow which may not always be involved in the early stages of disease (see Chapter 4). However, occasionally a bone marrow may be taken which can prove informative, particularly if there is some question as to whether bone marrow involvement has occurred.

Bone marrow aspirates from the sternum or posterior iliac crest are usually successful, but occasionally a dry tap may occur, which can be due to the following:

- myelofibrosis, osteosclerosis in myelodysplasia
- secondary myelofibrosis, osteosclerosis in tumours
- compact cellular marrow
- reticulo-endotheliosis
- faulty technique.

In these cases, a peripheral blood can be sent to the laboratory as an alternative, although this will only be of use if blast cells are present in sufficient numbers to detect an abnormal clone. Clotting problems can be encountered when sampling a suspected APML and this may render the sample unsuitable for culture.

2.1.1 Transport of samples

Bone marrow must be heparinized immediately upon aspiration since clotting renders the sample useless for cytogenetic study. Thus, the sample should be transported in a sterile container containing one of the following according to preference:

- 0.3 ml of preservative-free heparin (stock solution 1000 U/ml), or lithium heparin
- 2.0 ml HBSS containing 0.3 ml of heparin as above
- 5 ml transport medium such as that recommended in *Table 1*.

The transport medium is normally discarded following centrifugation, before setting up the sample, and for this it is advantageous if a conical-based tube is used for transport of the bone marrow aspirate. Transport bottles can be supplied to the referring clinician by the laboratory; these should be dated and given an expiry date 1 month ahead, after which the bottle should be discarded. Instructions should also be enclosed informing the clinician of the requirement of storing the transport bottles in the refrigerator prior to use, and prior to dispatch to the laboratory.

It is preferable that the samples are received as soon as possible. If a delay is anticipated, such as that expected when the referring institution is some distance away from the laboratory, then the use of transport medium described in *Table 1* is strongly recommended to minimize drying out of the sample and to maintain cell viability.

Inevitably, there will be occasions when samples arrive at inconvenient times for the laboratory, or when some delay occurs in dispatch of samples. In these circumstances, samples should be stored at 4°C overnight, or for no longer than 3 days.

It must be remembered, however, that there may be considerable deterioration of the sample leading to a possible misleading result if normal cells have survived better than abnormal cells. Samples from patients with ALL and samples with high white cell counts are particularly adversely affected by delays. Every effort should therefore be made to ensure that the sample is set up in culture with the minimum delay.

2.1.2 Sample size

Optimum sample size depends, to some extent, on the disease type. A sample size of 1–2 ml is adequate in most cases, although less than this can be acceptable, particularly if the marrow is very cellular (as in the case of CGL, where the

Table 1 Recommended transport medium for bone marrow aspirates

Material	Stock solution	Volume (ml)
Basal medium (e.g. McCoy's 5A or RPMI 1640)	1×	100.0
Penicillin solution	10 000 IU/ml	1.0
Streptomycin solution	10 000 μg/ml	1.0
Preservative free heparin	1000 U/ml	1.0

white count is always raised). It is advisable to ensure that the sample is not the final exudate from the syringe, as this represents the initial tap which will contain a large number of erythrocytes.

2.1.3 Optimizing cell density

The optimum cell density for a bone marrow culture is 10^6 cells/ml. Although a cell density lower than this can yield adequate results, a culture containing significantly higher cell density is much more likely to fail. It is therefore essential to the success of the culture that the cell density is optimized, and this is most accurately achieved by performing a cell count on the sample as it is received. The simplest way of doing this is to use a haemocytometer, as described in *Protocol 1*. Alternatively, a Coulter counter could be employed, although a diluted aliquot of bone marrow must be used to prevent clogging the apparatus. Some laboratories rely on 'educated guesswork' to assess cell density based on the suspected diagnosis and the appearance of the sample. If guesswork is relied upon, the amount of blood present in the sample should be considered, as blood generally does not contain a large number of blasts (particularly in MDS) so a bloody sample should not automatically be considered as hypercellular. Hypercellularity is less common in AML than ALL but is a usual symptom of CGL. A range of cell densities should be attempted in the case of CGL, erring on the side of more rather than less dilution. In CGL patients receiving chronic phase therapy, hypercellularity is less extreme, and in blood samples at least, non-dividing granulocytes may be a major component of white cell excess, sometimes necessitating long term culture (3–4 days) to achieve an adequate mitotic index (MI).

Protocol 1

Counting cells with a haemocytometer

Equipment and reagents

- Class 1 or 2 microbiological safety cabinet
- Haemocytometer
- Medium (unsupplemented, e.g. McCoy's 5A)
- Graduated pipette, plastic, 10 ml

Method

1 Take 0.1 ml of the sample (either undiluted or diluted with medium according to the method of transport) and dilute to 2 ml using a graduated pipette.

2 Add 1 drop of this diluted suspension to each side of the slide of the haemocytometer.

3 Count the cells in the four outer corner squares.

4 Divide this total by four to obtain the average number of cells per square. This gives a number of cells $\times 10^4$.

Protocol 1 continued

5 Multiply this total by 20 to correct for the initial dilution. This gives the number of cells per millilitre of the original suspension.

6 Adjust the final concentration of cells to 10^6/ml per culture.

Table 2 gives appropriate dilutions of samples after obtaining a cell count on the Coulter counter.

2.1.4 Bone marrow culture regimes

A recommended complete medium is shown in *Table 3*. Basal media in common use for bone marrow culture are RPMI 1640, Ham's F10, Iscove's and McCoy's 5A.

A variety of culture vessels are used by different laboratories. In general, it appears that bone marrow cultures grow best when there is a large surface area and for this reason some laboratories use 25-cm^2 tissue culture flasks. The

Table 2 Dilution of samples after obtaining a cell count on the Coulter counter to obtain a final concentration of 10^6cells/ml[a]

Coulter counter reading for sample provided ($\times 10^6$/ml)	Volume of sample to add to tissue culture medium (ml)	Volume of tissue culture medium (ml)
1	Maximum possible 3–4	Maximum possible 3–4
5	1	4
10	0.5	4.5
15	0.33	4.67
20	0.25	4.75
50	0.1	5
100	0.05	5
200	0.025	5
500	0.01	5
1000	0.005	5

[a]This table was kindly supplied by B. Gibbons, North-east London Regional Cytogenetics Laboratory, Great Ormond Street Children's Hospital NHS Trust, London.

Table 3 Recommended complete culture medium for bone marrow culture

Material	Stock solution	Volume (ml)
Basal medium (e.g. McCoy's 5A or RPMI 1640)	1×	100.0
Fetal calf serum[a]	1×	20.0
L-Glutamine	200 mM (100×)	1.0
Penicillin solution	10 000 IU/ml	1.0
Streptomycin solution	10 000 µg/ml	1.0

[a]A low serum wash medium for releasing the block in synchronized cultures can be made as above but by reducing the serum concentration to 5%.

disadvantage of using these vessels is that the culture has to be transferred into conical-bottomed tubes for harvesting which may result in a loss of cells and is an extra step in the procedure which could be avoided. A useful compromise is to use flat-sided Leighton tubes, where the sample can be cultured and also harvested without transfer of bone marrow material. If these are not available, Universal containers can be used, although harvesting should be performed using conical-based tubes.

The selection of culture regimes is, to some extent, a matter of preference and experience, but in some cases is directly related to the disease being investigated. This is particularly important in the case of known or suspected APML, where the diagnostic t(15;17) translocation may only be detected in cultures of 24 h or longer. Further guidance on selection of appropriate culture regimes according to disease type can be found in subsequent chapters.

2.1.4.1 Unsynchronized cultures

There are three approaches to the unsynchronized culture:

- direct
- short term (usually 24 h)
- overnight with colcemid.

Protocol 2 summarizes the three culture regimes.

Protocol 2

Unsynchronized bone marrow culture

Equipment and reagents

As for *Protocol 9* plus:

- Class 1 or 2 microbiological safety cabinet
- Incubator, 37°C
- Culture tubes e.g. flat-sided culture tubes (Nunc)
- Graduated pipettes, plastic, 10 ml
- Automatic pipette filler
- Complete culture medium (*Table 3*)
- Colcemid[a] working solution 10 µg/ml

Method

1 Centrifuge the sample at 200 **g** for 10 min and remove the transport medium from the pelleted bone marrow using a graduated pipette fixed to an automatic pipette filler.

2 Add 5 ml of complete culture medium to the number of culture vessels required.

3 Seed with an appropriate amount of bone marrow to give a final concentration of 10^6 cells/ml (See *Table 2*).

4 For direct cultures add 0.1 ml of colcemid immediately to give a final concentration of 0.02 µg/ml and incubate at 37°C for 1 h. For short term cultures incubate at 37°C

Protocol 2 continued

overnight; the following morning add colcemid as above and incubate for 1-3 h. For overnight with colcemid cultures add colcemid as above as late in the afternoon as possible, and incubate at 37 °C overnight.

5   Harvest cultures using *Protocol 9*.

[a] Caution: colcemid is toxic, a chronic poison and a possible teratogen. It is harmful by ingestion, inoculation and skin contact.

2.1.4.2 Synchronized cultures

Cell division can be blocked at various points in the cell cycle and subsequently released at a controlled time, producing synchronization of cell division. This enables colcemid exposure to be greatly reduced, consequently giving longer chromosomes than produced by unsynchronized cultures. However, despite the fact that one would expect a bottleneck of cells awaiting release, and possible large numbers of cells in division, MI is normally reduced, probably owing to the toxicity of the substances involved. The precise mechanisms are subject to debate, but practically these techniques have found great application in haematological cytogenetics. Three blocking agents have been found to be effective in bone marrow cultures:

- MTX
- FdU
- FdU and BrdU used in conjunction with one another.

2.1.4.2.1 Methotrexate synchronization

This technique has occasionally been found to be detrimental when used in the culture of bone marrow from patients with known or suspected ALL, and occasionally in high white cell count CMLs. Since the length of the cell cycle of the various cell types involved in malignancy is unpredictable, the timing of MTX treatment often requires some experimentation. *Protocol 3* describes a general method, but it is advisable to set up duplicate cultures, where possible, with different MTX timings.

Protocol 3

Synchronization of bone marrow cultures with MTX

Equipment and reagents

As for *Protocols 2* and *9* plus:

- MTX[a] working solution (final concentration 10^{-7} M)
- Low-serum culture medium (*Table 3*)
- Thymidine[b] working solution: 1.2 μg/10 ml = final concentration 10^{-5} M

Protocol 3 continued

Method

1   Set up a bone marrow culture as described in *Protocol 2*, steps 1–3.

2   Incubate at 37°C for 3 h to enable the cells to acclimatize to their environment prior to the addition of MTX.

3   Add 0.1 ml of MTX and incubate at 37°C for 14–17 h.

4   Centrifuge the culture tube at 200 **g** for 5 min. Discard the supernatant and add 5 ml of low-serum medium to wash the cells.

5   Centrifuge the culture tube at 200 **g** for 5 min.

6   Remove the supernatant and add 5 ml of low-serum medium.

7   Add 0.1 ml of thymidine and incubate at 37°C for 5–7 h.

8   Add 0.1 ml of colcemid to give a final concentration of 0.02 μg/ml for the final 15 min of culture time.

9   Harvest using *Protocol 9*.

[a] Caution: MTX is cytotoxic, may be a mutagen and cause reproductive disorders. It is harmful by ingestion, inhalation and skin contact. It may harm the unborn child.

[b] Caution: thymidine is toxic and harmful by ingestion, inhalation and skin contact.

2.1.4.2.2 FdU synchronization

Protocol 4 describes a technique based on that reported by Webber and Garson (8). It is thought that FdU is less toxic to the cells than MTX since it acts at only one point in the cell cycle as opposed to the several points blocked by MTX. It is therefore more suitable for cases of known or suspected ALL and also high white cell count CGL.

Protocol 4

Synchronization of bone marrow cultures with FdU

Equipment and reagents

As for *Protocols 2* and *9* plus:

- FdU[a] working solution:12.3 μg/10 ml = final concentration 0.1 μM
- Uridine[b] working solution: 0.488 mg/10 ml = final concentration 4 μM
- Thymidine[c] working solution:1.2 μg/10 ml = final concentration 10 μM

Method

1   Set up a bone marrow culture as in *Protocol 2*, steps 1–3.

2   Incubate at 37°C for 2–3 h to acclimatize cells prior to FdU addition. This step is optional if time is limited.

Protocol 4 continued

3 Add 0.1 ml FdU and 0.1 ml uridine[d] to the culture

4 Incubate at 37 °C for 14–17 h.

5 Add 0.1 ml thymidine[e].

6 Incubate at 37°C for 5–7 h.

7 Add 0.1 ml colcemid to give a final concentration of 0.05 μg/ml for the final 15 min of culture.

8 Harvest using *Protocol 9*.

[a] Caution: FdU is toxic, a chronic poison and a possible teratogen. It is harmful by ingestion, inoculation and skin contact.

[b] Caution: uridine is toxic and harmful by ingestion, inoculation and skin contact.

[c] Caution: see *Protocol 3* for risk information.

[d] Excess uridine ensures that RNA does not incorporate fluorodylate which may be formed from FdU (9).

[e] Note that unlike the MTX procedure, there is no necessity to wash the cells free of the blocking agent.

2.1.4.2.3 *Synchronization with a BrdU/FdU cocktail*

Protocol 5 describes our own adaptation of a BrdU synchronization method (10) using a cocktail of BrdU and FdU. Of all the synchronization methods available, the best results have been obtained with the method below.

Protocol 5

Synchronization of bone marrow cultures using a BrdU/FdU cocktail

As for *Protocols 2* and *9* plus:

- Incubator, 37°C
- Aluminium foil
- FdU[a] working solution (final concentration 4×10^{-3} M): 10 mg in 10 ml distilled water (Solution A)
- Uridine[a] working solution (final concentration 3×10^{-3} M): 10 mg in 10 ml distilled water (Solution B)
- Low-serum medium (*Table 3*)

- BrdU[b] working solution (final concentration 10^{-1} M): 30 mg plus 0.1 ml Solution A, 2 ml of Solution B and make up to 10 ml of distilled water
- Thymidine[a] working solution (final concentration 10^{-3} M) 2.5 mg in 10 ml of distilled water

Method

1 Set up a bone marrow culture as described in *Protocol 2*, steps 1–3.

2 Add 0.1 ml of the FdU–BrdU–uridine mixture.

Protocol 5 continued

3 Protect the cultures from light by wrapping in aluminium foil and incubate at 37 °C for 14–17 h.

4 Centrifuge the culture tube at 200 **g** for 10 min. Remove the supernatant.

5 Resuspend the pellet in 5 ml of low-serum medium.

6 Centrifuge the culture tube at 200 **g** for 10 min. Remove the supernatant.

7 Resuspend the cell pellet in 5 ml of low-serum medium and add 0.1 ml thymidine.

8 Incubate the culture tube at 37 °C for 5–7 h.

9 Add 0.1 ml of colcemid, to give a final concentration of 0.02 μg/ml for the final 15 min of culture.

10 Harvest using *Protocol 9*.

[a] Caution: see *Protocol 4* for risk information.

[b] Caution: BrdU is cytotoxic and may be a mutagen and cause reproductive disorders. It is harmful by ingestion, inoculation and skin contact. It affects the immune system and may harm the unborn child.

2.2 Peripheral blood culture

Peripheral blood can be used to study the cytogenetics of malignant conditions only if dividing leukaemic cells are present. A blood sample is required if the constitutional karyotype is to be checked. A constitutional change can be suspected if a novel rearrangement is observed which does not correspond to any of the known abnormalities associated with the disease type being studied, or when all the cells contain the same balanced abnormality.

Transport medium is not necessary for blood samples and can be detrimental to the sample in transit. Blood should be transported in a bottle containing 0.3 ml of preservative-free heparin, or alternatively a lithium heparin bottle may also be acceptable (N.B. not the beaded type of lithium heparin, as this appears to adversely affect the blood sample in transit and subsequent cultures often fail to grow).

All protocols used for bone marrow samples may be applied to unstimulated peripheral blood cultures. However, mitogens can be added to stimulate the proliferation of lymphocytes, where appropriate. Mitogens are employed in the cytogenetic study of malignancy when lymphoid diseases are known or suspected to be of B or T cell type, and are discussed further in Chapter 4. The T cell lymphocyte mitogen PHA is used for the investigation of constitutional karyotype.

The culture medium described in *Table 3* can also be used for blood culture.

2.2.1 White cell count

A Coulter counter is normally used to obtain a white cell count from a blood sample. If this apparatus is not available, then the cell counting method described in *Protocol 1* should be used.

Protocol 2 can be applied to unstimulated blood culture with a white cell count in the range of 4–$10 \times 10^9/l$ (adults). If the white cell count is significantly greater than this, it is advantageous to separate the white cells from the other blood components as described in *Protocol 6*.

Protocol 6

Separation of white cells from whole blood

Equipment and reagents

- Class 1 or 2 microbiological safety cabinet
- Universal containers, plastic 30 ml
- 1 ml Syringe without a needle or siliconized Pasteur pipette
- Graduated pipettes (plastic 10 ml)
- Lymphocyte separation medium (e.g. Ficoll-Hypaque or lymphoprep, Pharmacia)
- PBS or serum-free RPMI
- Complete culture medium (*Table 3*)

Method

1 Place 10 ml[a] lymphocyte separation medium into a sterile Universal container.

2 Layer 10 ml[a] fresh heparinized blood onto the surface by gently running the blood down the side of the inclined container with a pipette.

3 Centrifuge the Universal container at 700 **g** for 20 min. The red cells will settle into a pellet at the bottom of the tube leaving the white cells in a layer between the separation medium and the serum.

4 Carefully remove the white cells with a siliconized Pasteur pipette or a 1 ml syringe without a needle. Ensure that as little of the separation medium as possible is taken with these cells.

5 Place the cells in a fresh container and add 10 ml PBS or serum-free medium.

6 Centrifuge the container at 450 **g** for 10 min.

7 Remove the supernatant and resuspend in 10 ml PBS or serum-free medium.

8 Centrifuge the container at 150 **g** for 10 min.

9 Resuspend the cells in culture medium and count using *Protocol 1*.

10 Set up cultures at a final concentration of 10^6 cells/ml.

[a] These volumes can be adjusted according to the amount of blood available, but generally the amount of lymphocyte separation medium is equal to the amount of blood used.

2.3 Stimulated blood culture for constitutional karyotype analysis

If confirmation of an obvious chromosome rearrangement is required, the simple culture method given in *Protocol 7* will produce adequate preparations. However, if a more subtle rearrangement is suspected, chromosomes for higher resolution banding are obtained by using the synchronization method described in *Protocol 8*. This 'thymidine-block' method does not produce good results with bone marrow and should only be applied to blood cultures.

Protocol 7

Stimulated blood culture for constitutional analysis

Equipment and reagents

As for *Protocol 9* plus:

- Class 1 or 2 microbiological safety cabinet
- Incubator, 37°C
- Culture tubes, e.g. 30 ml plastic universal or flat-sided culture tube
- Automatic pipette filler
- Pipettes, plastic 10 ml
- Complete culture medium (*Table 3*)
- PHA[a] (reconstitute vial with 10 ml distilled water)
- Colcemid[b] working solution (as *Protocol 2*)

Method

1 Add 0.5 ml of heparinized blood or an appropriate amount of separated cell suspension to 5 ml culture medium.

2 Add 0.2 ml PHA.

3 Incubate at 37°C for 72 h.

4 Add 0.1 ml colcemid to give a final concentration of 0.02 μg/ml for 1–2 h.

5 Harvest using *Protocol 9*.

[a] Caution: PHA is a T lymphocyte mitogen. It is toxic and harmful by ingestion and inhalation.

[b] Caution: see *Protocol 2* for risk information.

Protocol 8

Synchronized blood lymphocyte culture using a thymidine block

Equipment and reagents

As for *Protocols 7* and *9* plus:

- Class 1 or 2 microbiological safety cabinet
- Thymidine[a] working solution: 1 g in 67 ml PBS

Method

1 Set up blood cultures as in *Protocol 7*, steps 1 and 2.

2 Incubate at 37°C for 48 h.

3 Add 0.1 ml thymidine working solution to the culture tube and incubate for a further 16 h.

4 Centrifuge the culture tube at 200 **g** for 8 min.

5 Remove the supernatant and resuspend the blood in 7 ml prewarmed PBS.

Protocol 8 continued

6 Centrifuge the culture tube at 200 *g* for 8 min.

7 Remove the supernatant and resuspend the blood in approximately 7 ml pre-warmed culture medium. Incubate at 37 °C for 3 h and 45 min.

8 Add 0.1 ml colcemid to give a final concentration of 0.05 μg/ml for a further 15 min of incubation.

9 Harvest using *Protocol 9*.

[a] Caution: see *Protocol 4* for risk information.

2.4 Harvest and slide-preparation of bone marrow and blood cultures

2.4.1 Harvest

The harvesting of bone marrow and blood cultures is described in *Protocol 9*.

Protocol 9

Harvest of bone marrow and blood cultures

Equipment and reagents

- Class 1 or 2 microbiological safety cabinet
- Graduated pipettes, plastic, 10 ml
- 0.075 M KCl (5.5 g in 1 l of distilled water). The solution should be prewarmed to 37°C in the incubator
- Disposable plastic pipettes, 1 ml
- Fixative: absolute methanol[a]–glacial acetic acid,[b] 3:1, freshly prepared and placed in the freezer prior to use

Method

1 Following colcemid treatment (*Protocol 8*, step 8), centrifuge the culture tube at 200 *g* for 10 min.

2 Remove the supernatant using a plastic disposable pipette and resuspend the cell pellet in 5–7 ml KCl solution for 10 min at 37 °C (blood) or 15 min (bone marrow).[c]

3 Following incubation, add a few drops of chilled fixative, mixing well.

4 Centrifuge the culture tube at 200 *g* for 10 min.

5 Remove the supernatant leaving a small amount just above the pellet. Gently tap the centrifuge tube to resuspend the cell pellet in the remaining supernatant.

6 Carefully add chilled fixative a few drops at a time, initially, with constant agitation to avoid clumps forming. If clumps do start to form, mix the cell suspension thoroughly with a disposable plastic pipette. Add further fixative to the tube (to three-quarters full).

7 Centrifuge the culture tube at 200 *g* for 10 min.

8 Remove the supernatant and replenish with fresh fixative, agitating the tube to obtain an even cell suspension.

Protocol 9 continued

9 Repeat steps 7 and 8 a further three times.

10 Prepare slides as in *Protocol 10*, or alternatively store the cell suspension at −20°C until slide preparation is required.

[a] Caution: methanol is highly flammable and toxic by inhalation.

[b] Caution: glacial acetic acid causes severe burns and is harmful in contact with the skin.

[c] Although the time of this treatment may vary according to cell type, cells should not be left in KCl for more than 20 min, as this may be detrimental to chromosome morphology.

2.4.2 Slide preparation

There are many different methods of preparing slides and each laboratory has a favourite technique. The aim is to produce well-spread chromosomes which remain as intact metaphase spreads. Any shortcomings in technique will either produce chromosomes that overlap with one another in a tangle (under-spreading) or metaphase spreads containing less than the complete modal number (over-spreading). An extreme case of over-spreading will appear on the slide as 'chromosome soup' with chromosomes having been scattered across the slide.

With practice, spreading stimulated blood chromosomes is simple. Bone marrow chromosomes, and to some extent unstimulated blood cultures, however, can be difficult to spread. *Protocol 10* outlines a method which should overcome even the most stubborn of cases. Spreading methods are also provided in Human Cytogenetics: constitutional analysis, Chapter 2.

Protocol 10

Slide preparation

Equipment and reagents

- Disposable Pasteur pipettes, plastic, 1 ml
- Forceps
- Slide rack (optional)
- Hotplate and/or oven at 70°C

- Fixative[a] (as *Protocol 9*)
- Microscope slides. Thoroughly clean the slides either by sonication or in methanol. Store in distilled water at 4°C prior to use (bone marrows) or 60°C (bloods)

Method

1 If the cell suspension has been stored at −20°C, apply steps 2 and 3. If the cell suspension has been freshly prepared, proceed directly to step 4.

2 Centrifuge the culture tube at 200 **g** for 10 min, remove the supernatant and replenish with fresh fixative.

3 Centrifuge the culture tube at 200 **g** for 10 min and remove the supernatant to just above the cell pellet.

Protocol 10 continued

4 Add a few drops of fixative to the pellet (approximately 0.5 ml, depending on the size of the pellet).[b]

5 Hold a wet slide horizontally with forceps and drop the cell suspension at each end of the slide to give a total of two drops from a Pasteur pipette held just above the slide.

6 Label the frosted glass on the slide with a pencil. Wipe the excess water from the back of the slide and immediately place upon a hotplate at approximately 70 °C (60 °C for blood cultures).

7 Either leave the slides to dry on the hotplate overnight, or put into a slide rack and place in an oven at 60 °C overnight.

[a] Caution: see *Protocol 9* for risk information.

[b] This does vary a great deal; occasionally, with a very low cell count as found in patients with pancytopenia, it may only be possible to produce one slide from the culture. In such cases, the supernatant should be taken down as far as possible without disturbing the pellet, and one slide made from the remaining mixture.

3 Banding methods

All banding techniques can be applied to bone marrow and leukaemic blood chromosomes; these are described in detail in Human Cytogenetics: constitutional analysis, Chapter 4.

Chromosomes prepared from malignant cells are particularly sensitive to various treatments involved in G-banding and chromosome morphology can often be fuzzy, with indistinct bands. *Protocol 12* gives a G-banding technique which has been modified for use with malignant chromosomes using Leishman's stain (*Protocol 11*), which appears to produce sharper banding than Giemsa stain.

Protocol 11

Preparation of Leishman's stain

Equipment and reagents

- Fume hood
- Conical flask, glass, 2 l
- Filter funnel
- Filter paper (24 cm filter speed medium fast—Qualitative 1) (Whatman)
- Hotplate 70 °C
- Parafilm (or aluminium foil)
- Universal containers, 30 ml
- Methanol (absolute, Analar grade, BDH)[a]
- Leishman's stain powder[b]

Method

1 Add 0.3 g powdered Leishman's stain to 200 ml methanol in a conical flask. This should be done gradually, preferably in a fume hood, agitating the flask periodically, to ensure that the stain is completely dissolved.

Protocol 11 continued

2   Cover the neck of the conical flask with Parafilm or aluminium foil and leave on a hotplate overnight at 70 °C.

3   Filter the solution through two layers of filter paper into sterile Universal containers, or as appropriate.[c,d]

4   Store in a dark cupboard.

[a] Caution: see *Protocol 9* for risk information.

[b] Caution: Leishman's stain powder is harmful by ingestion, inhalation and skin contact.

[c] Small aliquots are preferable to large ones as the staining power of Leishman's decreases with exposure to air.

[d] Caution: complete Leishman's stain will have the same risks as methanol. See *Protocol 9* for risk information.

Protocol 12

G-banding

Equipment and reagents

- Coplin jars
- Absorbent paper towels
- Forceps
- Hotplate, 70 °C
- Coverslips (64 × 24 mm, No. 1 1/2)
- Staining rack for horizontal staining
- Buffer, pH 6.8, prepared from Gurr's buffer tablets (Merck)
- Leishman's stain[a] prepared as *Protocol 11*. Use freshly prepared diluted 1:5 with buffer, pH 6.8

- 10 ml syringe with plastic quill for applying stain
- Saline solution: 8.5 g of NaCl in 1 l of distilled water
- Trypsin solution:[b] reconstitute a vial of Bacto-trypsin (Becton Dickinson) with 10 ml deionized water
- Glacial acetic acid (in a plastic wash bottle)[c]
- Absolute methanol (in a plastic wash bottle)[c]
- DPX or Xam mountant[d] (Merck)

Method

1   Prepare the following Coplin jars in the order given:
   (a) 1–2 ml trypsin solution in 50 ml saline solution.
   (b) 50 ml saline solution
   (c) two Coplin jars of 50 ml buffer, pH 6.8
   (d) 50 ml distilled water
   (e) 50 ml buffer, pH 6.8 (for diluting Leishman's stain).

2   Stain the slide horizontally with buffered Leishman's stain for 1 min.[e]

3   Dry the slide on a hotplate and then destain by flushing first with glacial acetic acid, by holding the slide tipped downwards with forceps and washing into the sink, and

Protocol 12 continued

then with methanol.[f] Keep the tap water running while washing the slides to drain away excess acetic acid and methanol.

4 Dry the slide on a hotplate then dip into the Coplin jar of trypsin for 20–50 s (depending on the preparation).

5 Rinse the slide in the Coplin jar containing saline.

6 Rinse the slide in the Coplin jar containing buffer, pH 6.8.

7 Stain the slide horizontally for 1 min with buffered Leishman's stain.

8 Rinse the slide in the second jar of buffer, pH 6.8.

9 Finally rinse the slide in the distilled water jar.

10 Mount a coverslip on the wet slide to allow examination of banding. This enables further re-banding if necessary. It must be remembered that the banding will not look as crisp and clear under water as it would in mountant, and hence the examination is only a rough guide to the quality.[g]

11 If banding has been successful, remove the coverslip and dry the slide on a hotplate. If further banding is necessary, repeat the procedure from step 1. Mount the slide with a coverslip using DPX or Xam mountant.

[a] Caution: Leishman's stain contains methanol. See *Protocol 9* for risk information.

[b] Caution: trypsin is an irritant which is harmful by ingestion, inhalation and skin contact.

[c] Caution: see *Protocol 9* for risk information.

[d] Caution: DPX contains xylene, which is highly flammable and toxic.

[e] If the slides are more than 2 days old, steps 2 and 3 can be omitted and the slide can be dipped directly into the trypsin solution.

[f] Caution: acetic acid is corrosive and methanol is easily absorbed through the skin. When flushing the slide, goggles are recommended to avoid splashes into the eyes; gloves are also recommended.

[g] Always be cautious when trying a first batch of slides. Under-band initially if unsure of the optimum trypsin treatment time which again can vary depending upon the conditions and the sample: under-banded slides can be rescued, over-banded slides cannot.

4 Preservation of bone marrow and whole blood for chromosome analysis

During the course of chromosome analysis of patients with haematological disorders, it is sometimes necessary to set up additional cultures.

Samples stored in the refrigerator for long periods degenerate and fail to grow in culture. Long-term preservation of bone marrow and blood samples is advantageous where:

(1) Repeated samples from the same individual are not always possible, as the first sample is taken at diagnosis prior to treatment and would be the sample of interest; subsequent samples of the patient's blood or bone marrow, following treatment, would be depleted of leukaemic cells.

(2) Repeated examination is required to check a translocation or abnormality, or if the original culture failed for any reason; on the second culture, high-resolution techniques could be carried out which were perhaps not possible at the time of sampling.

A simple technique to carry out the preservation of blood or bone marrow cells has been developed (11,12) and is described in *Protocol 13* (kindly supplied by D. M. Lillington, ICRF Department of Medical Oncology, St Bartholomew's Hospital, London, UK.

Protocol 13

Viable cryopreservation of blood and bone marrow

Equipment and reagents

For freezing:

- Cryopreservation bin
- Freezing vials, 1 ml
- Graduated pipettes, 10 ml
- Automatic pipette filler
- Water bath, 37 °C
- Freezing medium: RPMI 1640, FCS and DMSO,[a] 2:2:1
- Serum-free culture medium (neat)

- Liquid nitrogen freezer
- Thick heavy-duty protective gloves[b]
- Eye-shield or visor[b]
  For thawing:
- RPMI 1640 medium, supplemented with 10% FCS, antibiotics, and L-glutamine (See *Table 3* for concentrations)
- Centrifuge tube (10 ml)

Method

A. Freezing

1 Use 1 ml heparinized whole blood or bone marrow suspended in serum-free culture medium to a concentration of 2×10^7 cells or $2{-}10 \times 10^7$ lymphocytes separated as described in *Protocol 6*.

2 To 0.5 ml cell suspension, add 0.5 ml freezing medium drop-wise with continuous agitation. The final concentration to be added to a freezing vial should be $1{-}5 \times 10^7$ cells in 10% DMSO.[c]

3 Cool or freeze cells immediately. Most cryopreservation bins incorporate a mechanism to introduce vials gradually into the liquid nitrogen. Alternatively, any method using intermediate steps of gradual cooling at temperatures from 4 °C to -70 °C can be employed before freezing in liquid nitrogen.

B. Thawing

1 Prepare 30 ml of RPMI 1640 supplemented with 10% FCS per vial to be thawed.

2 Remove a vial from the liquid nitrogen and immediately quick-thaw in a 37 °C water bath or by hand.[d]

3 Transfer the cells to a sterile 10 ml tube using a pipette.

Protocol 13 continued

4 Add a drop of medium with FCS every 10 s for 2 min, then gradually increase the number of drops every 10 s to a total of 5 ml.

5 Top up to 10 ml and centrifuge at 600 **g** for 5 min.

6 Remove the supernatant and wash the cells twice more.

7 Resuspend the cells in 2 ml medium and perform a cell count (*Protocol 1*). Set up cultures in complete medium using the appropriate protocol.

[a] Sterilize the DMSO prior to use by filtering through a 0.2 μm filter.

[b] Gloves and eye shield are recommended for handling liquid nitrogen.

[c] DMSO is toxic to cells at room temperature at this concentration; to minimize the effects of this, vials must be immediately cooled or frozen.

[d] It is advisable to thaw one vial at a time and care must be taken at this stage to maintain viability.

5 General guidelines for analysis

5.1 The detection of abnormal and normal clones

The aim of cytogenetic investigation of malignant and related disorders is to detect any visible chromosome abnormality which may have occurred specifically in the neoplastic cells. These neoplastic cells often coexist with normal cells. Thus, most abnormal cases also show normal metaphases if sufficient cells are examined. Although the presence or definite absence of karyotypically normal cells may be of prognostic significance, the proportion of normal to abnormal cells is subject to both the effects of culture conditions and considerable sampling error. Caution should be exercised if the proportion of normal cells is used to assess clonal growth and regression. However, chromosome abnormalities are not detected in all malignant cells; in some cases, DNA studies show that genetic changes have occurred, but only at a molecular level and so cannot be detected by light microscopy. An example of this is the *BCR/ABL* gene rearrangement in apparently Philadelphia chromosome-negative CGL. Moreover, it is not yet clear whether all neoplastic cells have resulted from genetic rearrangement. In short, the detection of an apparently normal karyotype does not necessarily mean that the cell line from which it derives is itself normal.

This is further complicated by the fact that proliferation of normal cells may be favoured by particular culture regimes or delays in transport of the sample, as discussed previously and detailed in the next three chapters. The final factor influencing the result is the approach to analysis.

The effect of analysis on the detection of chromosomal abnormality in neoplastic cells is dependent on three factors:

- quality of metaphase spreads
- number of spreads analysed
- experience of the cytogeneticist.

5.1.1 Quality of metaphase spreads

The chromosomes of neoplastic cells often seem to have a predisposition to poor morphology and indistinct banding. This observation is undoubtedly more true of ALL cultures than of any other type of leukaemia. However, the abnormal metaphase spreads in myeloid conditions are not, as a rule, markedly inferior, although exceptions do arise. Thus, careful selection of the best metaphase spreads on the slide may bias the analysis towards cells with a normal karyotype. It is therefore of the utmost importance that a representative sample of metaphase spreads of all qualities are analysed. In other words, if there is a mixed population of spreads on the slides, an abnormality is more likely to be found in those of the poorest quality. The point is further discussed and demonstrated in Chapter 3.

5.1.2 The number of metaphase spreads to be analysed

Logically, the more spreads analysed, the greater the chance of detecting an abnormal clone. There are tables which show the number of cells that must be analysed to exclude mosaicism at various confidence limits and these can prove extremely useful (13).

Time and adequate material permitting, 30 cells fully analysed is probably the best criterion to adopt. In practice, a heavy work load often reduces this to between 15 and 20. Less than 10 cells is normally considered an inadequate result, unless of course, an abnormality has been detected. It is common practice for a normal result to be based on examination of 30 cells with a minimum of 10 analysed. Abnormal results can often be confidently determined on fewer than 30 cells, particularly if mosaicism is not an important issue. It is notable that centres claiming higher than average abnormality rates sometimes detect very low levels of mosaicism by virtue of their extensive analysis, which may not be considered practical in current diagnostic laboratories. Extended analysis is warranted, however, if low level mosaicism is anticipated and up to 100 cells could be examined with confidence limits for detecting a small clone given for the benefit of the referring clinician (13). Extended analysis is advisable when cytogenetics is required for confirmation of remission or relapse of acute leukaemia, where a known abnormality is being assessed. Although cytogenetics can be useful for detecting minimal residual disease following extensive examination of the sample, other molecular techniques are probably more useful because of the vast number of cells used in, for example, PCR, which is 100 000 times more sensitive than non-molecular cytogenetic techniques. For patients in treatment trials, there are particular requirements laid down by the organizing body, and the appropriate number of cells should be analysed in these cases.

If a specific abnormality has been identified in 20 cells, it would be acceptable to scan further cells for this without full analysis of the other chromosomes. This approach would also be appropriate where certain clones have already been identified in varying degrees of progression such as t(9;22)/t(9;22),i(17q)/t(9;22),+8,i(17)(q10). In such a case, the proportion of each clone could be established relatively quickly. This is also a good way to determine whether a small number of apparently normal cells coexist with an abnormal clone.

5.1.3 Experience of the cytogeneticist

It would be an omission not to discuss the experience of the cytogeneticist when one is referring to detection of abnormalities. It can take even an experienced cytogeneticist some time to get used to an approach to analysis which requires selection of inferior quality metaphase spreads, as discussed in Section 5.1. It is also a great advantage to have seen the abnormalities previously and to recognize the derivative counterparts in a translocation, as these may exist in a plethora of other changes such as those that occur in MDS transformed or transforming to AML. Familiarity with the appearance of the abnormal chromosomes is of great benefit when untangling the bizarre and complex karyotypes that can occur in certain types of malignant disease. Counting the cells is also most important; it may appear to be obvious, but it is surprising how easy it is to miss something truly simple such as trisomy 8. It is essential to have a checking system overseen by an experienced cytogeneticist specializing in bone marrow analysis. The learning process is always continuous and to recognize all the artefacts that one might come across in this field of work requires a number of years' experience. The more subtle changes may sometimes only be observed by the keen and trained eye and even the most experienced cytogeneticist can make an error. The advent of FISH and other forms of molecular technologies have proved extremely useful in sorting out complex changes or even detecting subtle changes such as the t(12;21) in ALL (see Chapter 3).

5.1.4 The definition of clonal abnormality

By convention laid down by the Fourth International Workshop on Chromosomes in Leukaemia (14), an abnormal clone is said to exist if:

- two or more cells have the same structural abnormality
- two or more cells have acquired the same chromosome (trisomy)
- three or more cells have lost the same chromosome (monosomy).

When chromosome abnormalities occur in single cells, they can virtually be ignored, as random changes do occasionally arise in all types of cells. However, if a single cell shows an abnormality which is known to be associated with a particular disease type (for example t(9;22) in a case of suspected or known CML) one could argue that some information has been obtained. However, a repeat sample, if possible, would be advisable. If the abnormalities remain as single cell findings, they should be reported with an explanation on the report, but will require confirmation before being considered as a genuine abnormal clone. Exceptions to this could be made in the case of a highly specific abnormality such as the t(15;17) in a case of known or suspected APML.

An apparently balanced chromosome rearrangement not commonly associated with the disease type being examined should alert the cytogeneticist to the possibility of a constitutional anomaly. In such cases, it is advisable to study a PHA-stimulated peripheral blood sample.

The interpretation of chromosomal loss must be approached with great caution. The smaller chromosomes, in particular, are often lost as an artefact of spreading. It is important to note whether a particular slide has been subject to over-spreading, with a large number of incomplete metaphase spreads, prior to drawing any conclusions about a particular lost chromosome. If there is any doubt about the significance of an apparent monosomy, it is wise to scan a large number of cells before making any interpretation. Opinion is divided as to the wisdom of reporting presumptive artefactual findings. It is our policy to avoid this since, in our experience, clinicians tend to misconstrue the significance of these anomalies and perpetuate this in the patient's notes. (The same problem arises when innocuous polymorphic variants are reported in constitutional karyotypes.) Once a patient has been erroneously assigned an 'abnormality' it is difficult to rectify the situation.

From the above, it is clear that the detection of abnormality in neoplastic cells is not straightforward and can amount to 'looking for a needle in a haystack'. However, with an educated application of both culture technique and also analysis, the results of haematological cytogenetics can be very rewarding.

6 Complementary techniques in cancer cytogenetics

Karyotype analysis in cancer cytogenetics is sometimes hampered by failure in culture and a paucity or complete absence of metaphase spreads, particularly in cases of severe pancytopenia, and those patients who have been subjected to chemotherapy. In such cases, it is sometimes possible to turn to molecular DNA techniques in order to proceed with the investigation. This is of particular value in the detection of minimal residual disease as many cells can be screened very rapidly. Such technology is also applied to cases where known submicroscopic rearrangements have occurred, such as the t(12;21) in B-lineage childhood ALL. The main approaches are FISH, RFLP/Southern blotting and PCR.

6.1 Fluorescence *in situ* hybridization

This topic is covered in detail in Chapter 6, and also in Human Cytogenetics: constitutional analysis, Chapter 6, so the following information is a simple overview.

FISH is a method of visualizing genetic material. It may be used to

- demonstrate the presence/absence of specific gene sequences on metaphase chromosomes or interphase cells
- indicate genetic rearrangement (including submicroscopic) in metaphase chromosomes or interphase cells
- identify the origin of chromosome material in markers or unbalanced translocation products

The basic principle of FISH is the hybridization of a fluorochrome-labelled DNA 'probe' with a complementary target DNA sequence in cells, tissue sections or metaphase spreads. This is achieved by denaturation of probe and target sequences, hybridization, and washing procedures. A fluorescent counterstain is then applied and the preparation is viewed using a fluorescence microscope with an appropriate set of filters. Specialized microscopic equipment using CCD cameras and computerized image analysis systems for the various FISH technologies are available. Many of the probes and other FISH reagents, together with recommended protocols are commercially available. These kits are generally reliable and simple to use in a busy routine laboratory. A typical kit-based technique is given in *Protocol 3* in Chapter 8.

FISH protocols include the following basic steps:

(a) **Slide pretreatments.** These may include an enzyme treatment to remove proteinaceous material which may interfere with hybridization, dehydration through an ethanol series to 'age' the cells and SSC washes to clean the preparation, and to render chromosomes less sensitive to over-denaturation.

(b) **Probe preparation.** Some probes may require labelling with a fluorochrome. Many are now supplied pre-labelled. In some cases, a denaturation step may be necessary.

(c) **Chromosome denaturation.** This is normally performed in hot formamide/SSC and halted by incubation in ice-cold 70% ethanol, followed by dehydration through an ethanol series.

(d) **Hybridization.** Denatured probe is applied to the denatured chromosome material and temporarily sealed with a coverslip. This is incubated at 37 °C in a 'humid chamber' (generally a sealed box containing moist tissues).

(e) **Post hybridization washes.** This is a series of washes to remove excess and loosely bound probe and is generally performed in SSC/detergent mixtures. The concentration of SSC determines the stringency of the washes, which varies according to the probe type used.

(f) **Counterstaining.** This is to provide an overall staining of the chromosomes or cells. Either DAPI (blue) or propidium iodide (red) are normally used, depending on the colour of the fluorochrome (obviously, the counterstain must be a different colour from the fluorochrome). Slides are mounted directly with the counterstain and may be viewed after a few minutes.

Some procedures may require additional steps, such as signal amplification.

Chapter 6, Section 6 summarizes the use of FISH for the detection of some of the specific translocations and other rearrangements associated with the leukaemias. In most cases, these are detected using a unique sequence probe from each of the genes involved in the rearrangement (sometimes used in association with chromosome-specific subtelomeric probes). In some cases, whole chromosome 'paints' are used (a cocktail of chromosome-specific probes which cover the entire length of the chromosomes). In these situations, the FISH investigation is specific to the chromosome rearrangement suspected on the basis of clinical indications.

It is important to ensure that the clinician is aware of the limitations of this approach – this laboratory occasionally receives referral forms requesting simply 'FISH' with no clinical details! Another example is the case of a t(9;22)-positive patient being monitored following therapy: further karyotypic changes can herald the approach of an accelerated phase from CML to acute leukaemia, and these would be missed if FISH were not complemented by a full karyotypic analysis.

The more advanced FISH technologies are currently applied mainly in research laboratories and are used for the identification of complex chromosome abnormalities which cannot be interpreted by non-molecular cytogenetic techniques. These include the multicolour FISH techniques, namely M-FISH and SKY (See Chapter 6, Section 3). These assign individual colours to each chromosome pair, plus X and Y, such that the composition of the derivative chromosomes from complex rearrangements can be ascertained. Comparative genomic hybridization (see Chapter 6, Section 5) provides a way of identifying losses or gains of heterozygosity of individual chromosome pairs from either cultured or uncultured samples (particularly solid tumours).

6.2 Restriction fragment length polymorphism analysis and Southern blotting

Restriction fragment length polymorphism analysis consists essentially of digesting DNA into fragments using restriction endonucleases so that individual fragment lengths can be measured. Southern blotting is the method used to achieve this. Any mutation resulting in a change in a restriction site for a given endonuclease will alter known fragment lengths. This, in turn, provides information about the nature of the mutation. Thus, the method can be used for the detection of reciprocal translocations, small deletions and loss of alleles at specific loci. Protocols for Southern blotting can be found in the volume by Maniatis *et al.* (15).

The ability of this technique to detect submicroscopic chromosome translocations was instrumental in the demonstration of the *BCR/ABL* rearrangement in microscopically Philadelphia-negative cases of CML. In some cases, the classic Ph chromosome may be masked by a complex translocation involving more than two chromosomes. Price *et al.* (16) recently described a rare case of AML in which there was a complex translocation involving 1, 9 and 22. DNA digested with the restriction enzyme XABL and hybridized to a 4.8 kb probe for the *BCR* region *(PHL/BCR3)* gave a 6.8 kb rearranged band in addition to the normal germline band of 9.8 kb: thus the *BCR* region was involved in the translocation.

6.3 Polymerase chain reaction

The polymerase chain reaction is 10 000 times more sensitive than Southern blotting, and 100 000 times more sensitive than conventional cytogenetic techniques. As such, it is a powerful tool for the detection of submicroscopic chromosome rearrangements.

DNA polymerase enzymes catalyse the copying of DNA from an appropriately primed template. Short lengths of complementary DNA (20–40 bp), termed primers, are required to start the reaction. One primer is selected from the region upstream of the translocation breakpoint; this should be complementary to one strand of the DNA double helix. The other primer, selected from the region downstream from the breakpoint, should be complementary to the other DNA strand. Detailed protocols for PCR are provided by Erlich (17).

Primers are normally selected for a single region of DNA. However, when PCR is to be used for the detection of a translocation, primers must be selected for the individual components of the translocation, which originate from different chromosomes. Accordingly, in the absence of a translocation, no amplified fragment would be obtained. Thus, for an investigation of an apparently Ph-negative CML, sense primers would be selected for the *BCR* region, and antisense primers would be selected for the *ABL* region. This would result in amplification of the fragment DNA representing the translocation. If no such amplified fragment is observed, it would mean the absence of the translocation. Clearly, it is essential to know the DNA sequence of the region surrounding the breakpoints.

6.3.1 Reverse transcriptase polymerase chain reaction

Reverse transcriptase (an RNA dependent DNA polymerase) can be used to make a DNA copy that is complementary in base sequence to mRNA, and this copy is termed cDNA. The mRNA populations differ in various cell types, as they may be devoted to synthesizing a specific type of protein for a particular function. Hence, cDNA from whichever cell type is chosen would be enriched in a particular protein synthesis function, thus facilitating the isolation of that protein.

The method of RT-PCR, using mRNA from patients with a disease affliction, relies on at least some mRNA being present in accessible cells e.g. blood cells. Conversion to cDNA can then be used as a template for pairs of exon-specific primers to generate overlapping DNA fragments. Screening of mutations requires the testing of DNA samples from a panel of patients and controls. If a candidate gene is intimated in a disease process, it must be shown to be mutated in affected individuals. This requires the design of pairs of specific primers for use in amplifying portions of the coding DNA either from genomic DNA (only if the exon/intron boundaries are known) or from cDNA.

The products of the individual amplification reactions are then subjected to one or more rapid mutation screening procedures designed to detect point mutation. The aim is to demonstrate a variety of patient-specific mutations which would be expected to have a deleterious effect on gene expression.

7 Summary

It is hoped that this chapter has guided the reader into the fundamentals of the cytogenetic analysis of cancer cytogenetics, and that the following chapters will expand upon the knowledge obtained from working with different disease types. Analysis of chromosomes from neoplastic cells can be fraught with difficulties, and often frustrations, but can also be extremely interesting and rewarding. With the aid of the information imparted by the chapters in this volume it is hoped that the reader will approach the task presented with renewed insight and vigour.

Acknowledgements

With thanks to 'Dudley' and his 'omnipresence' he has the force to help (but he hides it well).

References

1. Hoffbrand, A. V. and Pettit, J. E. (1984). *Essential haematology.* Blackwell Scientific Publications, Oxford.
2. Goldman, J. M. and Preistler, H. D. (eds) (1984). *Leukaemia.* Butterworths International Medical Reviews, London.
3. McDonald, G. A., Dodds, T. C., and Cruikshank, B. (1978). *Atlas of haematology.* Churchill Livingstone, Edinburgh.
4. Mufti, G. J., Flandrin, G., Schaefer, H-E., Sandberg, A. A., and Kanfer, E. J. (eds) (1996). *An atlas of malignant haematology, cytology, histology and cytogenetics.* Martin Dunitz Ltd, London.
5. HMSO (1988). *Control of substances hazardous to health regulations (COSHH).* HMSO, London
6. HMSO (1987). *Code of practice for the prevention of infection in clinical laboratories and post-mortem rooms.* HMSO, London.
7. Croner (1997). *Croner's Laboratory Manager* Croner Publications Ltd, Kingston-on-Thames.
8. Webber, L. M. and Garson, O. M. (1983). *Cancer Genet. Cytogenet.* **8**, 123.
9. Taylor, J. H., Haut, W. F., and Tung, J. (1962). *Proc. Natl. Acad. Sci. USA* **48**, 190.
10. Grezschik, K., Kim, M. A., and Johansmann, R. (1975). *Hum. Genet.* **29**, 41.
11. Kondo, K. and Sashki, M. (1981). *Jpn. J. Hum. Genet.* **26**, 225.
12. Nakagome, Y., Yokochi, T., Matsubara, T., and Fukada, F. (1982). *Cytogenet. Cell Genet.* **33**, 254.
13. Hook, E. B. (1977). *Am. J. Hum. Genet.* **29**, 94.
14. *Fourth international workshop on chromosomes in leukaemia, 1982* (1984). *Cancer Genet. Cytogenet.* **33**, 254.
15. Maniatis, T., Fritsch, E. F., and Sambrook, J. (1990). *Molecular cloning, a laboratory manual.* Cold Spring Harbor Laboratory Press, New York.
16. Price, C. M., Rasool, F. M., Shirji, K. R., Gow, J., Tew, C. J., Haworth, C. *et al.,* (1988). *Blood* **72**, 1829.
17. Erlich, H. A. (ed.) (1989). *PCR technology: principles and applications for DNA amplification.* Oxford University Press, Oxford.

Chapter 2
Cytogenetics in myeloid leukaemia

A. M. Potter and A Watmore

North Trent Cytogenetics Service, Sheffield Children's Hospital Trust, Western Bank, Sheffield S10 2TH, UK

1 Introduction

This chapter covers three haematological disorders of myeloid cells: AML, MDS and MPD. Both MDS and MPD have a propensity to evolve to acute leukaemia. Indeed, the diagnosis of AML in these cases may be simply based on the blast count. The poorly defined boundaries between disorders is reflected in the commonality of the chromosome findings in the three conditions.

The majority of chromosome changes in myeloid leukaemia, although characteristic of the disease, can also be observed elsewhere. This chapter attempts to identify those abnormalities considered exclusive to myeloid leukaemia (usually having a limited distribution within AML subtypes) and those strongly associated with myeloid disorders but occasionally appearing in other diseases. A third type of chromosome abnormality is also included. These are findings which are recurrent in myeloid disease, but frequently observed outside the myeloid lineage. These should not be considered as reliable lineage markers when seen alone. As with all malignancies, a proportion of myeloid leukaemias show only random changes. These confirm the neoplastic nature of the disease but provide no further information.

In some instances, particular combinations of abnormalities suggest the myeloid nature of the disease. These patterns probably represent the accumulation of characteristic secondary changes as the malignancy develops.

Although many abnormalities are seen more commonly in some disorders than in others, apart from a small number of highly specific changes it is not possible to differentiate between categories of myeloid disease on the basis of cytogenetics alone.

2 Special considerations for chromosome culture and analysis in myeloid disorders

Myeloid malignancies generally produce good chromosome preparations which have allowed the precise identification of several specific abnormalities including some subtle rearrangements. Any of the protocols in Chapter 1 can be applied confidently and at least 95% overall success may be expected.

2.1 Culture and analysis

A suitable regime for most myeloid conditions would be one overnight colcemid-treated culture and one short-term culture as described in *Protocol 2,* Chapter 1. In addition, one of the synchronization techniques could also be applied. Knowledge of the haematological background of the disease and sometimes of the individual case will indicate any special requirements. A directed approach to analysis is necessary, assessing each referral individually with respect to the extent of the analysis required and any specific abnormalities to be excluded. It should be remembered that for any recognized rearrangement, variants involving multiple chromosomes can be seen and that complex secondary karyo-

Table 1 Abnormalities largely restricted to myeloid conditions (percentage of cases in which the abnormality has been found)

Structural rearrangements	AML and transformed MPD	MDS	MPD chronic phase
t(1;7)	< 1%	< 1%	< 1%
t(3;5)	< 1%	< 1%	Rare
t(3;21)	< 1%	< 1%	< 1%
t(5;12)	Rare	< 1%	< 1%
t(6;9)	< 1%	< 1%	Rare
t(8;13)	< 1%	Rare	Rare
t(8;16)	< 1%	Rare	Rare
t(8;21)	> 5%	< 1%	Rare
t(15;17)	> 5%	Rare	Rare
inv(3) etc	1–5%	1–5%	Rare
inv(16)	1–5%	< 1%	Rare
del(5)(q)	1–5%	> 5%	< 1%
del(7)(q)	1–5%	> 5%	1–5%
del(20)(q)	< 1%	1–5%	> 5%
i(17q)	< 1%	< 1%	1–5%
Aneusomies			
−7	> 5%	> 5%	1–5%
+4	1–5%	Rare	Rare
+8	> 5%	> 5%	> 5%
+9	< 1%	1–5%	> 5%
+11	1–5%	1–5%	Rare
+13	< 1%	Rare	Rare
+14	Rare	< 1%	< 1%
+19	< 1%	1–5%	Rare
+22	1–5%	Rare	Rare

Table 2 Abnormalities not restricted to myeloid disease (percentage of cases in which the abnormality has been found)

Abnormality	AML and transformed MPD	MDS	MPD chronic phase
Partial trisomy 1q	< 1%	< 1%	> 5%
del(9)(q)	1–5%	Rare	Rare
t(9;22)	1–5%	Rare	> 5%
11q23 abnormalities	1–5%	< 1%	Rare
12p abnormalities excluding t(5;12)	< 1%	Rare	Rare
del(13)(q)	Rare	< 1%	> 5%
+15	< 1%	< 1%	< 1%
+21	1–5%	1–5%	Rare

typic evolution may also, on occasion, obscure changes of primary importance. Certain secondary changes are frequently linked to particular rearrangements. If cytogenetic studies fail to reveal the abnormality suggested by the clinical picture but a characteristic secondary change is seen, molecular studies should be considered.

Table 1 shows the variety of chromosome abnormalities frequently associated with myeloid leukaemia and an indication of the likely distribution in AML, MDS and MPD. *Table 2* illustrates the same distribution in abnormalities not restricted to myeloid disease. These will provide confirmation when other haematological criteria suggest this diagnosis. The list is not complete and excludes some extremely rare recent findings. All unusual rearrangements need to be checked against current catalogues of chromosome abnormalities and publications to establish whether they are associated with a specific disease subset. Although relatively few aberrations are exclusively myeloid, the presence of combinations of changes which are less specific but nonetheless typical of the lineage provides a strong indication of myeloid disease.

Because on reception of a malignancy referral the cytogeneticist will rarely be aware the extent to which their findings will be required to establish a diagnosis, the referring haematologist should be the primary arbiter of how quickly results are required. In the absence of a specific request the need for rapid clinical intervention remains the best guide to prioritizing cases. In general, this will include all acute leukaemias and any situation suggesting disease relapse or transformation when a change in treatment is required.

2.2 Choice of tissue

In most cases, the tissue of choice is bone marrow. However, myelofibrosis is an important exception for which blood culture is more appropriate. The blood sample should be processed in the same way as marrow since it will contain considerable numbers of haemopoietic cells. Apart from myelofibrosis, blood culture need only be considered as an alternative procedure where a marrow sample has proved inadequate. Blood culture is usually not appropriate for MDS, MPD (except CGL and myelofibrosis) or pancytopenic AML.

2.3 The use of mitogens in myeloid disorders

Mitogenic stimulation using PHA is usually only necessary to investigate a possible constitutional abnormality. However, leukaemic blood may not contain normal numbers of T cells, and those present may not always have a normal response to standard culture conditions. Cell density and culture regime may therefore require some adjustment, and a range of different cultures should be prepared. Where blood contains circulating leukaemic cells, these may be evident in addition to T cells in PHA-stimulated cultures, sometimes in overwhelmingly large numbers. The interpretation of results in these circumstances may not be straightforward and may require discussion of the patient's blood picture with the referring clinician. Ideally, this analysis should be carried out when the blood picture is normal.

Although there are no specific mitogens of use in the investigation of myeloid disorders, myeloid activity can be increased by supplementing cultures with conditioned media obtained from growth factor producing carcinoma cell lines (e.g. 5637 cells). It is possible, however, that some such supplements may favour normal cell growth. It is known that lymphoid and perhaps undifferentiated cells are disadvantaged in this type of system. Therefore, it is important to be aware of this when selecting an appropriate medium for use in this way and samples should also be cultured without supplement, especially if the diagnosis is in doubt.

2.4 Culture times with special reference to t(8;21) and t(15;17)

Direct cultures are of no special value in myeloid disorders. They may provide an early result, but normal results from direct preparations are unreliable. The earliest dividing cells seen in culture may be normal erythroid precursors. This would not be a problem if the erythroid line were known to be part of the malignant clone, but if this is not the case it is advisable to examine more than one culture if no abnormality is immediately seen.

Direct culture is a particular problem in the cases of t(8;21) and t(15;17). Where these translocations are expected, especially t(15;17), marrow should be cultured for 24–48 h as well as the usual times, and all cultures should be analysed before the abnormality can be confidently excluded. To allow for this, the referring clinician should indicate those patients in whom these translocations are suspected.

2.5 Effects of therapy on culture success

In AML it is important to know if the patient is undergoing cytotoxic therapy as this will affect the chance of culture success. Pre-treatment samples are thus desirable. Myelosuppressive treatment given in MPD and supportive therapy in MDS do not, however, usually interfere with cytogenetic cultures.

3 Acute myeloid leukaemia

3.1 Clinical features

Acute myeloid leukaemia describes malignancies of adults and children affecting myeloid (or strictly non-lymphoid) progenitor cells. The cell involved is an immature blast cell and the disease is classified according to morphological and immunological features. The overall prevalence of AML in the UK is 2.6 per 100 000 and most cases are aged over 50 years. A significant proportion develop from myelodysplastic conditions and some from chronic myeloproliferative disorders, although most are of unexplained origin. In a few cases, the disease can be clearly attributed to the effects of cytotoxic therapy for a previous malignancy. These diseases are termed therapy related or secondary as opposed to *de novo*.

In *de novo* cases, intensive chemotherapy can produce a state of remission and return the bone marrow picture to normal. Periods of remission vary in length and number, but the majority of cases of secondary disease relapse into an intractable leukaemia. Remission is less readily achieved where there has been a preceding chronic disorder. The main clinical distinction between secondary and *de novo* disease is that secondary disease is more refractory to treatment.

3.2 The French–American–British system of classification of acute myeloid leukaemia

The FAB system provides a working classification based on blast cell morphology. *Table 3* summarizes the features of the six major categories and two other rare types, M0 and M7, which require immunological techniques as well as morphology for classification. Most cases can be assigned a FAB type and the classification usually remains the same in relapse as at diagnosis. Further details are given in

Table 3 FAB Classification of AML

M1	Myeloblastic without maturation
M2	Myeloblastic with maturation
M3	Promyelocytic (hypergranular)
M3 variant	Promyelocytic (hypo- or micro-granular)
M4	Myelomonocytic with both granulocytic and monocytic differentiation
M4eo	M4 with eosinophilia
M5a	Monoblastic
M5b	Promonocytic–monocytic
M6	Erythroblastic (includes < 30% blasts if > 50% erythroblasts)
M7	Megakaryoblastic
M0	Myeloblastic with minimal evidence of differentiation

Chapter 5, *Table 4*. Most frequent is M4, followed by M2; Ml, M5 and M6 are less common and M3 is rare (6%).

3.3 Cytogenetics of acute myeloid leukaemia

Of 1612 patients successfully karyotyped at presentation in the UK Medical Research Council AML 10 trial (1), 58% (54% of adults and 73% of children) showed a cytogenetically abnormal clone in the bone marrow. The majority of these abnormalities were non-random. Reports of higher abnormality rates are probably achieved by the detection of minor clones rather than improvement in the quality of spreads. A number of chromosome abnormalities are largely restricted to AML and have very specific clinical correlations. These are t(8;21), t(15;17), inv(16) and their variants (see *Table 4*). M0 and M7 have been excluded from the table as too few cases with chromosome abnormalities have been reported in these categories.

Others, although typical of AML, have less or no specific associations. They may be encountered in other myeloid disorders, often with greater or equal frequency than in AML, but are rarely seen outside the myeloid lineage. Some others are recurrent changes in AML and other myeloid disorders but not restricted to that

Table 4 Distribution of specific changes according to FAB type[a]

	t(8;21)	t(15;17)	inv(16)
M1	5	–	–
M2	99	–	1
M3	–	108	–
M4	–	–	31
M5	–	–	–
M6	–	–	–
Total	109	108	32

[a] Figure based on published series (2–4).

Table 5 Distribution of less-specific changes when seen as the sole abnormality, according to FAB type[a]

	+8	−7	del(7)(q)	11q23[b]	+21
M1	10	1	3	1	4
M2	21	14	8	3	2
M3	2	–	–	–	-
M4	17	4	8	9	5
M5	13	8	1	38	2
M6	2	2	1	–	1
Total	65	29	21	51	14

[a] Figure based on published series (2–4).
[b] Certain variants of 11q23 abnormalities show greater specificity.

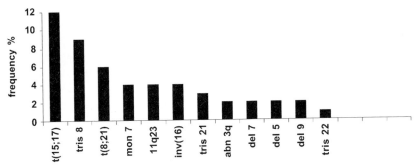

Figure 1 Frequency of chromosome abnormalities in AML as a percentage of all cases.

lineage. Important translocations in this group are t(9;22) and t(11;?)(q23;?). A number of complete and partial aneusomies are also seen (See *Table 5*).

The frequencies of the most common changes observed in the AML 10 Trial (with or without other changes) are shown in *Figure 1*. The distribution of the more common changes according to FAB type is shown in *Tables 4* and *5*. A significantly lower than average age distribution is seen for primary abnormalities t(15;17), t(8;21), 11q23 abnormalities and inv(16).

It is recognized that a visible cytogenetic event is not always needed to achieve the chimeric gene formation associated with non-random chromosome rearrangements and that an as yet undefined proportion will be detectable only by molecular methods. Most series suggest that with good cytogenetic studies, this population is relatively small but should not be overlooked.

4 The myelodysplastic syndromes

4.1 Clinical features

The MDS are a group of conditions of progressive bone marrow failure of normal maturation leading to peripheral cytopenias. More than one cell lineage is usually involved, and very often three. The prevalence is 1 in 100 000 and it is typically a disease of the elderly. Mild forms are often difficult to diagnose with certainty and cytogenetic analysis may be sought to confirm the condition as malignant. The rate of progression of the disease is variable and death is commonly caused by intolerable cytopenia, but there is a 20–40% risk of transformation to AML (*Table 6*). Although the duration of survival is related to the severity of the marrow dysfunction and to the blast count, there is as yet no reliable way of predicting transformation for an individual patient. When transformation to AML does occur, the leukaemia is almost always refractory to treatment. It is distinguished from *de novo* AML by myelodysplastic changes, but this may be an artificial distinction as early myelodysplastic changes are not always prominent enough to have been detected.

Table 6 FAB classification of MDS, excluding CMML

	% Of blasts in marrow	Other features
RA	< 5	< 15% Ringed sideroblasts in nucleated red cells
RARS	< 5	> 15% Ringed sideroblasts in nucleated red cells
RAEB	5–20	
RAEBt	21–29[a]	Also RAEBt if Auer rods present, irrespective of blast count or if ≥ 5% blasts in peripheral blood

[a]A blast count of ≥ 30% is a diagnostic criterion for AML.

4.2 The French–American–British classification of myelodysplastic syndromes

The FAB classification is currently in general use and subdivides MDS on the basis of percentage blasts and some morphological features. The figures are arbitrary but provide useful groupings in terms of prognosis as well as a background for interpretation of cytogenetic findings. CMML is conventionally included as part of MDS, although it has some features of a myeloproliferative disorder.

For the purposes of this chapter, the cytogenetics of CMML are considered under myeloproliferative disorders (Section 5) rather than here. *Tables 6* and *7* show the basis of the classification (a more detailed classification is shown in Chapter 5), the distribution of patients in FAB types, and the frequency of transformation to AML. Progression of the disease can lead to reclassification. Overall survival varies according to FAB type, with 5-year survival likely in 50% of RA or RARS but only 15% of RAEB. Most patients with RAEBt survive less than 2 years.

4.3 Cytogenetics of myelodysplastic syndromes

The clinical boundaries between MDS and AML are indistinct and a similar overlap occurs cytogenetically. Although many chromosome changes are non-random, none are specific for MDS and all also feature in AML and other myeloid diseases. Cytogenetics, therefore, is not useful for differential diagnosis. Some abnormalities are more frequent in certain FAB types but this relationship is not close enough to allow any patient to be assigned a FAB type on the strength of cytogenetics alone. Chromosome changes increase in frequency from 20 to 30% in RA and RARS to 60% in RAEBT.

Table 7 Approximate distribution of patients within FAB subtypes of MDS (excluding CMML) at presentation and frequency of transformation to AML

	% Of MDS patients at presentation	% Of patients transforming to AML
RA	35	15
RARS	23	10
RAEB	30	40
RAEBt	12	65

Table 8 Common chromosome changes in MDS

- del(5)(q11-q33)
- −7
- del(7)(q22-q36)
- +8
- del(11)(q14) or (q23)
- del(13)
- del(20)(q11)
- −Y

Chromosome changes may be expected in 40–50% of cases using current methods. *Table 8* gives the more common non-random findings. All these can be seen as single changes or in combination with each other or with other changes. More than half the abnormal cases show one of these simple changes, at least initially.

Recent evidence suggests that the karyotype can make an important contribution to evaluating likely clinical outcome. Patients with a normal karyotype, del(5)(q) and del(20)(q), as the sole abnormality have good survival rates. Other karyotypes, particularly those with multiple chromosome abnormalities, are thought to have poor outcomes (5).

Two or more chromosomally unrelated abnormal cell lines are seen more frequently in MDS than in other leukaemias. Any dual evolutions should be considered as complex karyotypes, and the appearance of a new but unrelated cell line taken as indication of an evolving clone.

5 Myeloproliferative disorders

5.1 Clinical features and classification of myeloproliferative disorders

The MPD are a group of related diseases characterized by increased proliferation of one or more of the erythropoietic, megakaryopoietic and granulopoietic components of the bone marrow due to a low grade malignant process. The four

Table 9 Classification of MPD

Disease	Major proliferative component
CML CGL CMML	Myeloid activity predominates
PRV	Red cell activity predominates
ET	Platelet activity predominates
MF	Reactive marrow fibrosis predominates

major myeloproliferative disorders are given in *Table 9* although other less well defined conditions also occur. They can be classified according to the major proliferative component.

Within this classification CML can be further categorized by morphology, karyotype and molecular analysis (6). (See also *Table 9*, Chapter 5) The categories considered here are chronic CGL, both Philadelphia-positive and -negative, and CMML. CGL is conventionally considered separately from other forms of MPD because of the distinctive nature of the disease.

There is extensive literature on the genetic changes in CGL, reflecting the importance of these studies in both the diagnosis and progression of the disease. In contrast, relatively few studies have been reported in the other forms of MPD where cytogenetics has been less helpful, although chromosome analysis may have a role in recognizing disease progression.

5.2 Incidence of cytogenetic changes in myeloproliferative disease

The chromosome abnormalities in MPD fall into the group generally associated with myeloid leukaemia. No chromosome changes found to date in MPD have been shown to be specific for the disease, apart from those in CGL. For this reason, it is not possible, on cytogenetic evidence alone, to distinguish MPDs from each other or from other forms of myeloid malignancies, with the exception of CGL.

The number of patients with chromosomally abnormal clones at diagnosis will depend on the specific disease studied. In CGL this will be over 95% of all cases. In myelofibrosis 50% will have a chromosome abnormality; 30% will have a chromosome abnormality in CMML, 13% in PRV and 5% in ET. The cytogenetics of CGL is considered in Sections 5.3.1 and 5.3.2. In other MPD, the following chromosome abnormalities are those most frequently observed: +1q (including +1,der(1;7)(q10;p10)), monosomy 7, del(7)(q), +8, +9, del(13)(q), and del(20)(q).

A number of other chromosome abnormalities have been reported in MPD as non-random findings, although these occur at low frequencies. This situation is analogous to that described in MDS: indeed, many of the abnormalities are common to both groups and include del(11)(q23), del(5)(q) and del(12)(p12).

5.3 Chronic granulocytic leukaemia: clinical features

Chronic granulocytic leukaemia is a well-defined disease associated with increasing splenomegaly and leucocytosis. There is a relatively benign chronic phase with a mean duration of about 3 years. The acceleration of the disease to an acute form occurs in the majority of cases and may be a rapid and easily recognized change (blast crisis) or, more commonly, a gradual clinical acceleration. Clinically, the symptoms of transformed CGL are similar to other forms of acute leukaemia and usually defined as more than 30% blasts in the peripheral blood or bone marrow. Although chromosome abnormalities accompany both forms of acute phase, cytogenetics may be of more use when distinguishing the onset of transformation in the absence of a blast crisis.

5.3.1 Cytogenetics of chronic-phase chronic granulocytic leukaemia

The specific chronic-phase finding in CGL is the Philadelphia (Ph) chromosome, found in 95% of all cases. This can normally be confidently identified on unbanded metaphases, although in a few reported cases the characteristic chromosome 22 product has been masked by additional material on the long arm.

Identification of a Ph chromosome confirms a suspected diagnosis of CGL. However, the absence of the Ph will not exclude such a diagnosis unless the associated molecular rearrangement of *ABL* on chromosome 9 with the *BCR* region on chromosome 22 has been excluded. Of the 5% of CGL cases without a Ph chromosome, approximately half have material from 9q34 inserted at 22q11 in a form which is not detectable by conventional cytogenetics but can be shown by molecular analysis. Philadelphia-negative cases without *BCR/ABL* rearrangement are classified as a separate disorder. If a *BCR/ABL* rearrangement is detected, then the course of the disease and associated chromosome findings will be similar to those described for Ph-positive CGL.

The most frequent cytogenetic pattern in the chronic phase is a single Ph chromosome. The following situations also occur in a minority of cases:

- normal cells may also be present; these are observed in 5% of diagnostic samples but tend to disappear during the course of the disease
- non-disjunction of the Ph chromosome
- loss of the Y chromosome.
- a further structural rearrangement or numerical change.

All these, when identified at diagnosis, are compatible with the chronic phase of the disease and there is little evidence that such findings, or variant forms of Ph (see Section 6.1.7), are of any prognostic significance. A possible exception may be the persistence of a normal cell line which has been associated with long survival (7) or the presence of i(17q), which is usually associated with transformation.

5.3.2 Cytogenetics of acute-phase chronic granulocytic leukaemia

The accelerated or blastic stage of CGL is usually accompanied by further non-random chromosome abnormalities. These changes often precede clinical deterioration and their detection can be useful in indicating the onset of transformation, particularly in the absence of a blast crisis.

More than 80% of transformed CGL cases show additional chromosome changes. These are mostly non-random and the most frequently observed are shown in *Table 10*. At least one of these can be seen in approximately 75% of transformed cases.

These chromosome changes may occur as the sole abnormality, in combination with each other, or accompanied by other abnormalities. Although there

Table 10 Common chromosome changes in transformed CGL

Additional change	Frequency (%)
+8	50
i(17q) and other abnormalities of 17p	35
+Ph	30
+19	15

appears to be a strong correlation between the presence of i(17q) and myeloid transformation (8), generally the identification of blast type is best done by the use of immunological markers.

However, as additional chromosome changes may also be seen during the chronic phase, in the absence of a clinically recognized acute phase, some caution should be exercised in suggesting transformation when new abnormal clones are first detected. The following points should be considered:

- chromosome changes seen at diagnosis should be distinguished from subsequent changes

- new abnormal clones appearing at a low level of mosaicism are not necessarily indicative of transformation

- any new chromosome finding including random changes present in the majority of cells or seen to be rapidly superseding the original clone suggests that the disease may be transforming

- trisomy 8 and, in particular, an extra Ph chromosome (sometimes in the form of an isochromosome) are often seen transiently in the chronic phase and are therefore not reliable indicators of transformation

- certain chromosome changes, e.g. i(17q) or other abnormalities of 17p and trisomy 19 are reliable indicators of transformation.

Some caution is also required when interpreting cytogenetic results after BMT. Although eradication of the Ph clone is a good prognostic indication, its persistence, particularly in small numbers, may be consistent with remission. The emergence of additional abnormalities suggest that if the patient has not relapsed, this will occur at some stage. Additional abnormalities seen at relapse after BMT are not those generally associated with transformed CML.

6 Cytogenetics of myeloid disease

6.1 Chromosome rearrangements

6.1.1 +1,der(1;7)(q10;p10)

This unbalanced rearrangement, resulting from the fusion of chromosome 1 and 7 centromeres giving rise to trisomy 1q and monosomy 7q, is an uncommon but well-documented finding mainly in MDS and AML (*Figure 2*). Half the reported

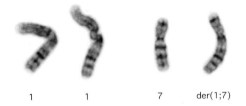

1	1	7	der(1;7)

Figure 2 +1,der(1;7)(q10;p10).

incidences are in therapy related leukaemia, and environmental mutagens have also been implicated. Prognosis is poor. There is usually a simple chromosome pattern (see Chapter 5, Section 2.9 for more details of therapy related disease).

6.1.2 Abnormalities of 3q21 and 3q26

A variety of rearrangements at 3q21 are seen throughout the range of myeloid diseases. The majority juxtapose 3q21 and 3q26 but less common translocations also occur. All are associated with trilineage dysplasia and megakaryocyte abnormalities, but not necessarily thrombocytosis. Survival is generally poor. Consideration of all abnormalities at 3q21 or 26 as a single category may be misleading as molecular studies have shown a variety of genetic events.

6.1.2.1 inv(3)(q21q26) and t(3;3)(q21;q26)

These equivalent rearrangements are seen in less than 1% of AML (most FAB types), MDS and CGL, usually in acceleration or transformation (*Figure 3*). Monosomy 7 is a recurrent additional abnormality particularly in *de novo* AML. *EV11* at 3q26 is dysregulated by this rearrangement. All other 3q21 or 26 abnormalities are less common.

6.1.2.2 Other rearrangements at 3q21

Translocation of 3q21 also occurs with chromosome 1 at p26 and chromosome 5 at a variety of reported breakpoints in the long arm. Although the reported cases have trilineage dysplasia and megakaryocyte abnormalities, it has not yet been established whether breakpoints are the same at the molecular level, indeed at least some cases of t(3;5) involve *MLF1* at 3q25.1.

6.1.2.3 t(3;21)(q26;q22)

The very subtle translocation resulting in *AML1/EAP* fusion is most commonly seen in therapy-related disease and transformed CGL (*Figure 4*) (9).

6.1.3 t(5;12)(q33;p13)

This rearrangement, although rare, occurs in a subgroup of myeloid malignancies having features of both MDS and MPD, commonly exhibiting eosinophilia and monocytosis. A variant involving t(10;12)(q24;p13) has been reported. This is one

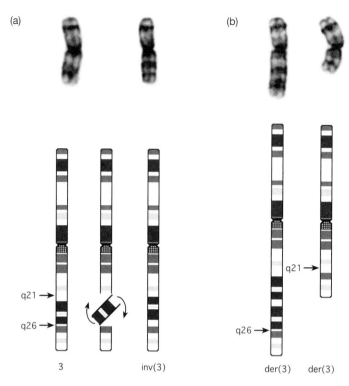

Figure 3 inv(3)(q21q26) and t(3;3)(q21;q26).

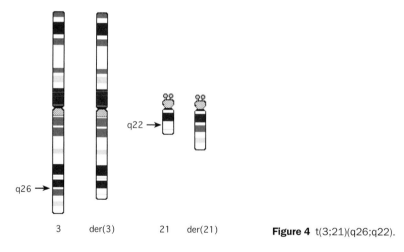

Figure 4 t(3;21)(q26;q22).

of the rearrangements involving the *TEL* gene. Other rearrangements are found in other disease types (10).

6.1.4 t(6;9)(p23;q34)

This is a very rare and subtle rearrangement (*Figure 5*). The resolution of t(6;9) breakpoints is difficult under the microscope. It results in a fusion of *DEK* and

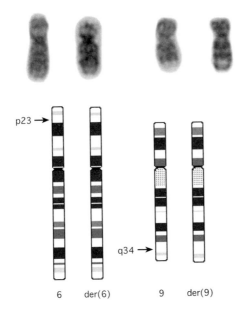

p23 →

q34 →

6   der(6)   9   der(9)   **Figure 5** t(6;9)(p23;q34).

CAN (which is distal to *ABL*). It is usually the sole change. Early reports suggested that t(6;9) marked a subset of AML, M2, or M4, with dyserythropoiesis and basophilia, but it has now been seen often enough in other myeloid conditions to refute this. The association with noticeable basophilia is by no means universal, but t(6;9) is usually seen in relatively young people with multilineage disease, suggesting that it originates in a multipotent stem cell. There is frequently a history of known toxic exposure (11).

6.1.5 Abnormalities of 8p

Rearrangement at 8p11 is extremely rare but well documented. Two distinct genetic and clinical entities have been observed (12).

6.1.5.1 t(8;16)(p11;p13)

Reported in less than 0.1% of AML, this translocation nevertheless defines a particular subtype (*Figure 6*). It fits uneasily into the current FAB M4/5 type. Patients are typically young with a high frequency of coagulation dysfunction and erythrophagocytosis or haemophagocytosis. Poor prognosis has also been reported. Occasional cytogenetic variants known to be related include t(8;22) (p11;q13), t(8;19)(p11;q13) and inv(8)(p11q13). Often, the rearrangement is seen as part of a very complex karyotype. t(8;16) and its variants show involvement of *MOZ* on 8p which distinguishes them from the rearrangements described below.

6.1.5.2 t(8;13)(p11;q12)

This translocation (*Figure 7*) is also rare and with its presumed variants t(8;9)(p11;q32) and t(6;8)(q27;p11) is associated with an unusual biphenotypic malignancy with myeloid hyperplasia, lymphadenopathy and eosinophilia. The

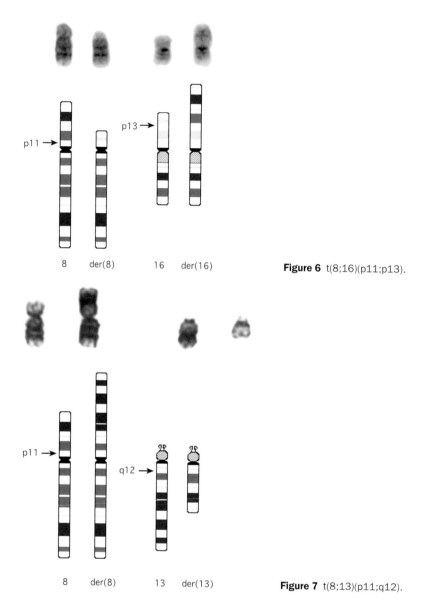

Figure 6 t(8;16)(p11;p13).

Figure 7 t(8;13)(p11;q12).

presentation is often T-cell lymphoblastic lymphoma rapidly transforming to AML (13).

6.1.6 t(8;21)(q22;q22)

This translocation (*Figure 8*) is seen in 8% of all cases of AML and is usually associated with a subgroup of AML M2 comprising young individuals with eosinophilia and a single Auer rod. The t(8;21) translocation also occurs in both M1 and M4. It has been reported occasionally in MDS, although these cases rapidly transform to AML.

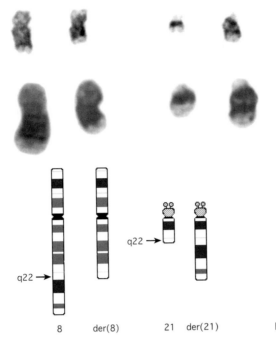

8 der(8) 21 der(21)   **Figure 8** t(8;21)(q22;q22).

The rearrangement is easily recognized down the microscope, although variant forms occur in about 4% of cases, usually involving a third chromosome. Variants have been reported which involve chromosome 8, but not chromosome 21, or vice versa, although chromosome 21 is more commonly involved (14).

Additional abnormalities are observed in 75% of cases. Most frequent are the loss of a sex chromosome, deleted 9q, trisomy 8 and monosomy 7. It remains unclear whether these additional abnormalities are of any clinical significance.

6.1.7 t(9;22)(q34;q11), the Philadelphia chromosome

The Ph chromosome is an abnormal chromosome 22 derived from a translocation which usually takes the form t(9;22)(q34;q11) (*Figure 9*); in about 5% of cases a variant translocation is present, either with translocation of 22 to a chromosome other than 9 (*Figure 10*) or showing complex rearrangement involving three or more chromosomes including 9 and 22. (*Figure 11*). However, molecular studies suggest that chromosome 9 is always involved, even though this may not be visible at the microscope (see Chapter 6, Section 6.1).

Although diagnostic for CGL the Ph chromosome is also seen in ALL (see Chapter 3) and is a rare finding in AML—usually either M1 or M2. As with other chromosome changes in AML, but in contrast to CGL, Ph is lost during disease remission. A Ph chromosome is an extremely unusual finding in MDS but rather more common in MPD, particularly in ET. Although many of these patients transform to a typical CGL in blast crisis, the significance of the Ph in other cases remains unclear.

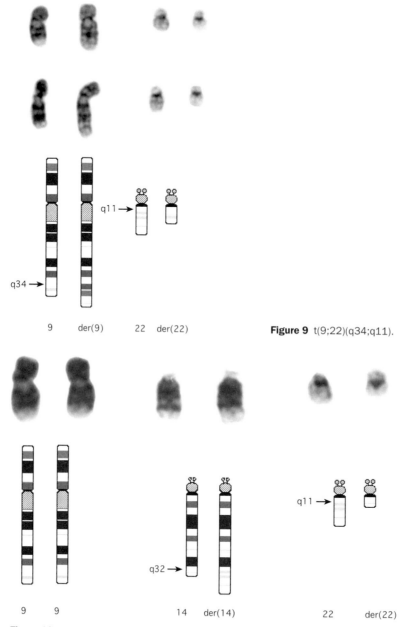

9   der(9)   22   der(22)

Figure 9 t(9;22)(q34;q11).

9   9   14   der(14)   22   der(22)

Figure 10 t(14;22)(q32;q11).

6.1.8 Abnormalities at 11q23

A range of abnormalities at 11q23 is seen throughout the spectrum of haematological disease (*Figures 12–15*). This reflects a variety of mechanisms of disruption of the *MLL (HRX, ALL1 OR HTRX)* gene. They are mainly seen in acute leukaemia, often in younger age groups and are particularly frequent in infant leukaemia.

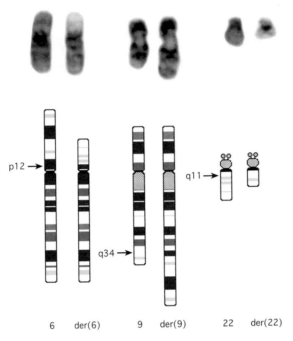

Figure 11 t(6;9;22)(p12;q34;q11).

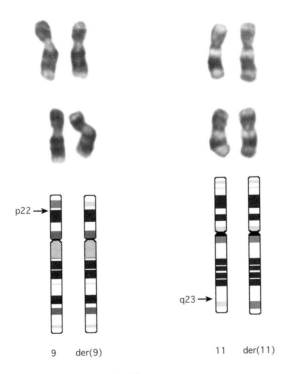

Figure 12 t(9;11)(p22;q23).

45

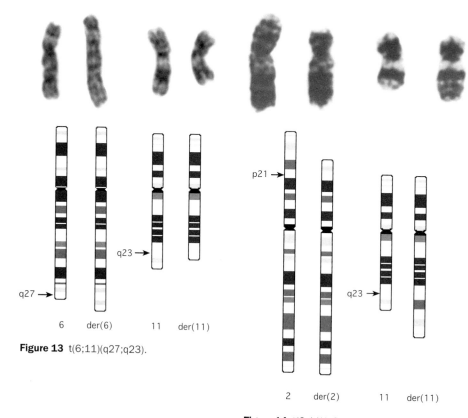

Figure 13 t(6;11)(q27;q23).

Figure 14 t(2;11)(p21;q23).

Secondary leukaemia following therapy with topoisomerase 2 inhibitors also has a high level of 11q23 involvement. Translocation producing novel *MLL* fusion genes is the main mechanism and although an ever increasing variety of partner sites is reported, the most frequent are shown in *Table 11*.

Less common partner sites are 1p32, seen equally in myeloid and lymphoid disease and 1q21, 2p21, 17q12~21, 17q25. Many others have been reported and are extensively reviewed by the European Workshop (15). Many of these rearrangements are subtle and can be more easily detected by chromosome paint-

Table 11 Partner sites involving 11q23

Rearrangements	% of all **11q23** rearrangements in study	Proportion of cases with myeloid disease
t(4;11)(q21;q23)	33.3	5%
t(9;11)(p21~22;q23)	22.7	>90%
t(11;19)(q23;p13.1) or (q23;p13.3)	9.6	p13.1, 100% p13.3, 22%
t(6;11)(q27;q23)	5.5	90%
t(10;11)(p12;q23)	3.6	80%

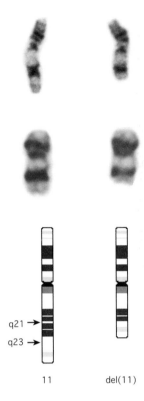

q21 →
q23 →

11   del(11)   **Figure 15** del(11)(q21q23).

ing. t(10;11), in particular, often takes a more complex form as an alteration of gene orientation is also required.

Although widely held to be of adverse prognostic significance, especially in infants and adults, there is less reliable information on particular subsets and it is possible that other parameters such as age may moderate this effect. Most 11q23 abnormalities in AML are in M4/M5, although biphenotypic or minimally differentiated disease is encountered in most of the common rearrangement groups. All subtypes of MDS are also represented and many transform rapidly to AML. t(2;11)(p21;q23) is relatively more common in MDS than AML, frequently with del(5)(q) as an additional abnormality.

Of the less common partners, 17q12 deserves special consideration as it could be confused with a cytogenetically similar rearrangement in AML M3 (see Section 6.1.9). Here, as elsewhere, molecular or FISH studies for *MLL* rearrangement can be valuable (see Chapter 6, Sections 4.6.2 and 6.4). Deletions at 11q23 have been reported in all disease types, with a higher incidence of MDS here than in the case of translocations. Possible translocations or insertions should be ruled out by FISH and *MLL* rearrangement should not be assumed.

Patients with trisomy 11 have been shown to harbour internal rearrangement of the *MLL* gene not detectable by currently available FISH probes. This trisomy as a sole abnormality is exclusive to myeloid disease although clinical and prognostic associations are not yet fully established.

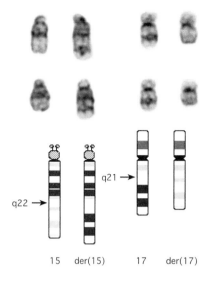

q21 →

q22 →

15   der(15)   17   der(17)

Figure 16 t(15;17)(q22;-q12~21).

6.1.9 t(15;17)(q22;q12~21)

This is one of the most common rearrangements and is found in 6% of AML (*Figure 16*). Breakpoints are difficult to determine under the microscope. This rearrangement has the most specific clinical association of all abnormalities in AML. It is present in almost all cases of acute promyelocytic leukaemia (M3 and M3v) with which it is pathognomically associated. Improvements in detection mean that very few cases of M3 are now reported without t(15;17). Outside M3, t(15;17) occurs in promyelocytic transformation of CML, suggesting that it is tightly restricted to promyelocytes.

It is clinically valuable to confirm M3 as this FAB type is responsive to combination therapy including ATRA, which is not effective in other subtypes and the prognostic implications are good with appropriate treatment.

Variant or complex translocations do not have known clinical significance provided that a *PML/RARα* (retinoic acid receptor-α) fusion is present. An important 'variant', however, is t(11;17)(q23;q12~21), which does not show the same response to ATRA in the few cases reported, despite M3 morphology. Here, *RARα* is fused with *PLZF*. The translocation should not be confused with the rare occurrence of t(11;17) involving *MLL* rearrangement (16).

The formation of an isochromosome from the chromosome 17 derivative of t(15;17) is also occasionally seen (*Figure 17*). In most cases, t(15;17) is the sole change, but about 30% also show trisomy 8 and other additional abnormalities can occur, particularly in relapse. It remains unclear whether secondary changes occurring at diagnosis are of any prognostic significance.

Although abnormal metaphase spreads in myeloid leukaemia are not normally inferior to those which are normal, cells with the t(15;17) are invariably poor. This observation, together with the fact that this translocation is rarely detected in short-term cultures (see Section 2.4) probably accounts for some of the reported cases of M3/M3v with normal karyotypes. Translocation (15;17) is

15   der(15)   17   ider(17)(q10)

Figure 17 t(15;17)(q22;q12~21),−17,+ider(17)(q10).

occasionally seen for the first time in relapse, presumably having been present but not detected at diagnosis, rather than occurring later in the disease.

6.1.10 Inverted 16 and other 16q abnormalities

A rearrangement of chromosome 16 at q22 has been reported in approximately 4% of all cases of AML. Almost all are pericentric inversions of chromosome 16 at pl3q22, resulting in *CBFβ/MYH11* fusion (*Figure 18*). However, a small number of patients with t(16;16)(p13;q22) are also seen (*Figure 19*). Some apparent deletions also result in *CBFβ/MYH11* fusion but deletions should not be assumed to be variants unless proven by molecular means.

Inversion of chromosome 16 can be difficult to spot in poor preparations and this may have accounted for differing estimates of its incidence. Although inv(16) often appears as the sole abnormality, trisomy 8 may also be present. Trisomy 22, otherwise rare in AML, is also frequently observed and its presence should therefore alert the cytogeneticist to the possibility of an inverted 16. Cryptic rearrangements are known to occur and probes are available for FISH analysis.

The abnormality is found in younger patients, frequently with organomegaly, hyperleukocytosis, eosinophilia and abnormal eosinophil granules. It has been specifically associated with M4Eo where it is seen in over 50% of cases. Although abnormal eosinophils may be a universal finding, inverted 16 has been seen in a

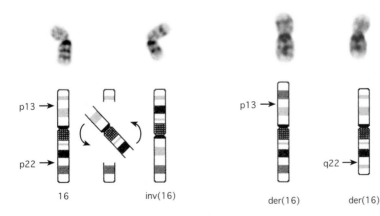

Figure 18 inv(16)(p13q22).

Figure 19 t(16;16)(p13;q22).

range of FAB types (17) and very occasionally in MDS (usually rapidly evolving to AML). Patients with this rearrangement in AML are thought to have a favourable prognosis.

6.2 Numerical abnormalities: trisomies

The most common and widespread abnormality in AML is trisomy 8. It is found in about 9% of cases overall but as the sole change in only 4% and is equally common in other myeloid conditions, but unusual as the only change in lymphoid malignancy.

Trisomy or partial trisomy 1q is a ubiquitous finding both in haematological disease and solid tumours. In myeloid disorders it is most often seen in MPD, but when seen in AML in association with der(1;7) it is of particular significance (see Section 6.1.1).

Other recurrent trisomies are 4, 6, 9, 11, 13, 14, 15, 19, 21 and 22 (18). (For details of +22 see inv(16) in Section 6.1.10.) Trisomy 4 is associated with AML M4 but the others are more widespread and are also encountered in chronic disease, indeed +9 and +14 are typical of MPD and MDS, respectively. Trisomy 11 is usually seen in acute leukaemia and is likely to be associated with *MLL* rearrangement (see Section 6.1.8). Most instances of +13 are in undifferentiated or minimally differentiated leukaemia, while +19 is a common secondary change in chronic disease, particularly transforming CGL. Trisomy 15 is an occasional finding in MDS but has also been seen in patients without confirmed haematological disease. Although extremely rare, trisomy 6 is seen in hypoplastic MDS and differentiates this from aplastic anaemia. Finally, trisomy 21 is not characteristic of any disease type and, like trisomies of chromosomes 19 and 9, is often a feature of chromosome evolution.

Other trisomies will be encountered but +12 and +7 are not expected. These are characteristic of chronic lymphoproliferative disorders and solid tumours, respectively.

6.3 Numerical abnormalities: monosomy

6.3.1 Monosomy 7

Monosomy 7 is seen in all myeloid leukaemias, both as a single abnormality or in more complex rearrangements. In all cases it appears to be associated with a poor prognosis and non-acute patients readily transform to AML. Although relatively common in AML (seen in 3% of cases as the sole abnormality and in 12% of cases overall) it does not appear to be associated with any FAB type. In MDS, monosomy 7 occurs more frequently in FAB types with high blast counts and secondary leukaemia and is characteristically associated with loss of either chromosome 5 or long arm 5.

Although monosomy 7 is found in myeloproliferative disease, particularly myelofibrosis, this finding has particular significance in childhood MPD, being associated with a recognizable disease entity resembling juvenile CGL. As in the other forms of myeloid leukaemia, this has been shown to have a poor prognosis. The disease appears to occur in siblings, which suggests a role for monitoring healthy family members.

6.3.2 Loss of sex chromosomes

Although loss of the X as the sole abnormality is a very rare finding, loss of the Y is frequently observed in all myeloid malignancies. It appears equally common in elderly males without haematological malignancy and should not be taken as evidence of a malignant change when seen alone. However, loss of the sex chromosomes is commonly observed associated with t(8;21) and, less frequently, loss of Y is associated with the t(9;22) translocation. In both cases, these changes are seen at diagnosis but have no apparent impact on prognosis.

6.4 Deletions

A number of recurrent deletions, sometimes in the form of unbalanced trans-locations, are seen in myeloid disease, mostly in conjunction with more specific changes or as part of a complex karyotype. Chromosomes involved are 5q, 7q, 9q, 11q, 12p, 13q, 16q, 17p, 20q. It has been recently demonstrated that some apparent deletions are in fact the result of subtle unbalanced translocations, and it may be important to distinguish between these in the future.

Many deletions are associated with evolving disease and involve the loss of tumour suppressor genes or putative tumour suppressor genes. This imbalance can also occur without concomitant cytogenetic disturbance and it may be that FISH would be a more sensitive method of establishing loss should it prove to carry prognostic significance.

The occurrence of some deletions in diseases of different lineage is consistent with loss of tumour suppressors with general influence. Alternatively it could simply reflect a variety of molecular lesions which are cytogenetically indistinguishable.

6.4.1 del(5)(q)

Deletion of 5q (*Figure 20*) is a well-recognized abnormality in myeloid leukaemia and, when seen as the sole abnormality, it marks a subset of MDS patients, usually with benign dysplasia. Typically, they are elderly patients, predominantly female, with refractory macrocytic anaemia and characteristic morphological abnormalities of the megakaryocytes. The risk of transformation to AML is low.

Apart from these cases, del(5)(q) occurring alone is a rare finding in AML (< 1%) and MPD but is commonly seen in complex karyotypes (3–4% AML), usually involving abnormalities of 3, 7, 12 and 17. In secondary leukaemias such combinations occur in approximately 80% of cases.

Although the breakpoint is variable, a consistently deleted region at 5q31.1 is found in cases of AML and MDS associated with secondary leukaemia and poor prognosis. However, the del(5)(q) syndrome (also referred to as 5q- syndrome) in MDS appears to have a common breakpoint at 5q32, apparently linked to a different gene (19).

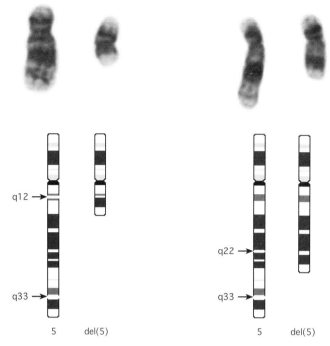

Figure 20 del(5)(q12q33) and del(5)(q22q33).

6.4.2 del(7)(q)

This is a common finding in AML and MDS, although more frequently observed in conjunction with abnormalities of chromosome 5 (see Section 6.4.1) in therapy-related disease. Breakpoints in the long arm are variable, with the most commonly reported deletions at 7q22-q36 and at 7q32-q36 (*Figure 21*). However, a substantial number of these 'deletions' have subsequently been identified as unbalanced translocations. All these abnormalities are usually associated with poor prognosis.

6.4.3 del(9)(q)

Although seen infrequently as the sole abnormality in myeloid leukaemia, particularly AML, del(9)(q) (*Figure 22*) is commonly observed as a secondary change, particularly in association with the 8;21 translocation. It is therefore desirable to rule out concomitant translocations by molecular means if t(8;21) is not apparent. The long arm deletion is variable in size and no common deleted segment has, as yet, been found.

6.4.4 del(12)(p)

These are usually secondary changes, also associated with abnormalities of chromosomes 3, 5, 7 and 17. Such deletions or unbalanced translocations may be subtle and difficult to detect.

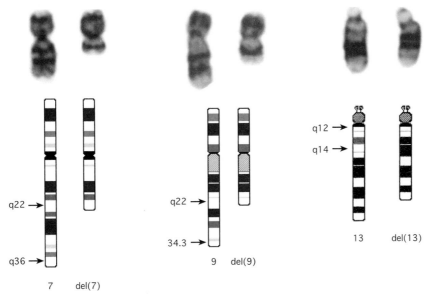

Figure 21 del(7)(q22q36).   **Figure 22** del(9)(q22).   **Figure 23** del(13)(q12q14).

6.4.5 del(13)(q)

Although characteristic of CLL, the deletion of chromosome 13 (*Figure 23*) is also observed in myeloid disease and is a particularly common finding (10%) in myelo-fibrosis. Although the deletion is variable, a common deleted segment at 13q14 has been demonstrated.

6.4.6 del(17)(p)

Although i(17q) (*Figure 24*) is an infrequent finding in all myeloid disease, it is particularly common in CGL where it is a reliable indicator of transformation, either alone or in conjunction with trisomy 8, trisomy 19 or an additional Ph chromosome. Occasionally, other abnormalities such as del(17)(p) or r(17) occur, suggesting that the loss of the short arms, possibly involving P53, may be the vital genetic event in isochromosomal formation. Its presence in either MDS or MPD suggests a poor prognosis.

6.4.7 del (20)(q)

The deleted 20 (*Figure 25*) is a common observation in myeloid disorders. Although most frequently associated with myeloproliferative disease, particularly PRV, this abnormality is also present in 5% of MDS patients and (on rare occasions) in AML, particularly AML M6. It is often difficult to define the breakpoints accurately and heterogeneity of breakpoints has been demonstrated. The deleted segment lies between 20q11 and 20q12 (20). Despite the diagnostic heterogeneity, patients with this abnormality show common morphological features of dysplasia in erythroid precursors and megakaryocytes.

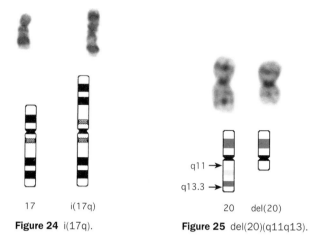

17   i(17q)

Figure 24 i(17q).

q11 →
q13.3 →

20   del(20)

Figure 25 del(20)(q11q13).

7 The role of chromosome analysis in myeloid disease

In AML, a limited number of highly specific associations provide not only a useful aid to FAB classification but, more importantly, serve as valuable prognostic indicators. For CGL, the Philadelphia chromosome is a specific disease marker but in other cases of MPD and MDS, cytogenetics has proved to be of little assistance in classification and few abnormalities have been shown to be of prognostic significance.

The karyotypic complexity found in AML has not yet been proved to modify prognosis. This is particularly true of additional chromosome abnormalities accompanying specific rearrangements. The same situation applies at diagnosis in CGL. However, in other forms of MPD and MDS, an increased number of chromosome abnormalities present indicates a poor prognosis. Similarly, chromosome evolution in these cases, and in CGL, characteristically occurs at disease progression and is therefore a useful marker of transformation.

In AML at remission, patients usually have normal karyotypes and this may prove useful in monitoring response to therapy, although this assessment may require extended counts. Relapse is characterized by a return of the original clone, sometimes with further evolution. Although in transformed MPD and MDS remissions are more difficult to obtain, when successful, the karyotype is more likely to revert to that seen during the chronic phase. Cytogenetics can provide additional confirmation of remission prior to bone marrow harvest for possible transplant, but this is only valuable when an abnormal clone has already been identified at diagnosis. In this case, extended analysis will again be required. The general applications of chromosome analysis in confirming engraftment and providing insight into the nature of post transplant relapse are covered in Chapter 5, Sections 2.14 and 2.15.

References

1. Grimwade, D. *et al.* (1998). *Blood,* **92**(7), 2322.
2. Berger, R. *et al.* (1987). *Cancer Genet. Cytogenet.,* **29**, 9.
3. Fourth International Workshop on chromosomes in leukemia 1982 (1984). *Cancer Genet. Cytogenet.* **11**, 251.
4. Fenaux, P. *et al.* (1989). *Br. J. Haematol.* **73**, 61.
5. Greenberg, P. *et al.* (1997). *Blood* **89**(6), 2079.
6. Griffin, J. D. (1986). *Semin. Hematol.* **23**(3), Suppl. 1 (July), 20.
7. Singer, C. R. J., Mc Donald, G. A., and Douglas, A. S. (1984). *Br. J. Haematol.* **57**, 309.
8. Heim, S. and Mitelman, F. (1987). *Cancer Cytogenetics.* Alan R. Liss, New York.
9. Secker-Waker, L. M., Mehta, A., and Bain, B. (1995). *Br. J. Haematol.* **91**, 490.
10. Wlodarska, I. *et al.* (1998). *Blood* **91**(4), 1399.
11. Lillington, D. N., McCallum, P. K., Lister, T. A., and Gibbons, B. (1993). *Leukaemia* **7**, 527.
12. Aguiar, R. C. T. *et al.* (1997). *Blood* **90**, 3130.
13. Abruzzo, L. V. *et al.* (1992). *Am. J. Surg. Pathol.* **16**, 236.
14. Minamihisamatsu, M. and Ishihara, T. (1998). *Cancer Genet. Cytogenet.* **33**, 161.
15. Secker-Walker, L. M. (1998). *Leukaemia* **12**, 776.
16. Chen, Z. *et al.* (1993). *Proc. Natl. Acad. Sci. USA* **91**, 1178.
17. Bernard, P. *et al.* (1989). *Leukemia* **3/10**, 740.
18. United Kingdom Cytogenetics Group (UKCCG) (1992). *Leukaemia Res.* **16**(9), 841.
19. Jaju, R. J. *et al.* (1998). *Genes Chromosomes Cancer* **22**(3), 251.
20. Asimakopoulos, F. A. *et al.* (1994). *Blood,* **84**, 3086.

Chapter 3

Cytogenetics in acute lymphoblastic leukaemia

B. Czepulkowski

King's College Hospital Cytogenetics Department, The Rayne Institute, 123, Coldharbour Lane, London SE5 9NU, UK

B Gibbons

North East London Regional Cytogenetics Laboratory, Level 2, Queen Square House, Queen Square, London WC1N 3BG, UK

1 Introduction

In the past, cytogenetic analysis of ALL has been hampered by the difficulty in obtaining good quality chromosomes for analysis. Poor spreading, fuzzy chromosomes and indistinct bands meant that only about 50% of cases analysed were found to have an abnormal clone, or because of metaphases that could not be analysed, a number of cases were classified as failures.

Improvements in cytogenetic techniques have increased the success rate and abnormality rates observed in ALL, and also given an insight into the importance of cytogenetic abnormalities in the pathophysiology and prognosis of haematological malignancies, including ALL. Abnormalities were detected in only about half of all ALL patients in initial banding studies (1) but now most centres report chromosomal abnormalities in 60–85% of ALL cases (2–6). In cases with a normal karyotype or in failed cases, interphase FISH provides an additional technique by which chromosome abnormalities of prognostic importance can be identified. Such cases are now routinely screened with panels of probes to detect cases of high hyperdiploidy, *BCR/ABL* fusion, *ETV6/AML1* fusion and splitting of the *MLL* gene. However, it should be noted that interphase FISH alone may give ambiguous results and confirmation from other techniques should always be sought (see Chapter 6).

That cytogenetic abnormalities confer important prognostic information in ALL was first reported by Secker-Walker *et al.* (7) in 1978 in a series of childhood ALL. It was noted that hyperdiploid karyotypes had better clinical outcomes than those with pseudodiploidy or hypodiploidy, the findings being confirmed in a follow-up study (8).

Acute lymphoblastic leukaemia is most common in childhood, with a peak incidence at about 2–5 years. There is second peak incidence at about 50 years of age which rises slowly with advancing age (9).

Most studies of karyotypic abnormalities have been performed in childhood ALL, adult ALL showing non-random abnormalities similar to those observed in childhood ALL, but their distribution and perhaps their biological significance differ somewhat (10). In infants, 85% show a *MLL* gene rearrangement, whereas hyperdiploidy and the t(9;22) translocation are seen in a very small percentage. In children, the hyperdiploid group comprises 25% of all abnormalities, while the *MLL* gene rearrangement is seen only in 5% of patients. The *ETV6/AML1* gene re-arrangement is observed in 25% of children. In adults, again the proportions of the different cytogenetic changes are altered, with the t(9;22) abnormality being observed in 25% of patients, hyperdiploidy only in 5% and the *MLL* gene rearrangement only in 5% (see *Figure 1*). This chapter deals with the difficulties in analysing and interpreting chromosome abnormalities in ALL, and also gives the major changes observed, with prognostic significance if known, and also any molecular associations which have been discovered to date.

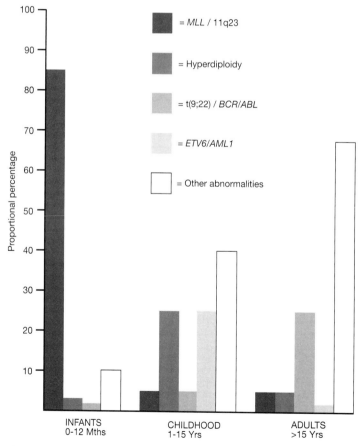

Figure 1 Cytogenetic subsets of ALL: chart showing varying proportions of major cytogenetic abnormalities.

2 Preparation of bone marrow samples from acute lymphoblastic leukaemia patients

A useful technique for high-quality direct bone marrow preparation has been given by Williams *et al.* (11). However, it is recommended that in addition to a direct method, other culture methods should be applied, including the one given for synchronization of bone marrow cultures in Chapter 1, since this will maximize the likelihood of successful culture, in addition to achieving preparations that yield chromosomes with good morphology.

2.1 Optimizing cell density in cultures from patients with a high white cell count

Patients with ALL have very wide-ranging white cell counts and it can be very difficult to produce successful cultures unless stringent procedures are carried out to ensure that cell density is approximately 10^6 cells per culture. It is advisable to use a Coulter counter or the cell counting method given in *Protocol 1* in Chapter 1 and the information in Chapter 1 *Table 2*.

2.2 Analysis guidelines

If careful attention is paid to the protocols described in Chapter 1, good-quality chromosome preparations should be achieved, but it is extremely important to ensure that the leukaemic cells are selected for analysis. Often, two morphologically different populations of metaphase cells are present in the preparation, and if this is the case, it is almost invariably true that the chromosomes with better spreading and crisper morphology have a normal karyotype. This variation in chromosome quality is undoubtedly more true of ALL than any other type of leukaemia, and this problem needs to be addressed when selecting cells for analysis. *Figures 2* and *3* illustrate the good-quality chromosomes of the normal metaphases and the poorer morphology of the abnormal metaphases in the same preparation. The difference in chromosome quality poses a problem because in order to detect and accurately characterize subtle chromosome abnormalities it is necessary to locate the best quality abnormal cells. It can be very tempting to select the best cells and hence only normal metaphases for analysis. Each laboratory therefore needs a scheme to ensure the analysis of cells with a wide-ranging morphology quality. Laboratories undertaking chromosome analysis for haematological malignancies should attempt to meet current standards of analysis as indicated by the abnormality detection rate reported in other recent studies (12). Awareness of the currently recognized non-random abnormalities is essential, and to aid the cytogeneticist a list of the major abnormalities is given in *Table 1*. More detailed consideration of the most important chromosome abnormalities is given in Section 4.

(a)

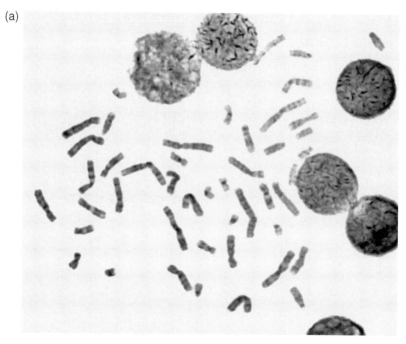

(b)

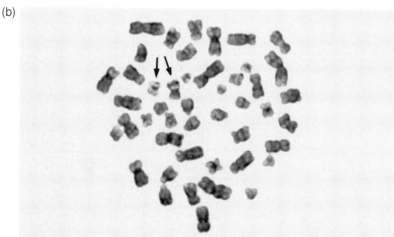

Figure 2 Cells from the same culture: (a) normal cell with good morphology; (b) leukaemic cell with poor morphology showing the t(11;19)(q23;p13.3) translocation (arrowed).

3 Classification of acute lymphoblastic leukaemia

Morphological evaluation has, for over a century, been the traditional method for classification of the various cytological types of acute and chronic leukaemia. Cytochemical stains assist in distinguishing the lymphoid from the myeloid leukaemias.

In recent years, immunocytochemistry has enhanced these methods and

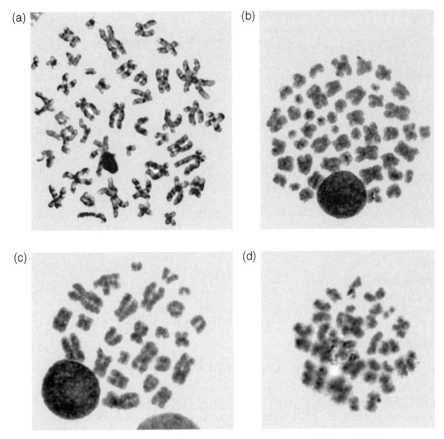

Figure 3 Cells from the same culture: (a) normal cell with best morphology; (b) high hyperdiploid cell with poor morphology; (c) and (d) near-haploid cells with variable morphology.

enabled further characterization of leukaemic blast cells. Certain immunocyto-chemical stains are sensitive to cell-specific antigens and these prove diagnostic-ally valuable when cytochemistry fails to provide an unequivocal result.

In addition to these immunological developments, advances in cytogenetics, such as high-resolution banding and the use of molecular probes, have enabled further characterization of the subgroups of ALL by the identification of consist-ent chromosomal changes. To understand the various cytogenetic changes that occur in ALL, it is important also to have an understanding of the morphological characteristics and their immunological features.

3.1 French–American–British classification system

The classification of ALL by the FAB cooperative group (13) has been used for a number of years as a means of distinguishing the three main subtypes of ALL (L1, L2 and L3). Chapter 5, *Table 6* expands upon the morphological criteria which give rise to the classification by the FAB system.

Table 1 Major non-random chromosome abnormalities in ALL

Early and Pre-B ALL	Mature B-cell ALL	T-lineage ALL
t(1;19)(q23;p13)	t(8;14)(q24;q32)	t(1;7)(p32;q35)
del(6)(q13–q23)	t(8;22)(q24;q11)	t(1;14)(p32;q11)
del(9)(p11–p13)	t(2;8)(p12;q24)	del(6)(q13–23)
dic(9;12)(p11–13;p11–12)		t(7;9)(q34;q34)
dic(9;20)(p11–13;q11)		t(7;11)(q35;p13)
t(9;22)(q34;q11)		del(9)(p11–13)
t(4;11)(q21;q23)		t(8;14)(q24;q11)
t(11;19)(q23;p13)		t(10;14)(q24;q11)
t(11;V)(q23;v)		t(11;14)(p15;q11)
t(12;21)(p12–13;q22) and del(12)(p11–13)		
Trisomy 8		
Trisomy 21		
Near-haploidy		
Severe hypodiploidy		
> 50 high hyperdiploidy		

3.2 Cytochemistry

Classification is enhanced by identifying various cytoplasmic constituents with cytochemical stains, which include MPO, NSE and PAS reaction.

Myeloperoxidase activity is located in the azurophilic granules present in granulocytes and monocytes but absent in lymphocytes, and is a useful tool in distinguishing lymphoid and myeloid leukaemias. An SBB stain gives similar information.

Lymphoblasts and myeloblasts contain non-specific esterases. In monocytes and monocytic precursors sodium fluoride inhibits the activity of NSE. These are not inhibited in lymphoblasts and myeloblasts so the test is helpful in distinguishing monocytic leukaemias from ALL.

The PAS test identifies cytoplasmic carbohydrate, carbohydrate coating protein and lipids. Myeloblasts are usually PAS-negative, and although increased amounts of PAS activity are detected in the cytoplasm of lymphoblasts, it is not specific as some do not contain PAS-positive material. It is more important to note the pattern of positivity. Typically, in ALL the PAS positive material appears as large block deposits around the nucleus of the leukaemic blast. *Table 2* shows the reactions of these various cytochemical stains in types of leukaemias.

3.2.1 Other stains

In T cell convoluted types of leukaemic lymphoblasts, acid phosphatase activity may appear in a localized paranuclear area. In other atypical lymphoblasts that contain azurophilic granules, stains for MPO, NSE and SBB are usually negative. In leukaemic lymphoblasts of all types, the cytoplasm has a high content of RNA and this may be intense in the L3 variant. The cell also has a perinuclear distrib-

Table 2 Cytochemical stain reactions

Stain/reaction	Positive	Negative
Myeloperoxidase (MPO)	M3 ++++ M1/M2 +++ M4 ++ M5 +	M7 L1 L2 L3
Non-specific esterases[a]	M5 ++++ (inhibited by NaF) M4 +++ M2 ++(not inhibited by NaF) L1 (not inhibited by NaF) L2 (not inhibited by NaF) L3 (not inhibited by NaF)	M1 M7
PAS test	Cytoplasm of lymphoblasts	Myeloblasts
AP activity	Paranuclear positivity in T-cell ALL Maybe positive in AML M1, M2 and M5	B-cell ALL[b]

[a] Note increased positivity with increasing maturation.

[b] The reaction in B-cell ALL can show weak positivity.

ution of vacuoles which are Oil Red O positive. Methyl green pyronine is also positive in L3 cells. β-Glucuronidase appears to have a distribution similar to that of acid phosphatase.

3.3 Immunology

The use of monoclonal antibodies has provided us with insights into the differentiation of leukaemia and has augmented further subdivision of lymphoid malignancies. Monoclonal antibodies are used to define cell surface antigens on normal and leukaemic blasts and the applications of immunophenotyping can be summarized thus:

- the distinction of ALL from AML, particularly in cases where morphology and cytochemistry results are equivocal
- the distinction of B-cell precursor ALL, B-cell ALL and T-cell ALL
- the detection of subtypes of AML
- diagnosis of AML M7 by detection of CD41a, CD42b and CD61
- recognition of chronic lymphoproliferative disorders of B- and T-cell type.

3.3.1 B-lineage acute lymphoblastic leukaemia

The majority of ALL cases are B-lineage in origin and are identified by positivity with monoclonal antibodies such as CD19 and CD20.

The four major immunological classes of B-lineage ALL represent the malignant counterparts of lymphoid cells at the premature, early and intermediate stages of differentiation. These are listed below:

- early B-precursor ALL or Pro-B ALL (previously Null-ALL)
- pre-pre-B ALL (previously common ALL)

- pre-B ALL
- B ALL.

The characteristics of the above are shown in *Table 3*.

Table 3 Immunological characteristics of ALL

Type of ALL	Cytogenetic abnormality	Antigenic profile (usual)	Comments	FAB type
Pro-B-cell ALL (Early B-precursor ALL)	t(4;11)(q21;q23) t(9;22)(q34;q11) t(11;19)(q23;p13.3)	HLA-DR TdT CD19	Often occurs in newborns and infants	L1/L2
Pre-pre-B-cell ALL	Near haploid del(12)(p) t(9;22)(q34;q11) del(6)(q)	HLA-DR TdT CD19 CD10 CD20	Most frequent type of ALL. 70% of non T-lineage ALL	L1/L2
Pre-B-cell ALL	t(1;19)(q23;p13) t(9;22)(q34;q11) t(12;21)(p12-13;q22)	HLA-DR TdT CD10 CD19 CD20 CD22 CD37 Cytoplasmic μ	15–20% of non-T-lineage ALL. Note cytoplasmic μ expression	L1/L2
B-cell ALL	t(8;14)(q24;q32) t(2;8)(p12;q24) t(8;22)(q24;q11) del 6q	HLA-DR CD10 CD19 CD20 CD22 CD24 SmIg	The three translocations account for 15–20% of ALL cases	L3
Early thymocyte ALL	9p abnormalities	CD7 CD5 CD71 CD38 CD2 TdT	Accounts for less than 1% of ALL cases	L1/L2
Intermediate thymocyte ALL	t or del 9p t(10;14)(q24;q11) t(11;14)(p13;q11)	CD7 CD5 CD2 CD1a CD3 CD4 CD8 CD45RB		
Mature thymocyte ALL	t or del 14q11 t(8;14)(q24;q11)	CD7 CD5 CD2 CD3 CD4 or CD8 CD6		

ALL represents approximately 50% of new acute leukaemias. Early B-precursor ALL and Pro-B ALL account for about 64% of the ALL cases, whereas pre-B ALL represents 20% of ALL cases and B ALL represents only 1% of ALL cases (for T ALL see Section 3.3.2).

3.3.2 T-lineage ALL

This group represents 15% of ALL cases, and patients usually display a high blast cell count, there is a predominance of older male patients with mediastinal mass. There are three types of T-cell ALL classes:

- early thymocyte T ALL
- common thymocyte T ALL
- mature thymocyte T ALL.

The characteristics and antigenic profile of all types of ALL are shown in *Table 3*.

3.4 Cellular differentiation

The phenotype of most leukaemic cells reflects the characteristics of normal cells. None of the markers described above are leukaemia-specific since they can be identified on normal as well as malignant cells.

The lymphocytes are the major cellular elements of the body's immune system. B-lineage lymphocytes are responsible for Ig-mediated immunity and the T-lineage lymphocytes play a role in cellular immunity, after conditioning in the thymus. They also regulate B cells, either enhancing or reducing the Ig-mediated immune response via helper T cells and suppressor T cells respectively.

During the maturation of B lymphocytes, somatic recombination of the Ig loci precedes Ig production. Newly synthesized molecules occur in the cytoplasm, and only following further maturation are Ig molecules expressed on the cell surface. These Ig loci are located at the following chromosomal bands:

- 14q32 Ig heavy chain gene
- 2p12 κ light chain gene
- 22q11 λ light chain gene (see Section 4.1).

In T-cell differentiation, the three loci below are essential in coding for components of the T-cell receptor:

- 14q11.2 α/δ chain locus
- 7q35 β chain locus
- 7p15 γ chain locus.

Figure 4 shows how lymphoid differentiation is associated with disease types and maturation levels. The most important markers for ALL are CD antigens specific for T and B cells, cIgμ, SmIg, CD10 (common acute lymphoblastic antigen, CALLA) and TdT. The five subtypes can be discriminated by their positive or negative expression of CD10, CD19, CD20, CD21, cytoplasmic CD22, CD34 and TdT, cIgμ, SmIg, HLA-DR and T-cell markers CD1 to CD8.

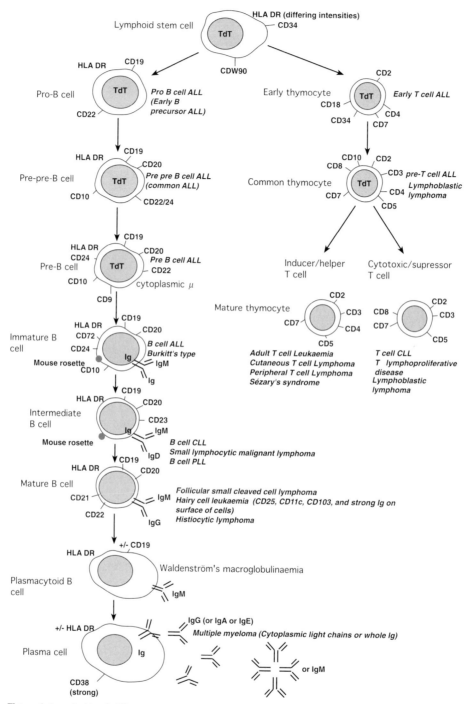

Figure 4 Lymphoid cell differentiation levels, showing immunological phenotype and associated disease categories. (With thanks to Keith Fishlock of the Immunophenotyping Department at King's College Hospital, London, UK, for his invaluable help in checking the contents and accuracy of this diagram.)

3.5 Morphology–Immunology–Cytogenetics classification

The MIC classification (14) uses all three disciplines to subdivide the different types of leukaemia. Cytogenetics is included in this categorization since it is apparent that certain chromosome abnormalities occur consistently in specific types of leukaemia. Karyotype has also been established as an independent prognostic factor in ALL.

The most common abnormalities, prognostic implications and associations are described in detail in Section 4.

3.5.1 Molecular mechanisms underlying chromosomal rearrangements in acute lymphoblastic leukaemia

The specific chromosome abnormalities associated with many types of leukaemia play a pivotal role in the development of the disease. In ALL structural chromosome abnormalities (translocation, deletion and inversion) are of prime importance in leukaemogenesis through two main mechanisms:

(1) Activation of a proto-oncogene through juxtaposition with a T cell receptor or immunoglobulin gene resulting in dysregulation and aberrant gene expression;

(2) Intragenic breakage followed by translocation resulting in the formation of a fusion gene encoding for a chimeric protein.

These structural chromosome rearrangements can be detected using FISH (see Chapter 6) which visualizes the juxtaposition of two signals from different chromosomes, or displays a split signal indicating the breakage of a targeted gene into two parts. Using single locus probes, results can be evaluated using interphase nuclei and this is a valuable tool where there is a paucity of metaphases.

4 Structural chromosome abnormalities

4.1 t(8;14)(q24;q32), t(2;8)(p12;q24) and t(8;22)(q24;q11)

The above translocations are highly specific to B-cell neoplasia, and are observed most frequently in mature B-cell ALL and Burkitt's lymphoma. They appear to be identical in both lymphomatous and leukaemic disease (see Chapter 4).

B-cell ALL patients tend to be male, with median age of 11 years in children and 40 years in adults. They present with bulky extramedullary disease and have frequent and early CNS involvement, an unusually high blast cell proliferative rate and, consequently, a rapidly progressive clinical course (15,16). The translocations are almost always associated with ALL L3 morphology. The frequency with which the three translocations occur is 85% for t(8;14), 10% for (8;22) and 5% for t(2;8). Three-way translocations, which are rare, but include chromosomes 8, 14 and a third chromosome, are also included in these values. Care should be exercised in order not to miss these variants during analysis. *Figure 5* illustrates these three translocations. One must be aware that in addition to the above chromosome abnormalities, mature B-cell ALL may also exhibit additional abnormalities the most common of which is dup(1q) (See *Figure 6*).

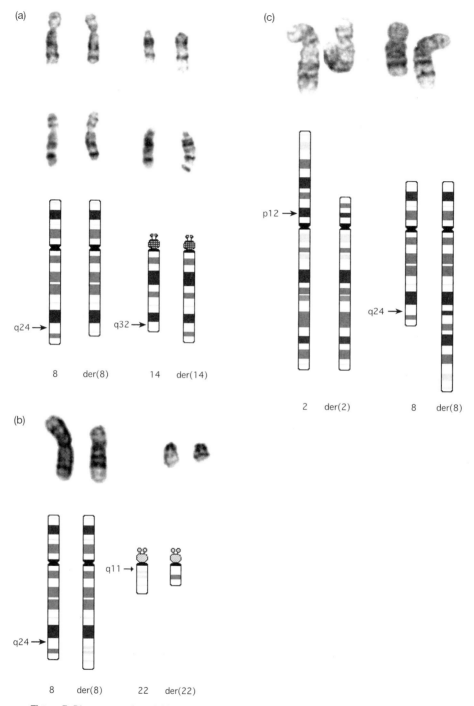

Figure 5 Diagrams and partial karyotypes of translocations: (a) t(8;14)(q24;q32); (b) t(8;22)(q24;q11). The homologue of the der(8) chromosome is shown as an iso(8)(q10) in the photograph, which was kindly supplied by the LRF and UKCCG database in ALL, Royal Free Hospital, London, UK. (c) t(2;8)(p12;q24).

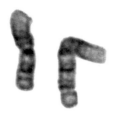

Figure 6 Partial karyotype showing duplication of 1q. The photograph of the dup(1q) was kindly supplied by the LRF and UKCCG database in ALL, Royal Free Hospital, London, UK.

4.1.1 Molecular events

In these classic translocations, the common denominator is the break at 8q24, where the oncogene *c-MYC* is located, and regulation of this oncogene is abnormal following translocation. The crucial event is the juxtapositioning of *c-MYC* with the immunoglobulin heavy chain gene locus at 14q32. In the variant translocations, *c-MYC* is brought into juxtaposition with the immunoglobulin κ light chain gene locus on chromosome 2p12, or the immunoglobulin λ light chain gene locus on chromosome 22q11 in the translocations t(2;8) and t(8;22), respectively. The rearrangements bring *c-MYC* under the influence of transcription-regulating sequences of the active immunoglobulin locus. This results in dysregulation of *c-MYC*, increased transcription and consequently neoplastic growth.

These translocations originally carried a poor prognosis, but the introduction of short-term dose-intensive regimens such as hyperfractionated cyclophosphamide, high-dose methotrexate and cytarabine have improved the clinical outcomes (16,17).

4.2 t(1;19)(q23;p13)

This translocation, and its rarer variant t(17;19)(q21–22;p13), is observed in about 25% of pre-B-cell ALL patients, 5–6% of ALL overall, and less than 5% of adult ALL (18,19). The cells usually have ALL L1 morphology.

The t(1;19) translocation is observed in two primary forms:

- as a balanced translocation t(1;19)

- as an unbalanced translocation, showing der(19)t(1;19) and two normal homologues of chromosome 1.

The latter unbalanced form is more common than the balanced rearrangement, (about 75%) and this can create a pitfall for the inexperienced cytogeneticist who may not recognize the derivative chromosome 19 in the presence of two normal homologues of chromosome 1. *Figure 7* illustrates the unbalanced form of this translocation, with diagrams showing both the balanced and unbalanced forms.

No differences in clinical presentation or prognosis exist between the two variants (20). ALL with the t(1;19) translocation is associated with high white cell counts, high LDH levels and the immunophenotype is positive for CD10, CD19, CD22 and cytoplasmic immunoglobulin and negative for CD21. The prognosis

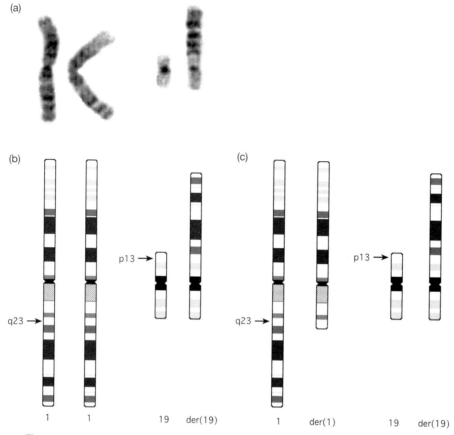

Figure 7 Partial karyotype (a) and diagram (b) of the unbalanced form of t(1;19)(q23;p13). The balanced form of t(1;19)(q23;p13) is shown in (c). The photograph in (a) was kindly supplied by the LRF and UKCCG database in ALL, Royal Free Hospital, London, UK.

tends to be poor and better responses have been gained with more intensified treatment.

4.3.1 Molecular events

The breakpoint on chromosome 19 has been mapped to band p13.2–p13.3 which contains a gene *E2A*, which encodes two transcription factors, E12 and E47. These genes are considered to be required for normal lymphopoiesis and regulation of B-cell development (21). The breakpoint on chromosome 1q23 is not as confined but the translocation disrupts the homeobox-containing 'pre-B-cell-leukaemia' gene (*PRL* or *PBX1*). The E2A/PBX1 fusion appears to function as a transcriptional activator.

4.3 T-lineage ALL

Both the clinical features and chromosome abnormalities seen in T-lineage ALL show a degree of overlap with those observed in the T-cell chronic lympho-

Table 4 Deregulation of proto-oncogenes in T-cell ALL

Proto-oncogene (location)	Deregulating gene	Chromosome abnormality
TAL1 (1p32)	*SIL*	Microdeletion 1p32
	TCR-α	t(1;14)(p32;q11)
	TCR-β	t(1;7)(p32;q35)
LCK (1p34)	*TCR-β*	t(1;7)(p34;q34)
c-MYC (8q24)	*TCR-α*	t(8;14)(q24;q11)
RBTN1 (11p15)	*TCR-δ*	t(11;14)(p15;q11)
RBTN2 (11p13)	*TCR-α/δ*	t(11;14)(p13;q11)
		t(7;11)(q35;p13)
HOX11 (10q24)	*TCR-α/δ*	t(10;14)(q24;q11)
	TCR-β	t(7;10)(q34;q24)
LYL1 (19p13)	*TCR-β*	t(7;19)(q35;p13)
TAN1 (9q34)	*TCR-β*	t(7;9)(q34;q34)[a]

[a] Note that *TAN1* is disrupted rather than deregulated.

proliferative disorders (see Chapter 4). T-lineage ALL is more common in males than females, and it typically affects older children and young adults. The disease is characterized by a high white cell count, lymphadenopathy, splenomegaly, mediastinal mass and CNS involvement, often with an aggressive course and short survival.

Approximately 25% of T-lineage ALL patients have translocations involving one of the T-cell receptor (*TCR*) genes located at 14q11.2, (*TCR-α/δ*), 7q35 (*TCR-β*) or rarely 7p14–15 (*TCR-γ*). The mechanism of oncogene activation is analogous to that observed in B-cell ALL; juxtaposition of a proto-oncogene with a *TCR* gene results in deregulation and aberrant expression (see *Table 4*).

4.3.1 Deregulation of *TAL1*

The proto-oncogene *TAL1* at 1p32 is deregulated in approximately one-third of paediatric cases. Most frequently, a microdeletion at 1p32 brings the promoter of *SIL* into juxtaposition with *TAL1* sequences. This microdeletion can be detected by PCR but is not visible by conventional G-banding techniques. The visible translocations t(1;14)(p32;q11) and t(1;7)(p32;q35) are less frequent mechanisms by which *TAL1* is deregulated by *TCR-α* and *TCR-β*, respectively.

4.3.2 Deregulation of *c-myc*, *RBTN1*, *RBTN2* and *HOX11*

Other proto-oncogenes are also deregulated via translocation into a position adjacent to a *TCR* promoter/enhancer; the most common rearrangements are t(8;14)(q24;q11) deregulating *c-MYC*, t(11;14)(p15;q11) deregulating *RBTN1*, t(7;11) (q35;p13) deregulating *RBTN2* and t(10;14)(q24;q11) deregulating *HOX11* (see *Figure 8*).

The t(8;14)(q24;q11) translocation is not solely specific to T-cell ALL, but has also been described in pre-B-cell ALL (22).

The t(10;14)(q24;q11) translocation is observed in 4–7% of T-cell acute

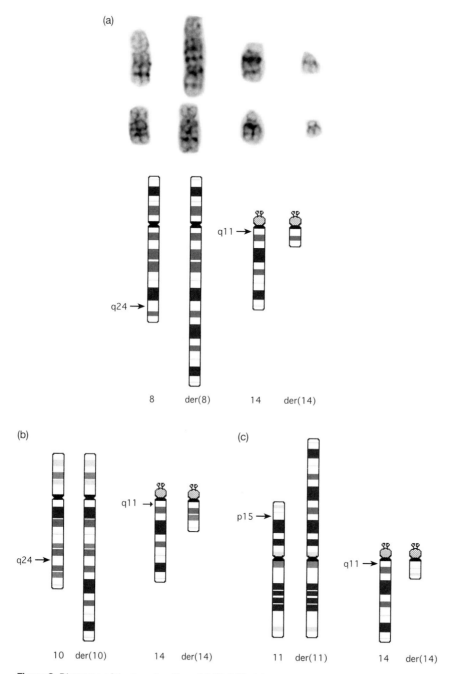

Figure 8 Diagrams of the translocations (a) t(8;14)(q24;q11), (b) t(10;14)(q24;q11) and (c) t(11;14)(p13;q11). The photograph of the t(8;14) was kindly supplied by A. Watmore, Centre for Human Genetics, Sheffield, UK.

leukaemias (23). This translocation appears to be associated with a favourable outcome, the CR being 100%, and 75% of patients achieve a disease free-survival rate of 3 years (3).

4.3.3 Disruption of *TAN1*

Although the translocation t(7;9)(q34;q34) brings *TAN1* into close proximity with the *TCR-β* locus, *TAN1* is disrupted rather than deregulated and a truncated protein is produced.

4.4 Deletion of 6q

Deletion of chromosome 6 occurs in about 4–6% of childhood ALL and less frequently in adults. The breakpoints are variable and occur between q14 and q21, and a more telomeric region distal to q23 (see *Figure 9*). Deletion 6q is observed in lymphoid disease and also solid tumours, and is often seen as a secondary change, although in one-third of cases it is observed as a sole change (1,15).

4.5 Abnormalities of 9p

Abnormalities of 9p, including deletions and unbalanced translocations with a p21-pter breakpoint result in loss of 9p sequences and hence reduction to hemi-

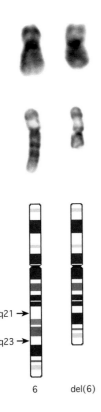

q21 →
q23 →

6   del(6)

Figure 9 Diagram and partial karyotype of deletion 6q.

zygosity. 9p abnormalities are present in approximately 10% of ALL, primarily in patients with T lineage ALL, but have also been observed in B-lineage ALL.

4.5.1 dic(9;12)(p11–13;p11–12)

The dic(9;12) is observed in approximately 1% of ALL (see *Figure 10*). It is almost exclusively seen in early B-lineage leukaemia and is most common in older children and young adults. Remission rates are very high and prognosis is good. Trisomy 8 is a frequent secondary finding associated with the dic(9;12).

4.5.2 dic(9;20)(p11–13;q11)

The dic(9;20) is a subtle chromosome abnormality, observed predominantly in early B-lineage ALL (see *Figure 11*). It often masquerades as monosomy 20, sometimes with apparent deletion of 9p. Trisomy 21 is a frequent secondary finding. In cases of apparent monosomy 20, FISH with either whole-chromosome paints or centromeric probes for chromosomes 9 and 20 is essential to confirm or exclude dic(9;20). Remission rates are high, although long-term prognosis has not been established to date.

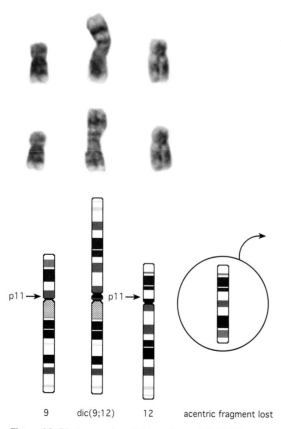

Figure 10 Diagram and partial karyotype of dic(9;12)(p11–13;p11–12).

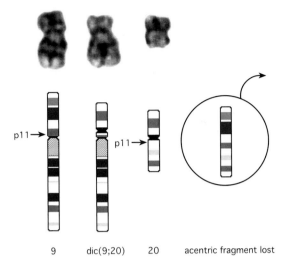

9   dic(9;20)   20   acentric fragment lost

Figure 11 Diagram and partial karyotype of dic(9;20)(p11–13;q11). The photograph of the dic(9;20) was kindly supplied by the LRF and UKCCG database in ALL, Royal Free Hospital, London, UK.

4.6 t(9;22)(q34;q11)

The translocation t(9;22) illustrated in Chapter 2 *Figure 9*, results in the Philadelphia chromosome, the der(22)t(9;22)(q34;q11). Although diagnostic for CGL, this translocation is present in 25–30% of adult ALL and approximately 5% of childhood ALL. It is rare in infants.

The t(9;22) is observed in ALL with varying degrees of immature B-cell differentiation but has also been observed in biphenotypic leukaemia expressing myeloid markers, or more rarely, T-cell markers.

In contrast to Philadelphia chromosome positive (Ph+ve) CGL, a normal cell population is present in most cases of ALL. In addition, up to 30% of Philadelphia chromosome translocations occur in hyperdiploid karyotypes of over 50 chromosomes (*Figure 12*). Full analysis is therefore important to avoid misclassification, as these patients do not belong to the high hyperdiploid group described in Section 5.2. It is particularly important to be aware of Ph+ve hyperdiploidy, because the presence of the t(9;22) translocation is associated with a poor prognosis, even in the presence of > 50 chromosomes, whereas typical > 50 hyperdiploidy is associated with a good response to conventional therapy, and carries a much better prognosis. An additional problem with analysis is that 5% of cases occur as variant or masked Philadelphia translocations that may be difficult to identify if metaphase spreads are of poor quality. In equivocal cases, FISH or RT-PCR should be used to confirm the presence or absence of a Philadelphia translocation.

Patients with Ph+ve ALL who have achieved apparent haematological remission often show persistence of the abnormal clone. In approximately 20% of

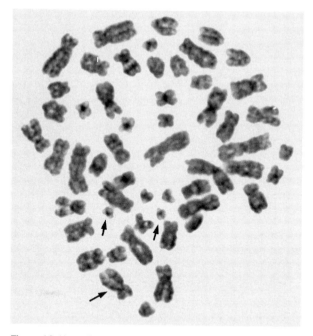

Figure 12 Hyperdiploid metaphase showing the t(9;22)(q34;q11) translocation (arrowed).

cases this can be detected at the cytogenetic level, however, interphase FISH can also be employed. Detection of residual disease is important, as its presence indicates that therapy should be continued for a longer period, particularly in patients being considered for bone marrow transplantation.

4.6.1 Molecular events

The molecular consequence of the t(9;22)(q34;q11) is the fusion of *ABL* at 9q34 with *BCR* at 22q11, forming a chimeric *BCR/ABL* gene which produces a chimeric protein with increased tyrosine kinase activity. Breakpoints at *BCR* cluster in two regions, the major breakpoint cluster region (*M-BCR*) which produces a 210 kDa protein and the minor breakpoint cluster region (*m-BCR*) which produces a 190 kDa protein. Either type of product can be observed in ALL, although, in contrast to CGL, the 190 kDa protein predominates. It is unclear whether Ph+ve ALL patients expressing the 210 kDa protein have a form of lymphoid acute-phase of CGL or a true *de novo* acute leukaemia. The *BCR/ABL* fusion gene can be detected by two-colour FISH or the chimeric mRNA can be detected by RT-PCR.

4.7 Abnormalities of 11q23 involving the *MLL* gene

The *MLL* gene at 11q23 is implicated in a large number of translocations, the most common of which in ALL are t(4;11)(q21;q23) and t(11;19)(q23;p13.3) (24). *MLL* is involved in most cases of infant or congenital leukaemia, and a smaller number of childhood and adult leukaemias that often display myelomonocytic or monocytic characteristics. It is also implicated in secondary leukaemia following therapy with DNA topoisomerase II inhibitors. Chromosome 11q should be examined with great care in all cases of infant, biphenotypic or secondary leukaemias as some of the translocations are subtle and easily overlooked. Involvement of *MLL* can also be detected by Southern blotting, or by FISH (see Chapter 6, Sections 4.6.2 and 6.4). The aberrant transcripts which result from these translocations can be detected by RT-PCR.

4.7.1 t(4;11)(q21;q23)

Translocation t(4;11)(q21;q23), illustrated in *Figure 13*, is observed in 40–50% of infants with ALL although it is less common in older children and adults. It is more common in females. Patients usually present with hepatosplenomegaly, CNS involvement and extremely high white cell counts with a high percentage of blasts. In such cases, it is particularly important to dilute both bone marrow and peripheral blood samples to give a culture concentration of approximately 10^6cells/ml.

The leukaemic cells are typically very immature blasts of early B-precursor or pro-B type, usually CD19+ve and CD10–ve. It is thought that the leukaemia arises in a stem cell with the ability to differentiate along both lymphoid and myeloid pathways; some cases appear to be biphenotypic with monocytic or myelomonocytic characteristics. Rarely, t(4;11)(q21;q23) is observed in AML.

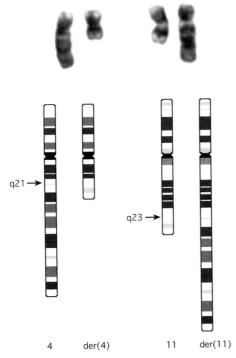

Figure 13 Diagram and partial karyotype of t(4;11)(q21;q23).

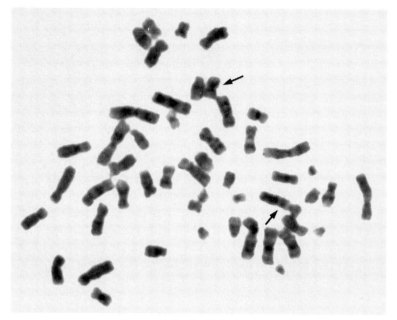

Figure 14 Hyperdiploid metaphase showing the t(4;11)(q21;q23) translocation (arrowed).

Prognosis is very poor, particularly for infants and adult patients. Remission, if achieved, tends to be short and relapse may occur while the patient is undergoing treatment.

t(4;11) appears most frequently as the sole abnormality, however, it may appear in more complex variant forms or rarely in a hyperdiploid karyotype, as shown in *Figure 14*. The molecular consequence of the t(4;11) translocation is *MLL/AF4* fusion.

4.7.2 t(11;19)(q23;p13.3)

Translocation t(11;19)(q23;p13.3), illustrated in *Figures 2* and *15*, is observed in approximately 10% of infants with ALL. In contrast to t(4;11), translocation t(11;19) involves a subtle exchange of only small chromosomal segments and thus there is a reduced likelihood of detecting the translocation in poor chromosome preparations. The clinical and immunophenotypic features of the disease are very similar to that observed in ALL with the t(4;11), except that biphenotypic leukaemia and AML are more common. Prognosis is poor for infants and adults, although older children tend to fare better having longer remissions.

The molecular consequence of the t(11;19) translocation is *MLL/ENL* fusion.

4.7.3 t(11;V)(q23;v)

Translocation t(1;11)(p32;q23), illustrated in *Figure 16*, is a less common structural rearrangement which is observed in the same type of disease as t(4;11) and t(11;19).

Translocation t(9;11), illustrated in Chapter 2 *Figure 12*, is primarily associated with AML/MDS and has been reported only rarely in ALL. Because of the

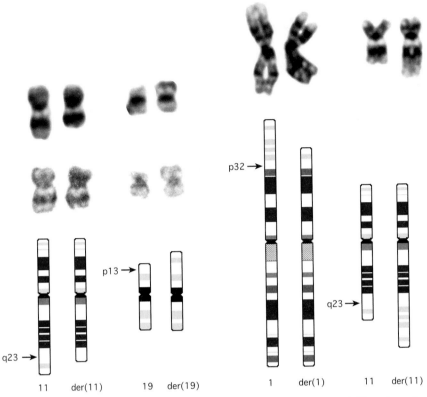

Figure 15 Diagram and partial karyotype of t(11;19)(q23;p13.3).

Figure 16 Diagram and partial karyotype of t(1;11)(p32;q23).

exchange of only small chromosomal segments it is a subtle abnormality that is easily missed.

A variety of other chromosomal rearrangements involving *MLL* have also been described, primarily in AML and biphenotypic leukaemia and rarely observed in ALL. These are described in more detail in Chapter 2, Section 6.1.8.

4.8 t(12;21)(p12–13;q22)

It is only recently that the cryptic translocation t(12;21)(p13;q22) has been identified using FISH techniques (25). Since the discovery of this translocation, which is not detected by conventional banding techniques, it has been observed in 20–30% of B-lineage childhood ALL and is the most frequent non-random translocation in this ALL subtype (26,27). In detecting the t(12;21) it should be noted that deletion of chromosome 12p is often a secondary change, and if deletion of 12p is seen it should be suspected that the other apparently 'normal' chromosome 12 may in fact be the der(12) of the t(12;21) translocation (i.e. neither chromosome 12 is normal). It should also be noted that when an apparent extra chromosome 21 or isochromosome 21q is present these may actually be the der(21)t(12;21) or the iso derivative chromosome 21. In such cases of suspected

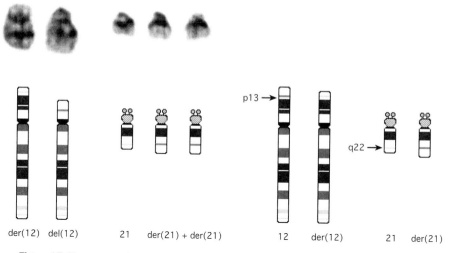

der(12)   del(12)   21   der(21) + der(21)   12   der(12)   21   der(21)

Figure 17 Diagrams and partial karyotype of the t(12;21)(p12-13;q22), showing the cryptic nature of this translocation. The G-banded photograph shows an extra copy of the derivative chromosome 21 and also a deletion of chromosome 12 in the p arm (i.e. both copies of chromosome 12 are abnormal). The photograph of t(12;21) was kindly supplied by the LRF and UKCCG database in ALL, Royal Free Hospital, London, UK.

t(12;21), it is essential to use FISH or RT-PCR techniques in order to reveal the t(12;21) exchange (see Section 4.8.1). It is also standard practice to test any apparently normal ALL case for the t(12;21) using FISH or molecular techniques (see *Figure 17* and Plate 1). See also Chapter 6, Section 6.4).

4.8.1 Molecular events

Molecular cloning has shown that t(12;21)(p12–13;q22) involves a reciprocal fusion of the *ETV6* gene on 12p13 to the *AML1* gene on chromosome 21q22 leading to a production of a *ETV6/AML1* fusion protein (28). The *ETV6/AML1* re-arrangement confers an exceptionally good clinical outcome in childhood B-cell ALL and provides prognostic information independent of the consensus workshop risk groups such as age and white cell count at presentation (29).

5 Numerical abnormalities

Approximately half of ALL cases exhibit numerical chromosome abnormalities, either alone or with structural changes. Historically, a number of ploidy groups have been identified but some of their importance has been superseded by the identification of specific translocations. The less heterogeneous ploidy groups with clear prognostic implications are:

- high hyperdiploid (> 50 chromosomes)
- severe hypodiploid (29–39 chromosomes)
- near-haploid (23–28 chromosomes).

5.1 High hyperdiploidy with > 50 chromosomes

Patients with hyperdiploidy of > 50 chromosomes typically have clones of 51–68 chromosomes. This type of leukaemia is common in children (20–30% of childhood ALL), predominantly female, peaking at 3–5 years old, although it is rare in infants and has a low incidence in adults (5% of adult ALL). High hyperdiploidy is associated with low white cell count, common ALL or early pre-B immunophenotype and FAB type L1 or L2. Prognosis is good, with long-term survival of 70–80% in children. Adults do less well, although event-free survival of 59% at 3 years has been reported. The good prognosis is thought to be related to leukaemic blast sensitivity to a number of anti-leukaemic drugs and the propensity of blast cells to respond by apoptosis. It is unclear why a proportion of patients fail to achieve long-term remission but there is some evidence that higher chromosome counts of > 56 chromosomes and the presence of trisomies 4 and 10 may be associated with a good prognosis whereas the presence of i(17q) is clearly associated with a poor prognosis (30). Although high hyperdiploid clones are rarely identical, they tend to show a pattern of chromosome gain with extra copies of chromosomes 4, 6, 10, 14, 18, 21 and X. The gains are thought to occur in a single step and, apart from chromosome 21, they tend to result in trisomy rather than tetrasomy for the chromosomes gained. This helps to distinguish typical high hyperdiploidy from the hyperdiploidy arising from doubling of a near haploid clone (see Section 5.2). Translocations and other structural chromosome abnormalities are present in approximately half of the high hyperdiploid cases. Duplications of 1q, deletion of 6q and random structural abnormalities have no known prognostic impact. However, the presence of non-random translocations such as the t(9;22), t(4;11), t(1;19) and t(12;21) signify that the translocation is likely to be the primary change and that the hyperdiploidy is probably a secondary event. In such cases, the leukaemia should be classified according to the translocation rather than the ploidy group in order to highlight the correct prognostic implications.

High hyperdiploidy can be detected by application of a panel of probes which will detect the characteristic pattern of gain (31). This technique can be applied to interphase cells but care must be exercised in interpretation and it is essential to exclude the non-random translocations by application of appropriate probes.

High hyperdiploidy should not be confused with near-triploidy/tetraploidy with > 68 chromosomes, which is rare in childhood ALL, although slightly more common in adults. The prognostic implications of near-triploidy/tetraploidy are unclear, although near tetraploidy (82–94 chromosomes) is often associated with T-lineage immunophenotype.

5.2 Near-haploidy

Near-haploidy is defined as < 30 chromosomes; the abnormal clone usually contains between 23 and 28 chromosomes. It is important not to mistake the near haploid cells for broken metaphase spreads. *Figure 3* shows four metaphase spreads from the same culture and illustrates the risk of missing a case of near-

(a)

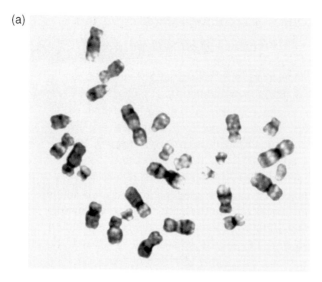

(b)

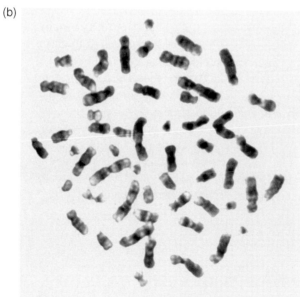

Figure 18 Two metaphases from the same preparation: (a) near-haploid cell with 27 chromosomes; (b) high hyperdiploid cell with 55 chromosomes.

haploidy if the smaller metaphases of often poor morphology are ignored (see also *Figure 18*). The pattern of chromosome loss in near-haploidy is not random, as there is preferential retention of two copies of chromosomes 6, 8, 10, 14, 18, 21 and the sex chromosomes. In addition to the near-haploid clone it is common to see a normal diploid clone and a cell line with double the near-haploid number of chromosomes, resulting in hyperdiploidy. Occasionally, the near-haploid clone is absent, but the hyperdiploidy is atypical, tending to have two or four copies of chromosomes, and can thus be distinguished from typical > 50 hyperdiploid ALL which often has three copies of chromosomes (32). The distinction is important as > 50 hyperdiploidy carries a good prognosis whereas near-haploidy defines a rare type of childhood ALL associated with short median complete remission duration and poor prognosis.

5.3 Severe hypodiploidy

ALL with severe hypodiploidy is rare and sometimes classed with near-haploidy as the prognosis is similar. The chromosome number ranges from 30 to 39 and the chromosomes commonly retained are copies of 1, 4, 5, 6, 8, 9, 10, 11, 18, 19, 21, 22 and the sex chromosomes. Patients with severe hypodiploidy tend to be adults whereas the near-haploid patients tend to be children or teenagers. Potential problems in analysis include the possibility of mistaking the hypodiploid clone for broken metaphases, and the presence of a population of cells with double the hypodiploid number, as this might be misinterpreted as a case of typical > 50 hyperdiploidy.

6 Summary

It is clear from the above examples that most, if not all, cases of ALL will have cytogenetic or molecular abnormalities. These changes may indicate early steps in the leukaemogenic process. Cytogenetics, molecular techniques, morphology and immunophenotyping have improved the classification in this heterogeneous group. Karyotypic changes provide valuable prognostic information, often independent of other variables, thus allowing high-risk and low-risk patients to be identified.

Treatment is tailored to specific risk groups and intensive therapy regimes including bone marrow transplantation can be reserved for those patients who have a high risk of responding poorly to conventional chemotherapy. Examples of the poor prognostic abnormalities include t(9;22), (11)(q23) abnormalities, t(1;19), near-haploidy and severe hypodiploidy. Patients with the more favourable indicators such as high hyperdiploidy and the t(12;21), can be treated with less intensive regimes. Once high-risk patients can be identified, their outcomes do improve with the appropriate treatment.

A great number of genes have now been identified and implicated in leukaemogenesis and study of them as well as of the transcription products will fundamentally enhance our understanding of these leukaemias.

Acknowledgements

The authors are grateful to LRF and UKCCG database in ALL at Cytogenetics Laboratory, Haematology Department, Royal Free and University College Medical School, London, UK, for *Figures 5b, 6, 7a, 11,* and *17.* B. C. would also like to thank David Jones for his help and support during the production of this chapter.

References

1. Heim, S. and Mitelman, F., (eds.) (1995), *Cancer cytogenetics*, 2nd edn, p. 20. Wiley-Liss, New York.
2. Third International Workshop on Chromosomes in Leukaemia (1983). *Cancer Res.* **43**, 868.
3. Groupe Francais de Cytogenetique Hematologique (1996). *Blood* **87**, 3135.
4. Fenaux, P., Lai, J. L., Morel, P., Nelken, B., Taboureau, O., Deminatti, M., and Bauters, F. (1989). *Hematol. Oncol.* **7**, 307.
5. Rieder, H., Ludwig, W-D., Gassman, W., Thiel, E., Loffler, H., Hoelzer, D., and Fonatsch, C. (1993). *Cancer Res.* **131**, 133.
6. Secker-Walker, L. M., Prentice, H. G., Durrant, J., Richards, S., Hall, E., and Harrison, G. (1997). *Br. J. Haematol.* **96**, 601.
7. Secker-Walker, L. M., Lawler, S. D., and Hardisty, R. M. (1978). *Br. Med. J.* **2**, 1529.
8. Secker-Walker, L. M., Chessells, J. M., Stewart, E. L., Swansbury, G. J., Richards, S., and Lawler, S. D. (1989). *Br. J. Haematol.* **72**, 336.
9. Mauer, A. M. (1990). In *Haematology* (ed. W. J. Williams, E. Beutler, A. J. Erslev, and M. A. Lichtman), p. 994. McGraw-Hill, New York.
10. Greaves, M. (1999). *Eur. J. Cancer* **35**(2), 173.
11. Williams. D. L., Harris, A., Williams, K. J., Brosius, M. J., and Lemonds, W. (1984). *Cancer Genet. Cytogenet.* **13**, 239.
12. Faderl, S., Kantarjian, H. M., Talpaz, M., and Estrov Z. (1998). *Blood.* **91**(11), 3995.
13. Bennett, J. M., Catovsky, D., Daniel, M. T., Flandrin, G., Galton, D. D. G., Gralnick, M. R., and Sultan, C. (1981). *Br. J. Haematol.* **47**, 553.
14. First MIC Co-operative Study Group (1986). *Cancer Genet. Cytogenet.* **23**, 189.
15. Sandberg, A. A. (ed.) (1990). In *The chromosomes in human cancer and leukemia* (2nd edn), p. 313. Elsevier, New York.
16. Cortes, J. E., Kantarjian H. M. (1995). *Cancer* **76**, 2393.
17. Fenaux, P., Lai, J. L., Miaux, O., Zandecki, M., Jouet, J. P., and Bauters, F. (1989). *Br. J. Haematol.* **71**, 371.
18. Pui, C-H., Crist, W. M., and Look, T. (1990). *Blood* **76**, 1449.
19. Copelan, E. A. and McGuire, E. A. (1995). *Blood* **5**, 1151.
20. Heim, S. and Mitelman, F (ed.) (1995). In *Cancer cytogenetics*, 2nd edn, p. 180. Wiley-Liss, New York.
21. Hunger, S. (1996). *Blood* **87**, 1211.
22. Erikson, J., Finger, L., Sun, L., Ar-Rushdi, A., Nishikura, K., Minowada, J. *et al.* (1986). *Science* **232**, 884.
23. Raimondi, S. C., Behm, F. G., Robertson, P. K., Pui, C-H., Rivera, G. K., Murphy, S. B., and Williams, D. L. (1988). *Blood* **72**, 1560.
24. European Union Concerted Action Workshop on 11q23, London, UK, May 1997 (1998). *Leukaemia* **12**, 776.
25. Romana, S. P., Le Coniat, and Berger, R. (1993). *Genes Chromosomes Cancer* **9**, 186.
26. Shurtleff, S. A., Buijs, A., Behm, F. G., Rubnitz, J. E., Raimondi, S. C., Hancock, M. L. *et al.* (1995). *Leukemia* **9**, 1985.
27. Raynaud, S., Cave, H., Baens, M., Bastard, C., Cacheux, V., Grosgeorge, J. *et al.* (1996). *Blood* **87**, 2891.
28. Golub, T. R., Barker, G. F., Bohlander, S. K., Hiebert, S. W., Ward, D. C., Bray-Ward, P. *et al.* (1995). *Proc. Natl. Acad. Sci. USA.* **92**, 4917.
29. Rubnitz, J. E., Downing, J. R., Pui, C-H., Shurtleff, S. A., Raimondi, S. C., Evans, W. E. *et al.* (1997). *J. Clin. Oncol.* **15**, 1150.
30. Raimondi, S. C., Pui, C. H., Hancock, M. L., Behm, F. G., Filatov, L., and Rivera, G. K. (1996). *Leukaemia* **10**, 213.

31. Ritterbach, J., Hiddemann, W., Beck, J. D., Schrappe, M., Janka-Schaub, G., Ludwig, W. D. *et al.* (1998). *Leukaemia* **12**, 427.
32. Onodera, N., McCabe, N. R., Nachman, J. B., Johnson, F. L., Le Beau, M. M., Rowley, J. D., and Rubin, C. M. (1992). *Cancer* **4**, 331.

Further reading

Bain, B. J. (ed.) (1999). *Leukaemia diagnosis.* Blackwell Science Ltd, Oxford.
Chessells, J. M., Swansbury, G. J., Reeves, B., Bailey, C. C., and Richards, S. M. (1997). *Br. J. Haematol.* **99**, 93.
Secker-Walker, L. M. (ed.) (1997). *Chromosomes and genes in acute lymphoblastic leukaemia.* R. G. Landes Co. (Texas) and Chapman and Hall, New York.

Chapter 4

The lymphomas and chronic lymphoid leukaemias

C. J. Harrison

Cytogenetics Laboratory, Academic Department of Haematology, Royal Free and University College Medical School, Rowland Hill Street, London NW3 2QG, UK

1 Introduction

Malignant lymphomas and chronic lymphoid leukaemias represent two highly heterogeneous groups of malignant disease. Both arise as a result of neoplastic proliferation of lymphoid cells. A number of chromosomal abnormalities have been associated with histopathology, disease staging, and prognosis. Although these are fewer than any of the other haematological disorders, cytogenetic information is increasing in importance as an aid to diagnosis and patient management. This chapter presents those techniques that have been the most successful in producing cytogenetic results and a summary of the important cytogenetic findings.

2 Lymphomas

Malignant lymphomas are a highly diverse group of localized tumours associated with abnormal proliferation of lymphoid cells. They usually arise in lymph nodes, thymus, spleen or mucosal associated lymphoid tissues, but they occasionally occur in other organs where lymphoid cells are found, for example, bone marrow, liver, skin or intestinal tract. Lymphoma tissue requires careful handling for chromosomal analysis. Details of the special requirements for successful chromosome preparations are presented here.

2.1 Culture of samples from lymphoma patients

Tissue dissected from surgical biopsies of the affected lymph node provides the best sample for successful chromosomal analysis of lymphomas. Culture of this tissue is more difficult to achieve than with leukaemic bone marrow since cell death *in vitro* may be considerable. Successful culture can be achieved on bone marrow samples infiltrated with tumour cells.

2.1.1 Culture medium

The preferred medium for use in the culture of lymph nodes, bone marrow, peripheral blood or other tissues from lymphoma patients is RPMI 1640 supplemented with 20% FCS, antibiotics—benzylpenicillin (sodium) BP, 100 000 units/l and/or streptomycin sulphate, 100 mg/l—and L-glutamine 292.3 mg/l. This will be referred to as RPMI. This medium is not exclusive, however, and other basal media may be substituted.

2.1.2 Lymph node biopsies

The lymph node tissue must be transported from the operating theatre as soon as possible following surgery. It is unusual for a whole lymph node to be provided, generally only material from a small biopsy is available. It is preferable to have a slice of tissue from the centre of the lymph node, avoiding the surrounding capsule material and fatty tissue. Place the tissue directly into culture medium immediately after surgery. This prevents drying out and provides a nutrient environment, in an attempt to maintain cell viability during transit. It is recommended that the sample be processed as soon as possible after arrival in the laboratory. Cultures are usually successful only if set up on the same day.

Protocol 1

The culture of lymph node biopsy material

Equipment and reagents

As for Chapter 1, *Protocols 1*, *2–5* (as appropriate), *9* and *10* plus:

- Class 2 microbiological safety cabinet
- Incubator, 37°C, humidified
- Petri dish, sterile plastic 35 mm
- Centrifuge tube, sterile, plastic
- Surgical knives or sharp scissors, sterile
- Flasks, 50 ml or universal tubes, 25 ml
- Trypan Blue[a], 0.4% solution (Sigma)
- Complete RPMI

Method

1   Transfer the tissue to a small Petri dish containing 1–2 ml RPMI and remove excess fat, blood, connective tissue, or necrotic areas with sterile surgical knives or sharp scissors. Retain the transport medium, as a large number of cells are often found in suspension. Pool these cells together with those obtained from the slice of tissue (in Step 3).

2   Chop up the tissue. The node tissue is usually soft and cells burst into the medium, giving it a milky appearance. Sometimes, the lymph node is of harder consistency. On these occasions, slice or mince the tissue into the smallest pieces possible.[b]

3   Collect the cells in suspension into a sterile centrifuge tube. Pool these cells with the retained transport medium (from Step 1) and top up to 10 ml with RPMI. Centrifuge at 200 **g** for 10 min and resuspend the cells in fresh RPMI. The remaining tissue fragments may be stored for future use in DNA analysis if required.

4   Determine cell viability using an exclusion dye; for example, Trypan Blue (this step

Protocol 1 continued

is important as a large number of cells may be damaged during the disaggregation process). Transfer 0.5 ml of 0.4% Trypan Blue solution (w/v) to a test tube and add 0.5 ml of the cell suspension. Mix thoroughly and allow to stand for 5–15 min. Live (viable) cells will not take up the dye, whereas the dead (non-viable) cells will do so.

5   Count the cells using *Protocol 1* in Chapter 1. Keep a separate count of viable and non-viable cells. Cell viability (%) = total viable cell (unstained)/total cells (stained and unstained) × 100.

6   Set up 10^6 viable cells/ml in 10 ml RPMI in 50-ml tissue culture flasks or 25-ml universal tubes. Incubate at 37°C in a humidified 5% CO_2 atmosphere. If this is not available, a closed culture system can be used. To increase the chance of a successful cytogenetic result, set up a range of cultures in the same way as described for bone marrow cultures (Chapter 1, *Protocols 2–5*, as appropriate). In order of preference, dependent on the number of cells available, set up the following cultures:

(a) Short-term culture, usually overnight incubation, including 30–60 min incubation with colcemid (0.05 μg/ml).

(b) Short-term culture with 4–16 h incubation with colcemid (0.05 μg/ml).

(c) Direct culture with 1 h incubation with colcemid (0.05 μg/ml).

(d) Synchronized culture.

(e) Stimulated cultures.[c,d]

7   Harvest the cultures and prepare metaphase spreads for chromosome analysis as described for bone marrow (Chapter 1, *Protocols 9* and *10*).

[a] Caution: Trypan Blue is a carcinogen and a teratogen.

[b] The yield of cells from hard tissue is usually low and the harsh mechanical disaggregation required further reduces cell numbers. Therefore, expect a lower success rate with this type of specimen.

[c] The stimulated cultures may produce metaphase spreads of improved quality, but it is essential to consider the results in conjunction with direct or short-term cultures, since evolution or selection of clones may arise over the longer culture period.

[d] Direct and short-term cultures may yield poor quality, poorly spread metaphases. Also, some B-lineage differentiated lymphomas require B-cell mitogens for cell proliferation. Therefore, since diagnosis is often unknown prior to cytogenetic investigations, set up lymph node cultures with polyclonal B-cell activators, as described for the chronic lymphoid leukaemias (Section 3.1).

2.1.3 Lymph node aspirates

An alternative method for collection of lymph node cells by fine needle aspiration biopsy has been developed by Kristofferson *et al.* (1) for cytogenetic analysis of lymphoma cells taken directly from the affected lymph node. Fine needle biopsy relies on the presence of a reasonable sized tumour at an accessible site. Although this method is not ideal for histological classification of lymphoma there are several advantages to using this procedure for cytogenetic investigations.

(1) The method is simple. It requires no surgical intervention and, as a result, causes little distress to the patient. This potentially increases the number of available samples;

(2) The cells are in suspension immediately following the aspiration, therefore, disaggregation is not required;

(3) It is an easy method for obtaining repeated biopsies. These may be from the same lymphoma over a specified period, from tumours at different sites, or additional biopsies if relapse occurs. Thus, cytogenetic analysis by means of fine needle aspiration is useful for the study of evolution over the course of the disease in relation to a range of clinical parameters.

Suitably qualified medical personnel would normally undertake the aspiration as follows. A cell suspension for aspiration is obtained from the tumour by using an aspiration gun. This is a special holder for a 10-ml disposal syringe with a 0.7 mm (22 gauge) needle 25 or 50 mm long, which provides a steady one-hand grip during aspiration, enabling fixation of the affected lymph node with the other hand. The skin is disinfected prior to puncture and local anaesthetic is not used. Aspiration is commenced when the needle has reached the target and terminated immediately when the needle tip leaves this site. Two or three aspirations are usually necessary.

Protocol 2

Culture of lymph node aspirates

Equipment and reagents

As for Chapter 1, *Protocols 1, 9* and *10* plus

- Class 2 microbiological safety cabinet
- Complete RPMI

Method

1   Suspend the aspirated cells in 5–10 ml RPMI immediately and count as described in *Protocol 1* in Chapter 1. Adjust the cell volume to 10^6/ml, resulting in a culture containing 5–10×10^6 in 5–10 ml medium. The cell number ($> 5 \times 10^6$) is the single most important factor for success with this technique.[a]

2   Incubate for 4–16 h, adding 0.05 μg/ml colcemid as in *Protocol 1* (this chapter), step 6.[b]

3.   Harvest the culture and prepare metaphase spreads for chromosome analysis as described for bone marrow preparations (Chapter 1, *Protocols 9* and *10*).

[a] When sufficient cells are obtained at sampling, successful cytogenetic results are achieved in 70% of cases (2). This is comparable to the success rate achieved for lymph node biopsies. On the other hand, samples with $<5 \times 10^6$ cells are $<10\%$ successful. These success rates are independent of tumour stage, or whether the sample is taken at diagnosis or relapse.

[b] Due to the small cell numbers obtained by this technique the disadvantage is that chromosome analysis normally relies on one culture only. The method shown to reliably produce >10 analysable metaphases is a short-term culture with 4–16 h incubation with colcemid (0.05 μg/ml) as described for lymph node biopsy samples in *Protocol 1*.

2.1.4 Lymphomas arising in organs other than lymph nodes

Tumours may be dissected from other organs, particularly spleen, liver, intestinal tract and skin. Handle these in the same way as described for lymph node biopsies in *Protocol 1*.

2.1.5 Bone marrow

In general, the cytogenetic analysis of bone marrow samples from lymphoma patients is uninformative. This is usually due to the low proportion of lymphoma cells present in the marrow in conjunction with their low mitotic index, which often results in failure to find an abnormal clone. However, in some lymphomas, particularly in childhood patients or those with advanced disease, a leukaemic phase occurs in which large numbers of tumour cells have infiltrated the bone marrow and blood. In these patients, samples of bone marrow and blood may be prepared for chromosome analysis as described for the other haematological malignancies (Chapter 1).

2.2 Classification of lymphomas

Malignant lymphomas are a heterogeneous group of tumours that may be broadly classified into Hodgkin's and NHL.

2.2.1 Non-Hodgkin's lymphoma

Non-Hodgkin's lymphoma is a highly diverse group of neoplasms, many of which still pose problems with regard to their precise histological classification. A variety of different systems have been used in the classification of NHL that made comparison between different studies difficult. This forced the development of an 'International Working Formulation' which allowed translation between equivalent terms of the other classification systems (3). This has now been replaced by a Revised European–American Classification of Lymphoid Neoplasms (REAL), proposed by the International Lymphoma Study Group, for both NHL and Hodgkin's disease (4). This includes immunological, clinical and pathological criteria. Cytogenetics and/or genetic rearrangements are also considered for their important role in confirmation of diagnosis and prediction of prognosis. The major categories of the REAL classification are listed in *Table 1*. At the time of writing, a new WHO classification is imminent.

2.2.2 Burkitt's lymphoma

One type of NHL that has been well classified clinically, histologically and genetically is Burkitt's lymphoma. It is endemic in children in Central Africa, although it also occurs in Europe, USA and Japan. It is known to have a viral aetiology involving EBV. The tumour is highly aggressive but potentially curable. Prognosis in children correlates with the bulk of disease at the time of diagnosis.

2.2.3 Hodgkin's disease

Hodgkin's disease is the most common type of malignant lymphoma, occurring most frequently in young males. The cytology is highly characteristic with the presence of Hodgkin's and Reed–Sternberg cells. The latter are thought to be the

Table 1 Summary of REAL classification

B-Cell Neoplasms

I   Precursor B-cell neoplasm: Precursor B-lymphoblastic leukaemia/lymphoma.

II   Peripheral B-cell neoplasms
    1   B-cell chronic lymphocytic leukaemia/prolymphocytic
       leukaemia/small lymphocytic lymphoma
    2   Lymphoplasmacytoid lymphoma/immunocytoma
    3   Mantle cell lymphoma
    4   Follicle centre lymphoma, follicular
       Provisional cytological grades: 1 (small cell), II (mixed small and large cell), III (large cell)
       Provisional subtype: diffuse, predominantly small cell type
    5   Marginal zone B-cell lymphoma
       Extranodal (MALT-type +/− monocytoid B cells)
       Provisional subtype: nodal (+/− monocytoid B cells).
    6   Provisional entity: splenic marginal zone lymphoma (+/− villous lymphocytes)
    7   Hairy cell leukaemia
    8   Plasmacytoma/plasma cell myeloma
    9   DLBCL[a]
       Subtype: primary mediastinal (thymic) B-cell lymphoma
    10 Burkitt's lymphoma
    11 Provisional entity: high-grade B-cell lymphoma, Burkitt-like[a]

T-cell and putative NK-cell neoplasms

I   Precursor T-cell neoplasm: precursor T-lymphoblastic lymphoma/leukaemia

II   Peripheral T-cell and NK-cell neoplasms
    1   T-cell chronic lymphocytic leukaemia/prolymphocytic leukaemia
    2   LGL
       T-cell type
       NK-cell type
    3   Mycosis fungoides/Sezary syndrome
    4   Peripheral T-cell lymphomas, unspecified[a]
       Provisional cytological categories: medium-sized cell, mixed medium and large cell,
       large cell, lymphoepithelioid cell
       Provisional subtype: hepatosplenic γδ T-cell lymphoma
       Provisional subtype: subcutaneous panniculitic T-cell lymphoma
    5   AILD
    6   Angiocentric lymphoma
    7   Intestinal T-cell lymphoma (+/− enteropathy associated)
    8   ATL/L
    9   ALCL, CD30[+], T and null-cell types
    10 Provisional entity: anaplastic large-cell lymphoma, Hodgkin's-like

Hodgkin's disease

Lymphocyte predominance
    Nodular sclerosis
    Mixed cellularity
    Lymphocyte depletion
    Provisional entity: lymphocyte-rich classical Hodgkin's Disease

---

[a] These categories are thought likely to include more than one disease entity. This table is extracted from reference 4.

malignant cells constituting up to 5% of the tumour. The remaining cells are benign histiocytes, lymphocytes, eosinophils and plasma cells. The histological categorization of Hodgkin's disease according to the REAL classification is given in *Table 1*.

2.3 Specific chromosomal changes in non-Hodgkin's lymphomas

Approximately 90% of NHL show clonal chromosomal abnormalities (5–8). This percentage is much higher than other haematological malignancies. In general, the karyotypes are highly complex, subclonal variation is common and many secondary chromosomal changes are present. This results in populations of cells with highly variable karyotypes occurring within the same patient, leading to difficulties in accurate interpretation of results. Despite this, several recurring karyotypic abnormalities have been identified that correlate with tumour histology, biological and clinical features of the disease, suggesting that genetic rearrangements play an aetiological role in lymphomagenesis (7,9). The well-established chromosomal abnormalities fall into two main groups: primary structural changes and secondary changes resulting in the gain or loss of chromosomal material. Their correlation with histology, immunophenotype and clinical outcome is summarized in *Table 2*. The primary chromosomal changes often involve one of the immunoglobulin genes (*IG*), located at 14q32, 2p12 and 22q11, and another chromosomal site, resulting in juxtaposition of genes and the consequent deregulation of the *IG* gene involved.

The important role of secondary chromosomal changes is emerging. It appears that the accumulation of secondary changes is linked to disease progression in which the increasing complexity of the karyotype is associated with an increasingly poor prognosis and shorter survival. Therefore, the identification of specific patterns of karyotypic evolution may provide a greater understanding of the mechanisms involved in tumour progression (10).

2.3.1 Primary chromosomal changes

2.3.1.1 t(8;14)(q24;q32)

The translocation, t(8;14)(q24;q32) (see Chapter 3 *Figure 5a*), is the important primary chromosomal rearrangement in Burkitt's lymphoma (11) and occurs in 80% of patients. The remaining 20% have one of the two variant translocations, t(8;22)(q24;q11) and t(2;8)(p11;q24) (see Chapter 3 *Figure 5b* and *c*). The chromosome band 8q24 is common to all. Additional secondary chromosomal abnormalities may also be present, resulting in a complex karyotype.

Owing to the highly specific nature of the chromosomal change, and the fact that Burkitt's lymphoma cells are known to be immunoglobulin producing, these tumours have been the subject of a large number of molecular studies. The chromosomes involved in the translocations with chromosome 8 carry the immunoglobulin heavy (*IGH*) (chromosome 14), κ (*IGK*) (chromosome 2), and λ (*IGL*) (chromosome 22) light chain genes, the location of which coincides with the breakpoints involved in the translocations. The oncogene *MYC* is located to chromosome band 8q24. As a result of the t(8;14)(q24;q32), *MYC* is inserted into the *IGH* locus on chromosome 14. In the variant translocations, *MYC* remains on chromosome 8 and *IGK* and *IGL* become juxtaposed with *MYC* on this chromo-

Table 2 Common chromosomal abnormalities in NHL

Abnormality	Related Abnormality	Genes Involved	Lymphoma
Primary changes			
t(8;14)(q24;q32)		*MYC/IGH*	Burkitt's
	t(2;8)(p12;q24)	*IGK/MYC*	Burkitt's
	t(8;22)(q24;q11)	*MYC/IGL*	Burkitt's
t(14;18)(q32;q21)		*IGH/BCL2*	Follicle centre cell
	t(2;18)(p12;q21)	*IGK/BCL2*	Follicle centre cell
	t(18;22)(q21;q11)	*BCL2/IGL*	Follicle centre cell
t(3;14)(q27;q32)		*BCL6/IGH*	DLBCL
	t(2;3)(p12;q27)	*IGK/BCL2*	DLBCL
	t(3;22)(q27;q11)	*BCL2/IGL*	DLBCL
t(11;14)(q13;q32)		*BCL1/IGH*	Mantle Cell
	t(11;22)(q13;q11)	*BCL1/IGK*	Mantle Cell
t(9;14)(p13;q32)		*PAX5/IGH*	LPL
t(14;15)(q32;q11~q13)		*BCL8/IGH*	DLBCL
inv(14)(q11q32)		*TCR/TCL1*	T-cell
	t(14;14)(q11;q32)	*TCR/TCL1*	T-cell
	t(X;14)(q28;q32)	*MTCP1/TCL1*	
t(2;5)(p23;q35)		*ALK/NPM*	ALCL
Secondary changes			
I Trisomies			
Trisomy 2			Follicular
Trisomy 3			T-cell
Trisomy 7			DLBCL
Trisomy 12			Small lymphocytic
Trisomy 18			Follicular
Trisomy X			Follicular
II Structural			
1p			T-cell
1q			DLBCL
6p			T-cell
del(6)(q)			DLBCL
del(11)(q)			Small lymphocytic
14q32			
17q		*BCL3*	Follicle centre cell
17p		p53	

some. Despite these differences, all three translocations activate *MYC* transcription constitutively.

2.3.1.2 t(14;18)(q32;q21)

The translocation, t(14;18)(q32;q21) is the most common chromosomal abnormality in NHL (see *Figure 1*). Variant translocations, t(2;18)(p12;q21) (see *Figure 2*) and t(18;22)(q21;q11) (see *Figure 3*), have been described. The *BCL2* gene has been mapped to the 18q21 breakpoint. As a result of these translocations, the *BCL2* is

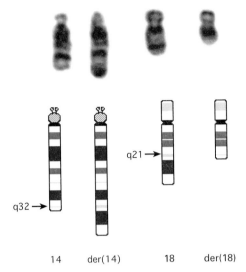

14   der(14)   18   der(18)

Figure 1 t(14;18)(q32;q21) is specifically associated with follicle centre cell lymphoma.

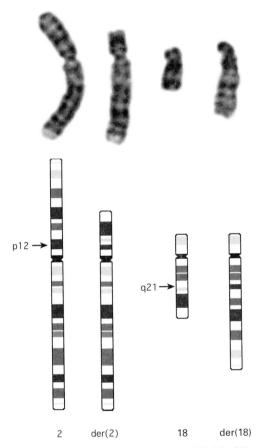

2   der(2)   18   der(18)

Figure 2 The variant translocation t(2;18)(p12;q21).

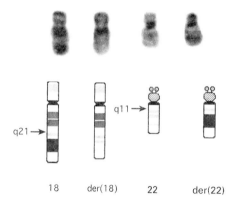

Figure 3 The variant translocation t(18;22)(q21;q11).

brought under the influence of the *IGH* gene enhancer in 14q32, *IGK* in 2p12 (12) or *IGL* in 22q11. In each case, this leads to dysregulation and overexpression of *BCL2*, resulting in tumour progression due to the prevention of apoptotic cell death (13). The t(14;18)(q32;q21) can be detected by dual colour FISH using locus-specific probes that encompass the breakpoints on chromosomes 14 and 18.

These translocations occur specifically in B-cell lymphomas of follicular centre cell origin, particularly the predominantly small cell type, and including large cell transformation of follicular lymphoma. They have also been reported in tumours with a non-follicular pattern but these have usually originated from a follicle centre cell lymphoma. In a small number of patients these translocations occur as the sole karyotypic change, in which case they are associated with a benign clinical course. It is more usual that they are accompanied by other chromosomal changes (5), for example, +X, +7, +12, +21 or + der(18)t(14;18) (q32;q21).

2.3.1.3 t(3;14)(q27;q32)

The breakpoint 3q27 is involved in the translocation, t(3;14)(q27;q32) (see *Figure 4*) or one of its variants, t(2;3)(p12;q27) (see *Figure 5*) or t(3;22)(q27;q11) (see *Figure 6*). These translocations are involved in the rearrangement of the *BCL6* gene at 3q27 with one of the *IG* genes, *IGH* (chromosome 14), *IGK* (chromosome 2) or *IGL* (chromosome 22) in a similar manner to *MYC* in t(14;18)(q32;q24) and the variants above (14,15). These translocations have been associated with DLBCL, occurring in ≈ 20% of cases. The presence of unidentified chromosomal material on 3q27 has also been reported.

2.3.1.4 t(11;14)(q13;q32)

The translocation, t(11;14)(q13;q32) (see *Figure 7*), leads to a rearrangement of the *BCL1* gene, located in 11q13, by its recombination within the *IGH* locus, leading to overexpression of cyclin D1. A variant translocation, t(11;22)(q13;q11), has been described which also leads to dysregulation of cyclin D1 as a result of the involvement of *IGL*. This abnormality occurs most frequently in mantle cell

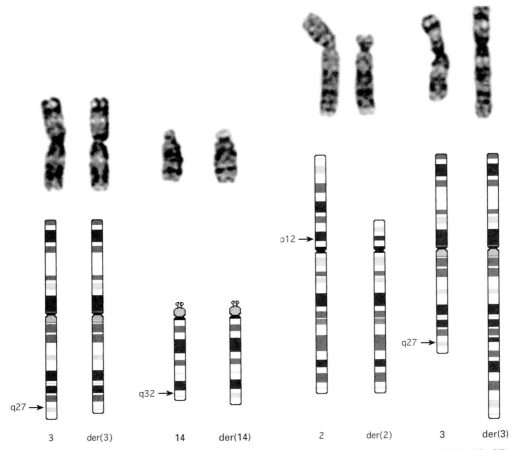

Figure 4 t(3;14)(q27;q32) involves *BCL6* and *IGH*.

Figure 5 The variant translocation t(2;3)(p12;q27).

lymphoma and is regarded as a diagnostic marker for this type of lymphoma (16,17), although it has been found in a small proportion of patients with PLL, SLVL and multiple myeloma (18).

2.3.1.5 t(9;14)(p13;q32)

The translocation, t(9;14)(p13;q32) involves rearrangement of *PAX5*, a transcription factor gene at 9p13, and *IGH* at 14q32. This abnormality is found in low-grade LPL (19).

2.3.1.6 t(14;15)(q32;q11~13)

The translocation, t(14;15)(q32;q11~13) involves *BCL8* and *IGH* and is associated with DLBCL (20).

2.3.1.7 Rearrangements of 14q11

Abnormalities involving 14q11 involve the α and δ T-cell receptor loci located in this band. These occur most frequently in lymphomas of T-cell type and are

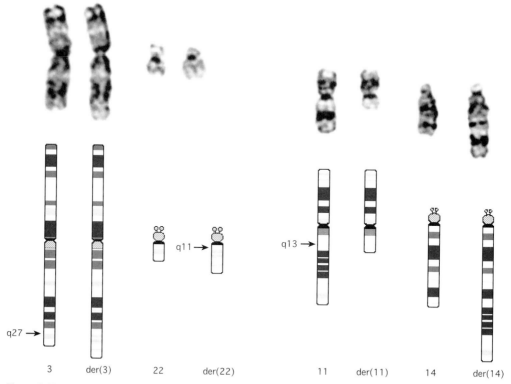

Figure 6 The variant translocation t(3;22)(q27;q11).

Figure 7 t(11;14)(q13;q32) involves *BCL1* and *IGH*. It is found in mantle cell lymphoma.

described in more detail in Section 3.2, in association with chronic lymphoid leukaemias.

2.3.1.8 t(2;5)(p23;q35)

The translocation, t(2;5)(p23;q35) (see *Figure 8*), is found in association with anaplastic large-cell lymphoma, alternatively known as Ki-1 positive lymphoma because of expression of CD30 (Ki-1) antigen (21). The translocation results in the fusion of the nuclear protein gene, nucleophosmin (*NPM*), in chromosome band 5q35 with the anaplastic lymphoma kinase gene (*ALK*) in chromosome band 2p23. This is often found as part of a complex karyotype and confers a relatively favourable prognosis.

2.3.2 Secondary abnormalities

2.3.2.1 Trisomies

(a) **Trisomy 2.** This abnormality occurs most frequently with other chromosomal gains in follicular lymphoma and has been associated with a poor prognosis.

(b) **Trisomy 3.** This is an established secondary change almost always associated with a T-cell phenotype and a diffuse histology involving large and small cells (5).

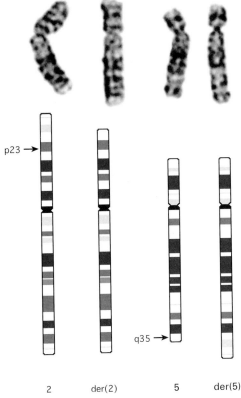

p23 →

q35 →

2   der(2)   5   der(5)

Figure 8 t(2;5)(p23;q35) is found in association with anaplastic large-cell lymphoma, alternatively known as Ki-1 positive lymphoma because of expression of CD30 (Ki-1) antigen.

(c) **Trisomy 7.** This trisomy has been variably reported in 5–15% of NHL. It occurs predominantly in DLBCL and is generally associated with a poor prognosis.

(d) **Trisomy 12.** Trisomy 12 correlates with small lymphocytic lymphoma, the counterpart of B-CLL (see Section 3.2) (5,9).

(e) **Trisomy 18.** This abnormality occurs in 10–15% of NHL and is usually accompanied by other numerical or structural changes. It occurs most frequently in low-grade follicular cases (5), as confirmed by CGH (22).

(f) **Trisomy X.** Trisomy X is a frequently occurring abnormality in NHL (8) and has been reported in approximately 21% of follicular lymphomas by CGH (22).

2.3.2.2 Other structural abnormalities

(a) **Chromosome 1.** Structural abnormalities of chromosome 1 occur in approximately 25% of NHL, usually in association with other secondary changes involved in clonal evolution. They arise in both the p and q arms in the form of translocations, deletions, duplications or isochromosome of 1q. The most frequent breakpoints in 1p are 1p22 and 1p36. Abnormalities leading to add(1) (p36) have been found in more than 10% of NHL. The most significant association of 1p abnormalities is with T-cell lymphomas.

Abnormalities of 1q, particularly those clustering in 1q21 in the form of deletions or translocations, have been associated with DLBCL (23). Chromosome 1 abnormalities in general are thought to be associated with a poor prognosis and a reduced survival (24).

(b) **Abnormalities of 6p.** Chromosomal abnormalities involving 6p21–p24 show a strong correlation with T-cell lymphomas (25). The proximity of the *HLA* locus points to the possibility that altered *HLA* expression may be a factor in lymphomagenesis in these cases.

(c) **Deletions of 6q.** Deletions of 6q (see *Figure 9*) have been found in up to 30% of NHL and specifically 17% of DLBCL. They are usually found in association with other abnormalities, in particular t(14;18)(q32;q21), as a secondary change (7). From cytogenetic analysis alone, the breakpoints on 6q have been found to be highly variable, largely due to the indistinct G-banding pattern of the 6q arm in poor-quality lymphoma preparations. LOH studies identified two RMD in NHL: RMD1 at 6q25–q27 and a RMD2 at 6q21–q23 (26). These were redefined by FISH studies and RMD2 was narrowed down to a 2 Mb region in 6q21 (27,28). A third RMD (RMD3) was later identified by LOH at 6q23 (29) which was associated with low-grade lymphoma lacking t(14;18)(q32;q21). In the same study, RMD1 and RMD2 were associated with intermediate and high-grade NHL, respectively. Rearrangements of 6q involving RMD1 may be linked to a significantly shorter survival than corresponding cases of intermediate-

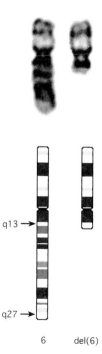

q13 →

q27 →

6   del(6)

Figure 9. Deletions of chromosome 6 have highly variable breakpoints. They are a characteristic marker of lymphoid malignancy, being found in all NHL types and chronic lymphoid leukaemia.

grade NHL without these abnormalities. The loss of these specific regions indicates the presence of tumour-suppressor genes, which may play an important role in the pathogenesis of NHL.

(d) **Deletions of 11q.** Abnormalities of 11q are frequently deletions involving 11q23–q25. They have been described in all NHL types but they appear to be most frequently associated with small lymphocytic lymphomas.

(e) **Other abnormalities of 14q.** Rearrangements of 14q represent the most common abnormality in NHL. They occur in approximately 50% of cases, and are heterogeneous with regard to their histopathological association. Although the well-established abnormalities described above are included in this group, the origin of the additional material on 14q is often unknown. It is of value to determine the involvement of *IGH* in the activation of an oncogene in these cases.

(f) **Abnormalities of chromosome 17.** Abnormalities of 17q, involving 17q21–q25 predominantly occur in follicular centre cell lymphoma (30). Rearrangements of the *BCL3* gene at 17q22 arise during clonal evolution and are correlated with transformation to a more aggressive disease. Abnormalities of 17p mainly involve deletions of 17p11 and p53. Loss of 17p has been confirmed as a frequent finding in follicular NHL by CGH (22).

2.4 Chromosomal changes in Hodgkin's disease

Reports of chromosomal abnormalities in Hodgkin's disease are scarce and no patterns of clinical and karyotypic associations have yet emerged (31). The main obstacles to cytogenetic investigations have been the low yield of metaphases and high proportion of normal cells when *in vitro* division is achieved. Thus, large numbers of cells need to be examined to detect an abnormal clone. Abnormal karyotypes are usually complex and ploidy changes in the triploid to tetraploid range are frequent (32). Abnormalities of certain chromosomal regions have been described in Hodgkin's disease, which are common to other malignancies, including NHL. These include trisomies of 3 and 7, deletions of 1p, 6q and 7q (32). The rearrangements, t(14;18)(q32;q21) and t(2;5)(p23;q35) have been found in Hodgkin's disease from molecular studies only, which requires further clarification (31). To date, no specific chromosomal change has been disclosed that indicates the genes involved in the aetiology of Hodgkin's disease. Deletion of 4q including the region 4q25–q27 is the only reported abnormality showing some specificity (32). Chromosomal abnormalities were thought to be restricted to the Reed–Sternberg and Hodgkin's cells, but evidence from FISH studies indicates that some of the morphologically normal cells were cytogenetically aberrant and may form part of the malignant cell fraction (33).

3 Chronic B- and T-lymphoid leukaemias

Chronic B- and T-lymphoid leukaemias belong to the group of diseases classified as the chronic lymphoproliferative disorders. They involve the mature cells of

Table 3 Chronic B- and T-lymphoid leukaemias

Disorder	Abbreviation
B-lineage disorders	
Chronic lymphocytic leukaemia	CLL
Chronic lymphocytic leukaemia, mixed cell type	CLL/PL
Hairy cell leukaemia	HCL
Plasma cell leukaemia	PCL
Prolymphocytic leukaemia	PLL
Splenic lymphoma with villous lymphocytes	SLVL
T-lineage disorders	
Adult T-cell leukaemia/lymphoma	ATL
Large granular lymphocyte leukaemia	LGLL
T-prolymphocytic leukaemia	T-PLL

the lymphoid lineage, which accumulate in bone marrow and peripheral blood. The classification is based on morphology, immunophenotype and histology (34). Cytogenetics and molecular genetics now play a role in diagnosis. The chronic lymphoid leukaemias are divided mainly into B- and T- lineages with a minority being of NK cell lineage. The main types are listed in *Table 3*. Details of their clinical, haematological and cytological features, histology and immunophenotypes are summarized by Bain (18).

3.1 Preparative techniques

The chronic lymphoid leukaemias have been the most difficult of the haematological disorders to analyse by cytogenetics. This has been due to their low spontaneous mitotic index, poor response to most common mitogens and unexplained problems of obtaining metaphases in cases with very high white cell counts. The use of FISH has improved the ability to detect numerical and structural abnormalities in the majority of patients by overcoming some of the difficulties in obtaining metaphases for karyotyping. Sets of DNA-specific probes have been developed for interphase FISH analysis of the most frequently occurring numerical and structural abnormalities in B-CLL (35).

Approximately 90% of chronic lymphoid leukaemias are of B-cell type. The identification of a group of mitogens (polyclonal B-cell activators) that primarily stimulate B cells considerably improved the success of cytogenetic analysis. Although PHA is the most commonly used mitogen, it primarily stimulates T cells. Therefore, normal cells found in chronic B-cell disorders stimulated with PHA probably represent the normal T cells. In a small number of these cases, T-cell dependent B-cell activation may occur, leading to the observation of chromosomal abnormalities. The mitogens that have been shown to provide maximum stimulation of malignant B cells are TPA (alternative name PMA) (36) and EBV (37).

The procedures in this chapter are restricted to the use of TPA, since this B-cell mitogen is the most commonly used. Because chronic lymphoid leukaemias arise in the more mature cells of the lymphoid series, the usual tissue for study is peripheral blood. If bone marrow is available, unstimulated cultures can be set up and processed for chromosome analysis as described in *Protocol 2* in Chapter 1.

3.1.1 Culture of peripheral blood samples

For culture, a 20 ml sample of peripheral blood should be collected in preservative-free heparin (100 units/ml). The cultures should be set up as soon as possible after collection using whole blood. If the white cell count is high it may be beneficial to separate the white cells from the other blood cells (see *Protocol 6* in Chapter 1). Although this is a time-consuming process, the advantage is that the B-cell population is enriched, thus increasing the chance of specific stimulation of the malignant clone. However, T-cell depletion of separated lymphocytes should be avoided as this adversely affects the response of the leukaemic B cells. Ideally, set up a series of cultures incubated with TPA over a range of times (*Protocol 3*); for example, 3 and 5 days, as the response time of the malignant cells varies between patients.

For known T-lineage lymphoproliferative disorders, a 'cocktail' of mitogens should be used, as the malignant T-cells are particularly difficult to stimulate into cell division. One successful combination is PHA (10 μg/ml) + PWM (20 μg/ml) + TPA (*Protocol 3*) added to each blood culture. Harvest the cultures and make chromosome preparations as described for other blood and bone marrow specimens (see *Protocol 9* in Chapter 1).

Protocol 3

The use of TPA as a mitogen

Equipment and reagents

As for Chapter 1, *Protocols 2, 7, 9* and *10* plus

- TPA Stock solution:[a] 100 μg/ml dissolved in absolute ethanol or DMSO, store frozen in the dark. Make a working solution of 2–5 μg/ml in RPMI immediately prior to use.
- Class 2 microbiological safety cabinet
- PBS

Method

1 Set up two bone marrow cultures (using *Protocol 2* in Chapter 1) and two blood cultures (using *Protocol 7* in Chapter 1, but omitting the PHA).

2 At the beginning of the culture period add 0.2 ml TPA working solution to each culture to give a final concentration of 50 ng/ml.

3 Incubate one blood and one bone marrow culture for 3 days, and one of each for 5 days.

4 Add colcemid as in *Protocol 7* in Chapter 1, but reduce the time of incubation to 15 min as TPA-stimulated cells are particularly prone to excessive chromosome contraction if over treated.

5 Prewash the TPA-treated cultures in PBS prior to hypotonic treatment to obtain cleaner chromosome preparations.

6 Incubate the TPA-treated cultures in hypotonic (as in *Protocol 9* in Chapter 1) but for an extra 10 min.

7 Continue to harvest following *Protocol 9* in Chapter 1 and make slides according to *Protocol 10* in Chapter 1. Be gentle when slide-making, as TPA potentiates bursting.

[a] Caution: TPA is a potential carcinogen therefore it must be handled with care to avoid user contamination and aerosols. For disposal of TPA it is recommended that the local code of practice for disposal of carcinogens is followed.

3.2 Specific chromosomal abnormalities

Published findings of cytogenetic abnormalities from cytogenetic studies in the chronic lymphoid leukaemias have been rather limited. Significant data were collected within the first and second meeting of the International Working Party on Chromosomes in Chronic Lymphocytic Leukaemia, which have pointed in the direction of those chromosomal regions that appear to be relevant in the pathogenesis of disease (38). Since CLL is the most common of the chronic lymphoid leukaemias, the majority of information on chromosomal changes relates to these cases. The other disorders are rare, therefore cytogenetic studies have been few and the true incidence of abnormal karyotypes remains uncertain. Some reported abnormalities relate to the initiation of CLL while others appear to have distinct clinical correlates and prognostic implications. Cytogenetic abnormalities, in general, in these diseases appear to be secondary events involved in the progression of the disease. Patients with complex karyotypes of more than three abnormalities usually show a more aggressive form of the disease. The most frequently occurring non-random chromosomal abnormalities in the chronic lymphoid leukaemias are summarized below.

3.2.1 Trisomy 12

Trisomy 12 is the most common numerical abnormality in CLL, arising in approximately 20% of cases. Although it occurs in other B-lymphoproliferative disorders, in general, it is characteristic of CLL. It may be the sole abnormality or found in association with other changes. Interphase-FISH with centromeric probes for chromosome 12 has become the method of choice for detection of this abnormality. It is highly sensitive and has been shown to reveal twice the number of trisomy 12 positive cases than cytogenetic analysis (39). A strong correlation exists between trisomy 12 and morphological changes in CLL. It is associated with an increased proportion of prolymphocytes in the variant form of CLL known as CLL, mixed type (CLL/PL). Trisomy 12 is more common in this mixed cell type than in CLL with typical cytological features (40). Trisomy 12 is related to a high proliferative activity and disease progression (41). The proportion of trisomy 12-positive cells increases as the disease progresses (42). Overall, patients with trisomy 12 show an unfavourable prognosis when compared with those with a normal karyotype. However, when the trisomy 12 group is sub-divided into patients in which trisomy 12 is the sole abnormality and those with trisomy 12 and additional changes, it is found that trisomy 12 alone is equivalent to a normal karyotype in relation to prognosis. Trisomy 12 with additional abnormalities shows a significantly shorter survival.

3.2.2 Abnormalities of 11q

Abnormalities of 11q are most frequently observed as interstitial deletions involving 11q21–q25, which have been found in 20% of CLL cases by FISH. Deletion of 11q has been associated with progressive disease and a poor prognosis in CLL (35,43). Notably, patients with this deletion were younger, had more advanced clinical stage, extensive peripheral abdominal and mediastinal lymphadenopathy and a significantly shorter median survival. The demonstration of a deletion at 11q23 may be the most important genetic parameter for prognosis in CLL.

3.2.3 Abnormalities of 13q

Rearrangements involving 13q usually involve 13q12–q14 (see *Figure 10*). Deletions of this region have been reported in approximately 10% of CLL cases, which increases to 53% when FISH is applied using probes specific for this region (42). From molecular and FISH studies the *RB1* (retinoblastoma) gene located at 13q14 has been shown to be deleted. In some cases, this loss was homozygous. More frequently, the *DBM* (deleted in B-cell malignancy) locus distal to *RB1* and, most frequently, *BRCA2* (breast cancer susceptibility gene) at 13q12.3 are deleted (44). There is a negative correlation between trisomy 12 and deletion of 13q, suggesting two independent mechanisms of leukaemogenesis.

3.2.4 Abnormalities of chromosome 14

Abnormalities of 14q are common findings in CLL and PLL, occurring in approximately 8% of cases. These may include the t(14;18)(q32;q21), as described in follicle centre cell lymphoma, although many different chromosomal regions

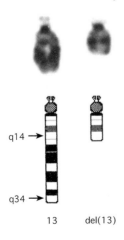

q14 →

q34 →

13   del(13)

Figure 10 del(13)(q14) occurs in approximately 10% of CLL cases.

have been identified as the donor segment on 14q32. The translocations, t(2;18) (p12;q21) and t(18;22)(q21;q11) occur more frequently in CLL than NHL (45).

3.2.5 t(11;14)(q13;q32)

This has been reported in a small number of cases in B-CLL, PLL, SLVL and PCL, in which the *BCL1* gene is involved, as described in Section 2.3.2. Some of these cases are thought to represent misdiagnosis of mantle cell lymphoma.

3.2.6 Abnormalities of 14q11

The most common rearrangements are inv(14)(q11q32) (see *Figure 11*) and t(14;14)(q11;q32). The 14q11 breakpoint is the site of the α and δ T-cell receptor gene loci, and *TCL1* is located to 14q32. *TCL1* becomes dysregulated as a result of its juxtaposition with the T-cell receptor, and when overexpressed inhibits apoptosis. The translocation t(X;14)(q28;q32), involving the *MTCP1* gene at Xq28, has been described as a variant. Other rearrangements involving 14q11 have been described, including t(8;14)(q24;q11) and t(11;14)(p13;q11). These abnormalities are specifically associated with LGL and various morphologies of T-cell lymphoma (7), including T-cell prolymphocytic leukaemia (T-PLL) and ATL/L.

3.2.7 Deletion of 6q

Deletions of 6q in the chronic lymphoid leukaemias involve the same range of breakpoints as the malignant lymphomas (Section 2.3.2). From cytogenetic

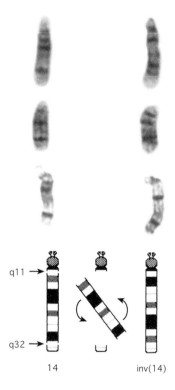

q11 →

q32 →

14   inv(14)

Figure 11 inv(14)(q11q32) is associated with T-cell disorders. The upper two partial karyotypes were kindly supplied by A. Watmore, Centre for Human Genetics, Sheffield, UK; the lower partial karyotype was kindly supplied by N. Bown, Department of Human Genetics, University of Newcastle-upon-Tyne, UK.

analysis approximately 6% of cases show deletions. This increases to 9% with a specific deletion of 6q21 detected by FISH. Although found in CLL and PLL, this abnormality is a reliable marker for lymphoid malignancy in general and is not preferentially associated with any disease type.

3.2.8 Isochromosome 8q

Trisomy 8q, generally occurring as an isochromosome 8q, has been found as a frequent abnormality in T-PLL, although the relevant biological consequences of the aberration have not been clarified (46).

3.2.9 t(6;12)(q15;p13)

This translocation may be a specific marker for PLL. Other rearrangements of 12p have also been described in T-PLL (47).

3.2.10 Abnormalities of 17p

Although p53 mutations are one of the most frequent genetic abnormalities in human cancer, the detection of cytogenetic changes at 17p is infrequent in CLL. However, when they are detected in the chronic lymphoid leukaemias they occur more frequently in mixed cell type, being associated with progression from CLL to CLL/PL and a significantly inferior prognosis (48). Mutations of p53 are more frequent in PLL (49).

4 Conclusion

Despite the difficulties in karyotypic interpretation and cell division *in vitro*, non-random chromosomal abnormalities have been identified in NHL and the chronic lymphoid leukaemias. The finding of primary chromosomal changes has pointed to the genetic pathways involved in the malignant process. They have associations with histology, clinical subgroups and prognosis. The accumulation of secondary changes linked to disease progression has provided additional prognostic information. These findings demonstrate that, although FISH and molecular techniques are being used increasingly in the accurate detection of known chromosomal changes, cytogenetics remains a vital tool to identify chromosomal interactions within complex karyotypes and in the discovery of new recurring abnormalities with prognostic significance in these diseases.

Acknowledgements

The author thanks Marie-Pierre Pinson for her help in preparation of the figures.

References

1. Kristoffersson, U., Olsson, H., Mark-Vendel, E., and Mitelman, F. (1981). *Cancer Genet. Cytogenet.* **4**, 53.
2. Kristoffersson, U., Olsson, H., Akerman, M., and Mitelman, F. (1985). *Hereditas* **103**, 63.
3. The Non-Hodgkin's Lymphoma Pathologic Classification Project (1982). *Cancer* **49**, 2112.

4. Harris, N. L., Jaffe, E. S., Stein, H., Banks, P. M., Chan, J. K., Cleary, M. L. *et al.* (1994). *Blood*, **84** 1361.

5. Fifth International Workshop on Chromosomes in Leukemia–Lymphoma (1987). *Blood* **70**, 1554.

6. Schouten, H. C., Sanger, W. G., Weisenburger, D. D., Anderson, J., and Armitage, J. O. (1990). *Blood* **75**, 1841.

7. Offit, K., Wong, G., Filippa, D. A., Tao, Y., and Chaganti, R. S. (1991). *Blood* **77**, 1508.

8. Hammond, D. W., Goepel, J. R., Aitken, M., Hancock, B. W., Potter, A. M., and Goyns, M. H. (1992). *Cancer Genet. Cytogenet.* **61**, 31.

9. Offit, K., Jhanwar, S. C., Ladanyi, M., Filippa, D. A., and Chaganti, R. S. (1991). *Genes Chromosomes Cancer* **3**, 189.

10. Johansson, B., Mertens, F., and Mitelman, F. (1995). *Blood* **86**, 3905.

11. Zech, L., Haglund, U., Nilsson, K., and Klein, G. (1976). *Int. J. Cancer* **17**, 47.

12. Hillion, J., Mecucci, C., Aventin, A., Leroux, D., Wlodarska, I., van Den Berghe, H., and Larsen, C. J. (1991). *Oncogene* **6**, 169.

13. Hockenbery, D. M. (1995). *Bioessays* **17**, 631.

14. Bastard, C., Tilly, H., Lenormand, B., Bigorgne, C., Boulet, D., Kunlin, A. *et al.* (1992). *Blood* **79**, 2527.

15. Ye, B. H., Rao, P. H., Chaganti, R. S., and Dalla-Favera, R. (1993). *Cancer Res.* **53**, 2732.

16. Leroux, D., Le Marc'Hadour, F., Gressin, R., Jacob, M. C., Keddari, E., Monteil, M. *et al.* (1991). *Br. J. Haematol.* **77**, 346.

17. Segal, G. H., Masih, A. S., Fox, A. C., Jorgensen, T., Scott, M., and Braylan, R. C. (1995). *Blood* **85**, 1570.

18. Bain, B. J. (1999). In *Leukaemia diagnosis.* (ed. Bain, B. J.), p. 158. Blackwell Science Ltd, Oxford.

19. Iida, S., Rao, P. H., Nallasivam, P., Hibshoosh, H., Butler, M., Louie, D. C. *et al.* (1996). *Blood* **88**, 4110.

20. Dyomin, V. G., Rao, P. H., Dalla-Favera, R., and Chaganti, R. S. K. (1997). *Proc. Natl. Acad. Sci. USA* **94**, 5728.

21. Mason, D. Y., Bastard, C., Rimokh, R., Dastugue, N., Huret, J. L., Kristoffersson, U. *et al.* (1990). *Br. J. Haematol.* **74**, 161.

22. Avet-Loiseau, H., Vigier, M., Moreau, A., Mellerin, M. P., Gaillard, F., Harousseau, J. L. *et al.* (1997). *Br. J. Haematol.* **97**, 119.

23. Cigudosa, J. C., Parsa, N. Z., Louie, D. C., Filippa, D. A., Jhanwar, S. C., Johansson, B. *et al.* (1999). *Genes Chromosomes Cancer* **25**, 123.

24. Whang-Peng, J., Knutsen, T., Jaffe, E. S., Steinberg, S. M., Raffeld, M., Zhao, W. P. *et al.* (1995). *Blood* **85**, 203.

25. Heim, S. and Mitelman, F. (1987). *Cancer cytogenetics.* Alan R. Liss, Inc. New York.

26. Gaidano, G., Hauptschein, R. S., Parsa, N. Z., Offit, K., Rao, P. H., Lenoir, G. *et al.* (1992). *Blood* **80**, 1781.

27. Menasce, L. P., Orphanos, V., Santibanez-Koref, M., Boyle, J. M., and Harrison, C. J. (1994). *Genes Chromosomes Cancer* **10**, 286.

28. Sherratt, T., Morelli, C., Boyle, J. M., and Harrison, C. J. (1997). *Chrom. Res.* **5**, 118.

29. Offit, K., Parsa, N. Z., Gaidano, G., Filippa, D. A., Louie, D., Pan, D. *et al.* (1993). *Blood* **82**, 2157.

30. Juneja, S., Lukeis, R., Tan, L., Cooper, I., Szelag, G., Parkin, J. D. *et al.* (1990). *Br. J. Haematol.* **76**, 231.

31. Bastard, C. (1996). *Leukemia*, **10** (Suppl. 2), S72.

32. Atkin, N. B. (1998). *Cytogenet. Cell Genet.* **80**, 23.

33. Jansen, M. P., Hopman, A. H., Haesevoets, A. M., Gennotte, I. A., Bot, F. J., Arends, J. W. *et al.* (1998). *J. Pathol.* **185**, 145.

34. Bennett, J. M., Catovsky, D., Daniel, M. T., Flandrin, G., Galton, D. A., Gralnick, H. R., and Sultan, C. (1989). *J. Clin. Pathol.* **42**, 567.

35. Dohner, H., Stilgenbauer, S., Dohner, K., Bentz, M., and Lichter, P. (1999). *J. Molec. Med.* **77**, 266.

36. Ross, F. M. and Stockdill, G. (1987). *Cancer Genet. Cytogenet.* **25**, 109.

37. Gahrton, G., Zech, L., Robert, K. H., and Bird, A. G. (1979). *New Engl. J. Med.* **301**, 438.

38. Juliusson, G., Oscier, D. G., Fitchett, M., Ross, F. M., Stockdill, G., Mackie, M. J. *et al.* (1990). *New Engl. J. Med.* **323**, 720.

39. Catovsky, D. (1997). *Hematol. Cell Ther.* **39** (Suppl. 1), S5.

40. Criel, A., Verhoef, G., Vlietinck, R., Mecucci, C., Billiet, J., Michaux, L. *et al.* (1997). *Br. J. Haematol.* **97**, 383.

41. Matutes, E., Oscier, D., Garcia-Marco, J., Ellis, J., Copplestone, A., Gillingham, R. *et al.* (1996). *Br. J. Haematol.* **92**, 382.

42. Garcia-Marco, J. A., Price, C. M., and Catovsky, D. (1997). *Cancer Genet. Cytogenet.* **94**, 52.

43. Fegan, C., Robinson, H., Thompson, P., Whittaker, J. A., and White, D. (1995) *Leukemia* **9**, 2003.

44. Garcia-Marco, J. A., Caldas, C., Price, C. M., Wiedemann, L. M., Ashworth, A., and Catovsky, D. (1996). *Blood* **88**, 1568.

45. Reed, J. C. (1998). *Semin. Hematol.* **35**, 3.

46. Matutes, E., Brito-Babapulle, V., Swansbury, J., Ellis, J., Morilla, R., Dearden, C. *et al.* (1991), *Blood* **78**, 3269.

47. Salomon-Nguyen, F., Brizard, F., Le Coniat, M., Radford, I., Berger, R., and Brizard, A. (1998). *Leukemia* **12**, 972.

48. Lens, D., Dyer, M. J., Garcia-Marco, J. M., De Schouwer, P. J., Hamoudi, R. A., Jones, D. *et al.* (1997). *Br. J. Haematol.* **99**, 848.

49. Lens, D., De Schouwer, P. J., Hamoudi, R. A., Abdul-Rauf, M., Farahat, N., Matutes, E. *et al.* (1997). *Blood* **89**, 2015.

Chapter 5

The role of cytogenetics in the diagnosis and classification of haematological neoplasms

B. J. Bain

Department of Haematology, St Mary's Hospital, Praed Street, London W2 1NY, UK

1 Introduction

Cytogenetic analysis is undertaken in patients with haematological disorders for two main reasons: firstly, to aid in the management of the patient and secondly, for the advancement of scientific knowledge. Often, both purposes are served simultaneously. The patient may benefit from confirmation of a provisional diagnosis and from the availability of prognostic information that can influence management. Cytogenetic analysis can be very useful during follow up, firstly for monitoring the response to therapy and secondly for detecting relapse and distinguishing relapse from a new therapy-related leukaemia. Cytogenetic analysis may also be required before patients are entered into therapeutic trials and may influence stratification within these trials.

The advances in scientific knowledge that have resulted from cytogenetic analysis have been fundamental. It was cytogenetic analysis, in cases of CML, that first permitted confirmation of the hypothesis that cancer resulted from mutation in a somatic cell with subsequent clonal expansion. The Philadelphia (Ph) chromosome was demonstrated in haemopoietic cells but not in other body cells and, when Ph-positive CML developed in one of identical twins, the other twin was found to be haematologically normal. Follow-up of individuals exposed to the atomic bombs at Hiroshima and Nagasaki also demonstrated that the Ph chromosome was an acquired cytogenetic abnormality, the appearance of which preceded the development of CML. More recently, cytogenetic analysis has led to the discovery of numerous oncogenes and a smaller number of cancer-suppressing genes and has led to the elucidation of their role in pathogenesis.

2 Information that can be gained from cytogenetic analysis

The information that can be gained from cytogenetic analysis of peripheral blood, bone marrow, lymph nodes or other tissues of patients in whom a haematological neoplasm is present or suspected is summarized in *Table 1*.

Table 1 Information that can be gained from cytogenetic analysis when a haematological neoplasm is present or suspected

At diagnosis

- Evidence of clonality and thus presumptive evidence of neoplasia
- Evidence as to which cell lineages are part of the neoplastic clone
- Confirmation of a diagnosis
- Information relevant to prognosis
- Demonstration of the close relationship of apparently different diseases
- Demonstration of a constitutional abnormality underlying the occurrence of neoplasia
- Demonstration of the likely sites of oncogenes and cancer-suppressing genes
- Demonstration that an apparently acquired disease has an intrauterine origin
- Demonstration of the likely etiological agent in therapy-related neoplasms
- Confirmation of the nature of transient abnormal myelopoiesis in Down syndrome
- Demonstration of a specific cytogenetic abnormality that permits subsequent molecular genetic monitoring for detection of minimal residual disease

During follow up

- Evidence of disease regression
- Evidence of disease recrudescence or evolution
- Evidence of engraftment following bone marrow or peripheral blood stem cell transplantation
- Distinction between relapse and either a secondary therapy-related neoplasm or a leukaemia resulting from neoplastic transformation of a donor stem cell

2.1 Evidence of clonality and thus presumptive evidence of neoplasia

2.1.1 Significance and usefulness of demonstration of clonality

The detection of a consistent cytogenetic abnormality in haemopoietic or lymphoid cells, which is not present in other body cells, provides strong evidence of neoplasia. Although clones of T and B lymphocytes may expand in response to an antigenic stimulus, such clones are cytogenetically normal. Similarly, although clones of haemopoietic cells may expand as a compensatory phenomenon following damage to and loss of haemopoietic stem cells, such cells are usually cytogenetically normal. (The demonstration of a cytogenetic abnormality in a case of aplastic anaemia is a cause for concern since it indicates the presence of a neoplastic clone and correlates with a worse prognosis.)

Proof of clonality by demonstration of a clonal cytogenetic abnormality is most important when it is not otherwise obvious that the condition is neoplastic. Cytogenetic analysis is not usually essential for demonstration of clonality of T and B lymphocytes, for which molecular and immunophenotyping techniques are available. However, it does have a role when transformation occurs in a very primitive lymphoid cell that is not expressing immunoglobulin and is not exhibiting rearranged immunoglobulin or T-cell receptor genes. In the case of NK cells and myeloid cells, demonstration of a cytogenetically abnormal clone may be the only way to demonstrate clonality. An alternative technique, analysis of X-linked polymorphisms, is less reliable and only applicable to females, although it may provide evidence of clonality in patients who lack a cytogenetic abnormality. These two techniques should therefore be seen as complementary.

Particular circumstances in which proof of clonality by demonstration of a cytogenetic abnormality has been found useful include:

- distinguishing the idiopathic hypereosinophilic syndrome from eosinophilic leukaemia
- distinguishing hypoplastic AML or MDS from aplastic anaemia
- distinguishing MDS from other causes of impaired bone marrow function
- distinguishing a large granular lymphocyte leukaemia of NK lineage from a reactive increase in large granular lymphocytes
- distinguishing PRV from secondary polycythaemia
- distinguishing essential thrombocythaemia from reactive thrombocytosis
- distinguishing early cases of CGL from reactive neutrophilia
- confirming a diagnosis of lymphoma when there are many inflammatory cells present, e.g. in case of angioimmunoblastic-lymphadenopathy-like lymphoma
- confirming a diagnosis of very low-grade lymphoma which may otherwise be diagnosed as 'pseudo-lymphoma'
- distinguishing a true large cell lymphoma from uncontrolled proliferation of lymphocytes in immunosuppressed patients with EBV infection
- confirming the presence of a neoplastic clone (of either myeloid or lymphoid origin) in patients with a proliferation of phagocytic histiocytes (haemophagocytic syndrome)
- demonstrating that, at least some cases, and by implication possibly all cases, of TAM in Down syndrome represent a neoplastic process
- demonstrating that rare cases of leukaemia or lymphoma in neonates result from transplacental passage of neoplastic cells.

2.1.2 Problems in using cytogenetic analysis for the demonstration of clonality

There are a number of problems in using cytogenetic analysis for the demonstration of clonality and for the presumptive identification of a neoplastic proliferation.

(1) Not all neoplasms have an identifiable clonal cytogenetic abnormality;

(2) Neoplastic cells may have a clonal cytogenetic abnormality but the cells that enter mitosis and are therefore analysed may be residual normal cells. This occurs quite commonly in CLL and was previously also often the case when suboptimal techniques were used to investigate acute hypergranular promyelocytic leukaemia;

(2) Some neoplasms, for example ALL associated with t(12;21)(p12;q22), have a cytogenetic abnormality that is very difficult to detect by non-molecular cytogenetic analysis;

(3) Neoplastic cells may have metaphases of poor quality so that recognition and characterization of any abnormality present may be difficult. Cytogeneticists must resist the temptation to analyse only good-quality metaphases since it may be the poor-quality metaphases that represent the leukaemic or lymphomatous cells;

(4) A cytogenetic abnormality detected in bone marrow cells may be irrelevant because it is a constitutional rather than an acquired abnormality;

(5) The demonstration of a clonal cytogenetic abnormality does not necessarily indicate that the most obvious cell population present is neoplastic. For example, in haemophagocytic syndromes the neoplastic clone may be of T lymphoid or NK origin rather than macrophage lineage. Similarly, a cytogenetically abnormal clone in the bone marrow of a patient with hyper-eosinophilia may be of lymphoid rather than myeloid origin, with the eosinophils being reactive. The latter problem can be further elucidated by investigating whether the abnormal metaphases are associated with eosinophil granules;

(6) Two cytogenetically-unrelated clones may be demonstrated, suggesting the possibility of two independent neoplasms. In at least some of these cases the two populations appear to be daughter clones, derived from a single cytogenetically normal parent clone.

2.2 Evidence as to which cell lineages are part of the neoplastic clone

Cytogenetic analysis can be used to determine which lineages are part of a neoplastic population. This is possible, to some extent, with non-molecular cytogenetic techniques but can often be done more readily by use of the technique of FISH. In the case of the megakaryocyte lineage, the demonstration of polyploid abnormal metaphases provides presumptive evidence of involvement of this lineage; this technique was used, for example, in demonstrating that megakaryocytes in CGL were Ph-positive. For other lineages, it is necessary to use a supplementary technique to demonstrate the lineage of the cells with the cytogenetic abnormality. With conventional techniques it may be possible to observe the association of abnormal metaphases with characteristically staining granules (eosinophils) or, by using a Perls' stain, with haemosiderin granules (erythroid cells). It is also possible to culture bone marrow and select individual colonies of a specific lineage for cytogenetic analysis. When FISH is used, immunophenotyping can be combined with cytogenetic analysis to demonstrate T, B or myeloid lineage of karyotypically abnormal cells. When there is myeloid differentiation, immunophenotypic analysis can be further refined to determine if the cytogenetically abnormal cells are of erythroid, granulocytic/monocytic or megakaryocytic lineage.

When an apparent lineage switch occurs, cytogenetic analysis can indicate that both phases of the disease represent proliferation of the same neoplastic clone. This is so, for example, when a switch from lymphoblastic to monoblastic lineage occurs in acute leukaemia associated with t(4;11)(q21;q23).

Examples of the use of cytogenetic analysis to determine which lineages are part of a neoplastic population are:

- in CGL the t(9;22)(q34;q11) rearrangement producing the Ph chromosome occurs in a pluripotent stem cell so that cells of all myeloid lineages are Ph-positive as are some cells of T lymphoid or B lymphoid origin

- in the rare myeloproliferative/lymphoproliferative disorder associated with t(8;13)(p11;q12) and related cytogenetic abnormalities, the mutation occurs in a pluripotent stem cell with the result that the karyotypic abnormality is demonstrable in myeloid cells and, during the acute phase of the disease, in myeloblasts, T lymphoblasts or B lymphoblasts

- in AML associated with various poor-prognosis cytogenetic abnormalities, e.g. monosomy 7, the karyotypic abnormality is demonstrable in all myeloid lineages

- in AML associated with several good-prognosis cytogenetic abnormalities, e.g. t(15;17)(q22;q12~21), the cytogenetic abnormality is confined to cells of granulocyte lineage

- in the rare cases of AML related to mediastinal germ cell tumours, the demonstration of i(12p) in both leukaemic blasts and the cells of the germ cell tumour indicates that the leukaemic clone is derived from the same multipotential mesenchymal cell that gave rise to the germ cell tumour

- in acute myelofibrosis and chronic idiopathic myelofibrosis, any cytogenetic abnormality is confined to myeloid cells with the fibroblasts being karyotypically normal and therefore reactive cells rather than part of the neoplastic clone

- in Hodgkin's disease, cytogenetic abnormalities are demonstrable in Reed–Sternberg cells and their mononuclear variants, providing evidence that this is the neoplastic population and that other cells, or at least the majority of other cells, are reactive.

2.3 Confirmation of a diagnosis

Some cytogenetic abnormalities are so strongly associated with a specific subtype of leukaemia or lymphoma that, when they are observed in a patient who has appropriate clinical and haematological features, their presence can confirm a provisional diagnosis. Other cytogenetic abnormalities, for example trisomy 8 or del(6)(q), are so lacking in specificity that their presence is of no value in precise diagnosis. Some of the cytogenetic abnormalities useful in confirming a diagnosis are shown in *Table 2*. It should be noted that the importance of a cytogenetic abnormality in the diagnostic process is determined by the ease of diagnosis using other criteria. Thus, the demonstration of t(15;17)(q22;q12~21) is rarely necessary for the diagnosis of classical hypergranular promyelocytic leukaemia, but is of more importance in confirming a diagnosis of the variant form of promyelocytic leukaemia, in which the cytological features are not always straightforward.

Table 2 Some cytogenetic abnormalities that confirm a provisional diagnosis if observed in a patient with appropriate clinical and haematological features

Cytogenetic abnormality	Diagnosis that may be confirmed
t(8;21)(q22;q22)	M2 AML with *AML1-ETO* fusion
t(15;17)(q22;q12~21)	M3 or M3 variant AML with *PML-RARα* fusion
inv(16)(p13q22) or t(16;16)(p13;q22)	M4Eo or other AML associated with *CBFβ-MYH11* fusion
t(9;22)(q34;q11)	Chronic granulocytic leukaemia
t(5;12)(q33;p13)	Chronic myelomonocytic leukaemia with eosinophilia with *PDGFβ-TEL* fusion
t(8;13)(p11;q12), t(8;9)(p11;q32) or t(6;8)(q27;p12)	Chronic myelomonocytic leukaemia with eosinophilia/T lymphoblastic lymphoma syndrome associated with rearrangement of *FGFR1* gene
t(14;18)(q32;q21), t(2;18)(p12;q21) or t(18;22)(q21;q11)	Follicular lymphoma or large cell transformation of follicular lymphoma
t(8;14)(q24;q32), t(2;8)(p12;q24) or t(8;22)(q24;q11)	Burkitt's lymphoma or L3 subtype of ALL
inv(14)(q11q32) or t(14;14)(q11;q32)	T-lineage prolymphocytic leukaemia
t(2;5)(p23;q35)	Anaplastic large cell lymphoma

The importance of cytogenetic analysis in confirming a diagnosis is also determined by the proportion of cases in which non-molecular cytogenetic techniques demonstrate the relevant cytogenetic abnormality. For both inv(16)(p13q22) and t(8;21)(q22;q22) molecular genetic analysis has been found to be considerably more sensitive. Occasional cytogenetic abnormalities are so difficult to recognize by standard cytogenetic analysis that it is much better to rely on molecular genetic analysis; this is the case in ALL associated with t(12;21)(p12;q22).

It should be noted that no chromosomal rearrangement, by itself, confirms a diagnosis. For example, t(9;22)(q34;q11) may be observed in CGL, AML, ALL and acute biphenotypic leukaemia. t(8;14)(q24;q32) may be observed not only in Burkitt's lymphoma and the L3 category of ALL but also in transformed follicular lymphoma. Even t(15;17)(q22;q12~21) which is almost pathognomonic of acute promyelocytic leukaemia has been observed, albeit rarely, in transformation of CGL and in acute leukaemia supervening in PRV.

2.4 Information relevant to prognosis

Cytogenetic analysis provides information of major prognostic significance in AML and ALL. This information is being increasingly used for stratification of patients for therapy. The most intensive forms of treatment are withheld in patients with better prognosis disease while patients with very poor prognosis disease may be treated more intensively, for example with bone marrow transplantation or with more experimental chemotherapeutic regimes.

Cytogenetic analysis also gives important prognostic information in MDS but since there is no very effective form of therapy yet available for these disorders, this prognostic information does not have much impact on patient management.

The presence and nature of any cytogenetic abnormality is also of prognostic relevance in CLL and in mantle cell lymphoma. In CLL, 13q14 abnormalities are of little prognostic import, whereas trisomy 12, del(11)(q) and complex cytogenetic abnormalities are indicative of a worse prognosis. In mantle cell lymphoma, tetraploid subclones have been shown to be associated with blastoid variants and with a worse prognosis.

2.5 Demonstration of the close relationship of apparently different diseases

Demonstration of identical cytogenetic (and molecular genetic) abnormalities has been useful in indicating the close relationship of apparently different conditions. The demonstration of t(15;17)(q22;q12~21) provided evidence that cases described as the hypogranular or microgranular variant of promyelocytic leukaemia were actually the same as hypergranular promyelocytic leukaemia, an observation that was subsequently confirmed by demonstration of the *PML-RARα* fusion gene and of responsiveness to administration of ATRA in both conditions. Similarly, there was initially controversy as to whether the small-cell variant of T-lineage prolymphocytic leukaemia was the same condition as the large-cell variant. The demonstration of the same primary cytogenetic abnormalities in both, either inv(14)(q11q32) or t(14;14)(q11;q32), suggested that they were indeed morphological variants of the same condition. This conclusion was further supported by observation of an identical secondary cytogenetic abnormality (trisomy or multisomy of 8q), an identical molecular genetic abnormality (dysregulation of *TCL1* by proximity to the T-cell receptor αδ locus) and an identical immunophenotype.

Even chromosomal rearrangements that are not totally specific for a particular entity can, nevertheless, provide evidence of the relationship of apparently different entities. For example, mantle cell lymphoma was initially described by different groups under a variety of names, including diffuse small centrocytic lymphoma, non-Hodgkin's lymphoma of intermediate differentiation and mantle zone lymphoma. The observation of t(11;14)(q13;q32) in all these conditions suggested that they might be identical, a suggestion that was made more likely by the demonstration of an identical molecular genetic defect (rearrangement of the *BCL1* gene which is brought into proximity to the immunoglobulin heavy chain gene) and an identical immunophenotype. However, this karyotypic abnormality is a reminder that diagnosis cannot rest on karyotype alone. Although it is likely that cases of 'chronic lymphocytic leukaemia' with t(11;14)(q13;q32) are actually mantle cell lymphoma this does not appear to be true of cases of splenic lymphoma with villous lymphocytes and prolymphocytic leukaemia with this cytogenetic abnormality, since they differ considerably from mantle cell lymphoma in other characteristics.

The observation of trisomy 12 in CLL, small lymphocytic lymphoma and some cases of lymphoplasmacytoid lymphoma suggests a relationship between these conditions. Knowledge as to whether this is a close relationship must await elucidation of the underlying molecular genetic defect responsible for leukaemogenesis since trisomy 12 is likely to be only a secondary cytogenetic abnormality in these conditions.

2.6 Demonstration of a constitutional abnormality underlying the occurrence of neoplasia

Cytogenetic analysis can provide evidence of an inherited or constitutional abnormality underlying a haematological neoplasm. A variety of techniques are applicable. A diagnosis of Fanconi anaemia as the underlying cause of AML is confirmed by demonstration of susceptibility to clastogenic agents. A diagnosis of underlying dyskeratosis congenita is supported by cytogenetic analysis of cultured fibroblasts. A diagnosis of Down syndrome underlying TAM or M7 AML is confirmed by conventional cytogenetic analysis.

The diagnosis of an underlying inherited or constitutional abnormality is of more than theoretical interest since it is relevant to choice of therapy. Patients with Fanconi anaemia are particularly susceptible to irradiation and to radiomimetic drugs so that pre-transplant conditioning must be modified. Patients with dyskeratosis congenita are particularly prone to post-transplant morbidity and mortality, a factor that should be considered when deciding on therapy.

The diagnosis of Down syndrome is important in differentiating TAM in neonates with Down syndrome from congenital leukaemia, for example associated with t(4;11)(q21;q23). The former has a relatively good prognosis and requires only supportive measures while the latter has a very grave prognosis and requires active management.

2.7 Demonstration of the likely sites of oncogenes and cancer suppressing genes

The investigation of breakpoints associated with translocations, inversions, insertions and other cytogenetic rearrangements has led to the discovery of many oncogenes (or proto-oncogenes) that not only contribute to oncogenesis when their function is perturbed but also have an important role in controlling proliferation, differentiation and death of normal cells.

The search for new cancer-suppressing genes in consistently deleted regions of chromosomes, for example in del(5)(q), del(7)(q) and del(20)(q), has so far been less productive, although deletions of known cancer-suppressing genes, such as p53 and *RB1* have been demonstrated in haematological malignancies.

The demonstration of activation of oncogenes or deletion or loss of function of cancer-suppressing genes has so far been only of theoretical interest. However, it is likely that this knowledge will eventually have practical applications. This view is supported by observations in acute promyelocytic leukaemia, in which the sensitivity to differentiating therapy with ATRA can be related to the rearrangement of the retinoic acid receptor (*RARα*) gene which is associated with t(15;17).

2.8 Demonstration that an apparently acquired disease has an intrauterine origin

Recent investigations of identical twins with ALL have provided evidence that this condition is sometimes of intrauterine origin. This has been shown for a number of twin pairs with t(4;11)(q21;q23) and for a smaller number of twins with t(12;21)(p12;q22). In these cases, not only was the same cytogenetic abnormality present in both twins, but the DNA rearrangement was the same at the molecular level. This suggests that the leukaemic clone arose in one twin and spread by a shared placental circulation to the other. This information is relevant to searches for leukaemogenic agents that might be operating in pregnancy.

2.9 Demonstration of the likely etiological agent in therapy-related neoplasms

The characteristics, including the typical cytogenetic abnormalities, of therapy-related leukaemia following alkylating agents are well known. More recently, therapy-related leukaemia following topoisomerase-II interactive drugs has been recognized. These leukaemias occur with a shorter latent period and fewer of them demonstrate myelodysplastic features. They have been found to be associated with a different range of cytogenetic abnormalities (*Table 3*). The prognosis is not always as bad as that of therapy-related leukaemia following alkylating agents. In particular, when acute leukaemia arises following topoisomerase II inhibitor therapy, and a cytogenetic abnormality that is usually associated with a relatively good prognosis is found, the leukaemia retains its usual relatively good prognosis. Recognition of therapy-related leukaemia is very important for planning optimal therapeutic regimes.

In addition to identifying likely cases of therapy-related leukaemia, cytogenetic analysis has provided evidence suggesting that exposure to pesticides and organic solvents may be oncogenic, leading to development of MDS. Cytogenetic abnormalities demonstrated in exposed individuals were similar to those seen in MDS and AML following therapy with alkylating agents, specifically complex karyotypic abnormalities, deletions and monosomies of chromosomes 5 and 7, trisomy 8, and abnormalities of 7p and 17p.

2.10 Confirmation of the nature of transient abnormal myelopoiesis in Down syndrome

Cytogenetic analysis has identified a number of neonates with Down syndrome and TAM in whom haemopoietic cells had a clonal cytogenetic abnormality, in addition to the constitutional trisomy 21 or equivalent. In a number of cases the extra clonal abnormality involved further copies of chromosome 21 or an abnormality of chromosomes 5 or 7. The clonal abnormality was confined to haemopoietic cells and disappeared on remission of the disorder. Analysis of

Table 3 Cytogenetic abnormalities associated with secondary (therapy-related) acute leukaemia[a]

Following alkylating agents and nitrosoureas	Following topoisomerase II-interactive drugs
Drugs incriminated:	
chlorambucil, busulphan, cyclophosphamide, melphalan, carmustine (BCNU), lomustine (CCNU)	etoposide, teniposide, doxorubicin, daunorubicin, epirubicin, mitozantrone, bimolane, razoxane
Chromosomal rearrangements:	
Complex chromosomal rearrangements including:	Chromosomal abnormalities with an 11q23 breakpoint:
−7	t(1;11)(q21;q23)
del(7)(q)	t(4;11)(q21;q23)
−5 and del(5)(q)	t(6;11)(q27;q23)
del(12)(p)	t(9;11)(p21;q23)
−17	t(10;11)(p11;q23)
del(17)(p)	inv(11)(p14q23)
del(13)(q)	t(11;16)(q23;p13)
−18	t(11;17)(q23;q25)
del(20)(q)	t(11;19)(q23;p13.1)
der(1)t(1;7)(q10;p10)	t(11;21)(q23;q22)
and other unbalanced translocations leading to loss of part of	Chromosomal rearrangements with a 21q22 breakpoint:
5q or 7q	t(3;21)(q26;q22)
and/or dup of 1q	t(7;21)(q31;q22)
inv(3)(q21q26)	t(8;21)(q22;q22)
t(3;3)(q21;q26)	Other
t(6;9)(p23;q34.3)	t(6;9)(p23;q34.3)
t(8;16)(p11;p13)	t(8;16)(p11;p13)
	t(9;22)(q34;q11)
	t(15;17)(q22;q12)
	inv(16)(p13q22)

[a] Modified from Bain BJ, (1999) *Leukaemia Diagnosis*, 2nd edn. Blackwell Science, Oxford, 1999.

X-linked polymorphisms of haemopoietic cells has similarly been used to demonstrate clonality. This evidence suggests that this condition is actually a transient leukaemia. Because remission occurs spontaneously, only supportive treatment is needed. Cytogenetic analysis is thus of very great importance in neonates with apparent leukaemia. This is so even in the absence of phenotypic features of Down syndrome since TAM has occurred both in neonates with mosaic Down syndrome, in whom phenotypic abnormalities were minor, and also in two infants with trisomy and pentosomy 21, respectively, in bone marrow cells, who showed no karyotypic abnormality after remission.

2.11 Demonstration of a specific cytogenetic abnormality that permits subsequent molecular genetic monitoring for detection of minimal residual disease

Cytogenetic analysis is unsuitable for monitoring minimal residual disease. However if a cytogenetic abnormality is detected on initial karyotypic analysis, this can indicate which specific molecular genetic abnormality could usefully be monitored for detection of minimal residual disease.

2.12 Evidence of disease regression

Cytogenetic analysis is not a very sensitive technique for demonstrating residual leukaemic cells in the bone marrow so that, although the persistence of karyotypically abnormal cells gives clear evidence that the leukaemia has not been eliminated, the reverse is not necessarily true. Nevertheless, there are circumstances in which monitoring has been clinically very useful.

Cytogenetic analysis is often used to demonstrate disease regression in patients with CGL being treated with interferon. A good cytogenetic response may indicate that, in that particular patient, continued interferon is a better therapeutic option than bone marrow transplantation.

2.13 Evidence of disease recrudescence or evolution

The reappearance of the initial karyotypic abnormality provides clear evidence of relapse while the appearance of new cytogenetic abnormalities within the original clone indicates disease evolution, often with a worse prognosis.

2.14 Evidence of engraftment following stem cell transplantation

Evidence of engraftment following bone marrow or peripheral blood stem cell transplantation can be easily achieved in patients with a cytogenetic abnormality in their leukaemic cells (which is not present in the normal donor cells) and also when there has been a sex-mismatched transplant, even if the leukaemic cells have a normal karyotype. When a same-sex transplant has been performed, it is also often possible to distinguish between host and donor chromosomes on the basis of cytogenetic polymorphisms.

2.15 Distinction between relapse and either a therapy-related neoplasm or leukaemia of donor cells

Cytogenetic analysis can be used when there is apparent recurrence of leukaemia in order to distinguish recurrence from development of a new therapy-related leukaemia. It was this type of analysis which led to the demonstration that etoposide and related drugs were leukaemogenic. Children with ALL subsequently developing AML were found to have karyotypic abnormalities different from those initially present and often with an 11q23 breakpoint. This provided clear evidence of a therapy-related leukaemia rather than of a phenotypic switch in the leukaemic clone. Conversely, phenotypic switch of the original leukaemic clone, often from early pre-B ALL to acute monoblastic leukaemia, was demonstrated in infants with t(4;11)(q21;q23).

Cytogenetic analysis can also be crucial in demonstrating the rare event of a

Table 4 The FAB classification of acute myeloid leukaemia

FAB category	BM erythroblasts as % of NC	BM blasts	Blast cytochemistry	Other criteria
M1	<50%	≥30% of NC; ≥90% of NEC	≥3% SBB or MPO positive	BM maturing granulocytic component ≤10% of NEC; BM maturing monocytic component ≤10% of NEC
M2	≤50%	≥30% of NC; 30–99% of NEC	≥3% SBB or MPO positive	BM maturing granulocytic component >10% of NEC; BM maturing monocytic component <20% of NEC and other criteria of M4 not met
M3	<50%	not specified	≥3% SBB or MPO positive	predominant BM cell is an abnormal promyelocyte, either hypergranular (M3) or hypogranular (M3 variant)
M4	<50%	≥30% of NC	≥3% SBB or MPO positive	BM granulocytic component ≥20% of NEC; significant monocytic component in BM, PB or both
M5	<50%	≥30% of NC	≥3% SBB or MPO or NSE positive	BM monocytic component ≥80% of NEC; M5a has monoblasts ≥80% of monocytic component; M5b has monoblasts <80% of monocytic component
M6	≥50%	≥30% of NEC	variable	
M7	<50%	≥30% of NC	variable	blasts identified as megakaryoblasts by ultrtastructural examination or immunological techniques
M0[a]	<50%	≥30% of NC	<3% SBB or MPO positive	blasts identified as myeloid or ultrastructural examination or immunological techniques

[a] Not included in original FAB classification.

Abbreviations: BM = bone marrow; NC = nucleated cells; NEC = non-erythroid cell (macrophages, lymphocytes, and plasma cells are also excluded from the count); SBB = Sudan black B; MPO = myeloperoxidase; PB = peripheral blood; NSE = non-specific esterase (e.g. alpha naphthyl acetate esterase).

leukaemia developing in a donor cell, either lymphoid or myeloid. Results of conventional karyotypic analysis must be interpreted with caution as it is possible that the cells entering mitosis and being analysed are the small proportion of residual normal donor cells, rather than the dominant leukaemic cells. FISH analysis can be very useful in this circumstance.

3 The role of cytogenetic analysis in the classification of haematological neoplasms

Haematological neoplasms have traditionally been classified on the basis of morphological features, supplemented in recent decades by immunophenotyping. For myeloid neoplasms the most widely used classifications are those proposed by the FAB cooperative group. The FAB classifications of AML and MDS are shown in *Tables 4* and *5*. The FAB group have also proposed a morphological classification of ALL (*Table 6*). The main importance of this last classification was the recognition of the L3 category of acute lymphoblastic leukaemia. The assigning of cases to the L1 or L2 categories was found to be of little significance.

Table 5 The FAB classification of the myelodysplastic syndromes

Category	Peripheral blood		Bone Marrow
Refractory anaemia (RA) or refractory cytopenia[a]	anaemia,[a] blasts ≤1%, monocytes ≤1 × 10⁹/litre	and	blasts <5%, ring sideroblasts ≤15% of erythroblasts
Refractory anaemia with ring sideroblasts (RARS)	anaemia, blasts ≤1%, monocytes ≤1 × 10⁹/litre	and	blasts <5%, ring sideroblasts ≤15% of erythroblasts
Refractory anaemia with excess of blasts (RAEB)	anaemia, blasts >1%, monocytes >1 × 10⁹/litre blasts <5%,	or and	blasts ≥5% blasts ≤20%
Chronic myelomonocytic leukaemia (CMML)	monocytes >1 × 10⁹/litre granulocytes often increased, blasts <5%		blasts up to 20% promonocytes often increased
Refractory anaemia with excess of blasts in transformation (RAEBT)	blasts ≥5% or Auer rods in blasts or in blood or marrow		blasts >20% but <30%

[a] Or, in the case of refractory cytopenia, either neutropenia or thrombocytopenia.
Reproduced with permission from Bain, B. J. (1999), Leukaemia Diagnosis, 2nd edn., Blackwell Science, Oxford, 1999.

Table 6 The FAB classification of acute lymphoblastic leukaemia

L1 Blasts are mainly small and relatively uniform in appearance. The nucleocytoplasmic ratio is high. The nuclei are predominantly round with nucleoli being either inconspicuous or not visible by light microscopy. The chromatin pattern is predominantly diffuse but with smaller blasts showing chromatin condensation. The cytoplasm is scanty and slightly to moderately basophilic; some cytoplasmic vacuolation may be present but vacuolation is not heavy.

L2 Blasts are larger than in L1 ALL and more heterogeneous. The nucleocytoplasmic ratio is lower. Nuclei are more pleomorphic with some nuclei being indented, cleft, or irregular. The cytoplasm is variable in amount but is often abundant. The degree of cytoplasmic basophilia is variable. Cytoplasmic vacuolation may be present but is not heavy.

L3 Blasts are large and homogeneous. The nucleocytoplasmic ratio is high, though not as high as in L1 ALL. The nuclei are predominantly round with a finely stippled chromatin pattern and usually prominent nucleoli. Cytoplasm is strongly basophilic and in at least some cells there is heavy vacuolation.

Table 7 Proposed MIC-M categories of acute myeloid leukaemia[a]

Cytogenetic abnormality	Molecular genetic abnormality	FAB category
t(1;11)(p32;q23)	*MLL-AF1p* fusion	M5
t(1;11)(q21;q23)	*MLL-AF1q* fusion	M4
inv(3)(q21q26) or t(3;3)(q21;q26)	*EV11* dysregulation	Various
t(3;5)(q25.1;q34)	*NPM-MLF1* fusion	Various
t(3;12)(q26;p13)	Fusion of various genes at 3q26 with *TEL* at 12p13	Various
t(3;21)(q26;q22)	Heterogeneous, mainly *AML1-EAP*, *AML1-EV11* and *AML1-MDS1*	Variable
t(4;11)(q21;q23)	*MLL-AF4* fusion	M5
t(5;17)(q32;q21)	*NPM-RARα* fusion	M3-like
t(6;9)(p23;q34)	*DEK-CAN* fusion	M2Baso
t(6;11)(q27;q23)	*MLL-AF6* fusion	M4 or M5
t(7;11)(p15;p15)	*NUP98-HOXA9* fusion	M2
inv(8)(p11;q13)	*MOZ-TIF2* fusion	M7
t(8;16)(p11;p13)	*MOZ-CBP* fusion	M4 or M5
t(8;21)(q22;q22)	*AML1-ETO* fusion	M2
t(9;11)(p21–22;q23)	*MLL-AF9* fusion	M5
t(9;22)(q34;q11)	*BCR-ABL* fusion	M0, M1 or M2
t(10;11)(p12;q23)	*MLL-AF10* fusion	M5
t(10;11)(p11.2;q23)	*MLL-AB11* fusion	AML
t(10;11)(p13;q14)	*CALM-AF10* fusion	M4
ins(11;9) (q23;p22p23)	*MLL-AF9* fusion	M5
inv(11)(p15q22)	*NUP98-DDX10* fusion	Various
t(11;16)(q23;p13)	*MLL-CBP* fusion	Variable
t(11;17)(q23;q21)	*MLL-AF17* fusion	M5
t(11;17)(q23;q21)	*PLZF-RARα* fusion	M3-like
t(11;19)(q23;p13.1)	*MLL-ELL* fusion	M4 or M5
t(11;19)(q23;p13.3)	*MLL-ENL* fusion	M4 or M5
t(11;22)(q23;q13)	*MLL-p300* fusion	AML
+11, 11q+ or normal	Partial tandem duplication of *MLL*	AML
t(12;22)(p13;q11)	*MN1-TEL* fusion	Variable
t(15;17)(q22;q12~21)	*PML-RARα* fusion	M3
inv(16)(p13q22) or t(16;16)(p13;q22)	*CBFβ-MYH11* fusion	M4Eo
t(16;21)(p11;q22)	*FUS-ERG* fusion	Variable
t(X;11)(q13;q23)	*MLL-AFX* fusion	M4 or M5

[a]Modified from Bain BJ, Interactive Haematology Imagebank, Blackwell Science, Oxford, 1999.

Shortly after the publication of the FAB proposals for the classification of acute leukaemia, another cooperative group proposed the addition of cytogenetic analysis so that classification would be based on morphology, immunophenotyping and cytogenetics (a MIC classification). The present author has proposed an updating of these classifications to include molecular genetic analysis with the classifications being designated MIC-M. There is already a large amount of data available that permits the classification of many cases of acute leukaemia in this manner. *Table 7* shows a proposal for such a classification. Proposals for a MIC-M classification have been advanced only quite recently and whether they will gain general acceptance remains to be seen.

At the time of writing, it appears likely that further proposals for the classification of the acute leukaemias and the MDS will be promulgated by an expert group working under the auspices of the WHO. It is likely that these classifications will use the terminology of the FAB group but will have different criteria for assigning cases to various categories. It is therefore of considerable importance that haematologists and cytogeneticists now state which classification is being used in any publication.

There is no generally agreed terminology or classification of the chronic myeloid leukaemias. The classification used by the present author is shown in *Table 8*. It is suggested that the term CML be used as a generic term with the designation CGL being used for cases which have a *BCR-ABL* fusion gene, whether or not a Ph chromosome is detected on cytogenetic analysis. It is also important to recognize that Ph-negative chronic myeloid leukaemias in children usually differ in their characteristics from myeloproliferative disorders in adults. They should therefore be categorized separately. The traditional term employed is juvenile chronic myeloid leukaemia but more recently the term juvenile chronic myelomonocytic leukaemia has also been used. There is no general agreement on criteria for the further categorization of other Ph-negative chronic myeloid leukaemias. The FAB group have suggested that adult cases with less than 10% granulocyte precursors in the peripheral blood be designated CMML, while cases with 10% or more of circulating granulocyte precursors are designated aCML. Others have suggested different criteria for making these diagnoses and for

Table 8 The chronic myeloid leukaemias

Chronic granulocytic leukaemia
Ph-positive, *BCR-ABL* fusion gene present
Ph-negative, *BCR-ABL* fusion gene present
Atypical chronic myeloid leukaemia
Chronic myelomonocytic leukaemia
Chronic neutrophilic leukaemia
Chronic eosinophilic leukaemia
Chronic basophilic leukaemia
Juvenile chronic myeloid leukaemia and other myelodysplastic/myeloproliferative disorders of childhood
Chronic myeloid leukaemia following other myeloproliferative disorders

Table 9 Some proposed MIC-M categories of chronic myeloid leukaemia[a]

Category of leukaemia	Cytogenetic abnormality	Molecular genetic abnormality
Chronic granulocytic leukaemia	t(9;22)(q34;q11)	*BCR-ABL* fusion
CGL with p210 protein		Typical CGL phenotype
CGL with p190 protein		Prominent monocytosis
CGl with p230 protein		Neutrophilic variant of CGL
Chronic myelomonocytic leukaemia	t(5;7)(q33;q11.2)	*HIP1/PDGFβR* fusion
Chronic myelomonocytic leukaemia with eosinophilia	t(5;12)(q33;p13)	*TEL-PDGFβR* fusion
Chronic myelomonocytic leukaemia with eosinophilia/T-lineage lymphoblastic lymphoma	t(6;8)(q27;p12)	*FOP-FGFR1* fusion
Chronic myelomonocytic leukaemia with eosinophilia/T-lineage lymphoblastic lymphoma	t(8;9)(p11;q32)	*FAN-FGFR1* fusion dysregulation
Chronic myelomonocytic leukaemia with eosinophilia/T-lineage lymphoblastic lymphoma	t(8;13)(p11;q12)	*ZNF198-FGFR1* fusion
Chronic myelomonocytic leukaemia	t(9;12)(p24;p13) or variant complex translocation	*TEL-JAK2* fusion

[a] Modified from Bain BJ, Interactive Haematology Imagebank (CD-ROM), Blackwell Science, Oxford, 1999.

defining the cut-off point used to distinguish between the myelodysplastic syndromes and the myeloproliferative disorders. It is recommended that, for the sake of uniformity and consistency, the FAB criteria should be employed until such time as there is an alternative internationally agreed classification.

It is also possible to classify chronic myeloid leukaemias by a MIC-M approach, although there are many Philadelphia-negative cases which cannot be classified in this manner because the molecular mechanism of leukaemogenesis has not yet been defined. Some common and some rare types of chronic myeloid leukaemia which could be classified in this manner are shown in *Table 9*.

Chronic lymphoproliferative disorders have been classified by the FAB group on the basis of cytology and immunophenotype. Numerous classifications have also been proposed which are based on histological features, often supplemented by immunophenotype. The most recent of these is the REAL classification which also incorporates some cytogenetic information (see Chapter 4 *Table 1*, for a summary). At the time of writing it appears likely that a new WHO classification, based on the REAL classification, will be promulgated. As for AML and MDS, it is important that publications relating to lymphoma and the chronic lymphoid leukaemias state which classification is being employed. It is likely that increasing use will be made of cytogenetic and molecular genetic information in classifying lymphoproliferative disorders.

4 Relationship between the cytogeneticist and the haematologist

A close relationship between the haematologist and the cytogeneticist is essential if maximum useful information is to be produced from cytogenetic investigation of patients with haematological disorders. Consultation is necessary in order that appropriate specimens are provided at a time when the laboratory can handle them. It is desirable for the cytogenetics laboratory to know whether any abnormal cells present are likely to be lymphoid or myeloid and whether any specific cytogenetic rearrangement is suspected since this may affect the techniques employed. It is often necessary to dispatch a bone marrow specimen to a cytogenetics laboratory before it is known whether there is a genuine diagnostic problem or whether the specimen contains abnormal cells. To avoid wasting resources, it is important that the haematologist examines a stained film promptly and contacts the laboratory if the investigation requested has become redundant or inappropriate. It is also necessary for the haematologist to inform the cytogenetics laboratory of the importance and degree of urgency of the investigation. The laboratory needs to know whether information, in order to be clinically useful, is required within days, weeks or months. Case conferences and audit are useful tools in promoting a useful interaction between cytogeneticists and those more directly involved in patient management.

Because of limitations of resources it may not be possible to carry out all the investigations that the haematologist would ideally wish to have done. Justifiable reasons for carrying out cytogenetic analysis include:

- the benefit of the individual patient
- the increase of knowledge and thus the benefit of future patients
- the increase of basic scientific knowledge
- the continuing education of haematologists, cytogeneticists and trainees in these disciplines.

When resources are limited, consultation is necessary to develop satisfactory policies so that the investigations performed are those that are most likely to be of benefit to patients. The benefit may be more accurate diagnosis or the provision of information that will influence treatment or permit disease monitoring. Treatment decisions may be influenced as follows:

- demonstration of a good-prognosis cytogenetic abnormality may be an indication to withhold the most intensive forms of treatment, as when bone marrow transplantation is withheld from patients in first remission with AML associated with t(8;21), t(15;17) or inv(16)

127

- demonstration of a poor-prognosis rearrangement may, in some circumstances, indicate that withholding intensive treatment is appropriate, as when a complex cytogenetic abnormality is found in an elderly patient with AML

- demonstration of a specific cytogenetic rearrangement may confirm a precise diagnosis and indicate that a very specific form of treatment is indicated, for example in M3/M3 variant AML, Ph-positive CGL or L3/B cell ALL

- demonstration of an underlying genetic abnormality may influence choice of treatment and also has implications for other family members, e.g. in Fanconi anaemia or dyskeratosis congenita.

Prognostic information may be of benefit to the patient, even if it does not immediately influence management. For example, although prognosis is always uncertain, it is desirable that a haematologist/oncologist discussing the diagnosis and management of a low- or intermediate-grade lymphoma with a patient has as accurate a diagnosis as is possible and can therefore make a realistic assessment of prognosis. The oncologist is likely to speak with more optimism to a patient with a follicular lymphoma than to a patient with mantle cell lymphoma. These diagnoses are usually based on histology but in some patients, for example those with circulating lymphoma cells, cytogenetic analysis can confirm a provisional diagnosis based on cytology and ensure that information given to the patient is appropriate.

If cytogenetic information is to be correctly interpreted and, in particular, if new knowledge is to be gained then it is important that any haematological disorder is as well characterized as possible. The advancement of knowledge for the ultimate benefit of future patients is likely to come particularly from centres that investigate and document their cases carefully and from cooperative multicentre trials. However, despite limited resources, the importance of continuing education and of maintaining the interest of medical practitioners in the disease as well as the patient should not be underestimated. Fully informed doctors are likely to be better doctors.

Chapter 6

Molecular cytogenetic technologies

L. Kearney
MRC Molecular Haematology Unit, Institute of Molecular Medicine, John Radcliffe Hospital, Headington, Oxford OX3 9DS, UK

D. W. Hammond
Institute for Cancer Studies, Sheffield University Medical School, Beech Hill Road, Sheffield, S10 2RX, UK

1 Introduction

The importance of cytogenetic analysis in the study of malignancy has been enhanced over the past decade by the incorporation of a range of techniques based around FISH. In the leukaemias, cytogenetic analysis provides the first step in the identification of genes involved in leukaemogenesis, by identifying consistent chromosomal rearrangements. FISH has added to this capacity by providing a rapid and accurate method for the identification of translocation breakpoints and commonly deleted regions. Progress in identifying consistent rearrangements in some solid tumours has been more laborious. The new multicolour karyotyping techniques M-FISH and SKY combine the screening potential of cytogenetics with the accuracy of molecular genetics. These promise to unravel complex karyotypes associated with many solid tumours, and to uncover new non-random rearrangements. However, these techniques still require metaphase chromosomes, and are not applicable to all tumour types. The advent of CGH has provided access to a range of tumour types, circumventing the need for metaphase chromosomes. Since its first description, the growth in CGH has been exponential, identifying new regions of amplification and deletion in a wide variety of tumour types (reviewed in ref. 1). The major limitation of CGH is the low resolution, owing to the reliance on metaphase chromosomes. This limitation has now been overcome, by replacing condensed metaphase chromosomes with cloned DNA arrayed in small spots and immobilized to the surface of a glass slide (2). It is envisaged that this matrix CGH will allow a whole genome screening for imbalance using clones spaced evenly over the entire genome.

The applications for FISH in malignancy cover an enormous range of clinical diagnostic and research situations. These include:

- the identification of non-random chromosome abnormalities with defined prognostic value
- the characterization of marker chromosomes
- interphase FISH for specific abnormalities in cases of failed cytogenetics
- monitoring disease progression/success of bone marrow transplantation
- gene mapping
- the identification of new non-random abnormalities
- the identification of translocation breakpoints
- the identification of commonly deleted regions
- the lineage involvement of clonal cells
- the study of 3D chromosome organization in interphase nuclei.

This chapter concentrates on the more specialized FISH techniques with an impact on the study of malignancy. The problems and pitfalls of implementing such techniques into diagnostic cytogenetics are also discussed.

2 Basic fluorescence *in situ* hybridization protocols

The sensitivity of FISH techniques is such that the detection of directly fluorochrome labelled probes is now feasible. Directly fluorochrome labelled probes are essential for any quantitative analysis, and are preferable for CGH and M-FISH. However, some dyes (e.g. Cy3.5 and Cy5.5) cannot be used as substrates for DNA polymerases, and therefore indirect labelling methods must be used. The following are a series of basic protocols for labelling, hybridization and detection, which can be adapted for a range of FISH applications. We find that labelling either indirectly with a hapten such as digoxigenin or biotin, or directly with fluorochrome requires essentially the same nick translation conditions. These methods have been used successfully for unique sequence probes, including cosmid, PAC, P1 and YACs, as well as repetitive sequence probes. An alternative method for labelling whole-chromosome paints is amplification using a degenerate oligonucleotide primer (DOP-PCR) (see *Protocol 3*).

Table 1 Stock solutions

20×SSC (3 M NaCl, 0.3 M sodium citrate). Add 175.3 g NaCl, 88.2 g sodium citrate to 800 ml distilled water and stir until dissolved. Adjust the pH to 7.0 with sodium hydroxide and make the volume up to 1 l

1×PBS. Dissolve 8 g NaCl, 0.2 g KCl, 1.4 g Na_2HPO_4, 0.24 g KH_2PO_4, in 800 ml distilled water. Adjust pH to 7.4 with HCL,[a] then make up to 1 l. Autoclave before use. Alternatively, dissolve 10 PBS tablets (Sigma P-4417) in 1 l distilled water

1 M Tris (various pH). Dissolve 121.1 g Tris base in 800 ml distilled water. Add concentrated HCL,[a] to the desired pH (e.g. 65 ml for pH 7.5, 42 ml for pH 8.0). Ensure that the pH meter has an electrode that is suitable for Tris buffer. Make up to 1 l and autoclave

Table 1 Continued

0.5 M EDTA,[b] pH 8.0. Add 18.6 g disodium EDTA.2H$_2$O to 80 ml distilled water. Stir and adjust pH to 8.0 with sodium hydroxide pellets. Keep stirring until the solution clears (it will only dissolve as it nears the correct pH). Make up to 100 ml and autoclave

TE (10 mM Tris, 1 mM EDTA).[b] Add 1 ml of 1 M Tris and 200 μl of 0.5 M EDTA to 99 ml distilled water

3 M sodium acetate. Dissolve 40.8 g sodium acetate.3H$_2$O in 80 ml distilled water. Adjust the pH to 5.2 with glacial acetic acid[c] (at least 15 ml will be necessary). Make up to 100 ml

10% SDS.[d] Dissolve 100 g of electrophoresis grade SDS in 900 ml of H$_2$O. Heat to 68°C to dissolve. Adjust the volume to 1 l. To avoid breathing the fine SDS oiwder, buy the correct amount of SDS and add the full amount of water in a fume hood

50% dextran sulphate.[e] To a 50 ml sterile tube containing 10 ml 2× SSC slowly add 10 g dextran sulphate (sodium salt mol wt ~500 000, Sigmal D-8906). Heat at 65°C and vortex frequently until the dextran sulphate has dissolved. This will take 20–30 min. Make up to 20 ml with 2× SSC, aliquot and freeze at −20°C

Hybridization buffer. Add 10 ml of formamide[f] AR (Fluka), 4 ml 50% dextran sulphate,[e] 2 ml of 20× SSC (pH 7.0), 2 ml of 10% Tween 20[g] and 2 ml distilled water. Mix well, aliquot and store at −20°C

10× TBE (electrophoresis buffer). 108 g Tris base (89 mM), 55 g boric acid[h] (89 mM), 40 ml 0.5 M EDTA,[b] pH 8.0 (2 mM) in 1 l

5× bromophenol blue (gel loading buffer). 10% (w/v) Ficoll, 0.1 M Na$_2$EDTA, 0.5% (w/v) SDS, 0.1% (w/V) bromophenol blue

Agarose gels. Use agarose Type I, low EEO (Sigmal A-6013). Add the desired amount to a volume of 1× TBE buffer sufficient for constructing the gel. Melt the agarose in a microwave over. Cool to 55°C in water bath before pouring the gel to prevent warping the gel apparatus

50% (v/v) formamide,[f] pH 7.0 (for formamide washes). Using 20× SSC pH 5.2 ensures that the resulting formamide solutions will be approximately pH 7.0. For enough wash solution for three coplin jars, add 75 ml Fluka formamide (purified), 15 ml 20× SSC, pH 5.2, and 60 ml distilled water, and mix well. Check pH is approximately 7.0 with pH paper

70% (v/v) formamide,[f] pH 7.0 (denaturing solution). 35 ml Fluka formamide (purified), 5 ml 20× SSC, pH 5.2, 10 ml distilled water, 25 μl 0.25 M. Check pH with pH paper

4% paraformaldehyde.[i] Make up on the day of use. In a fume hood weigh 10 g paraformaldehyde into 1 1 l glass beaker. Add 250 ml PBS, stir, and heat to 70°C to dissolve. Cool, and adjust pH to 7.4 with 1 M sodium hydroxide

Ethanol series. 70%, 95%, absolute ethanol. Make up weekly (change absolute daily)

Vectashield mountant.[j] For single colour hybridizations 9with FITC probes) use Vectashield containing 1.0 μg/ml DAPI (1 μg of 1 mg/ml stock) and 0.75 μg/ml PI (10 μg of 25 mg/ml stock). For single colour hybridizations with Texas Red probes or dual colour hybridizations with FITC and Texas Red probes use Vectashield containing 1.0 μg/ml DAPI only

---

[a] Caution: HCl is corrosive and a poison. Avoid skin contact and inhalation.

[b] Caution: EDTA is irritating to the eyes, respiratory system and skin.

[c] Caution: acetic acid causes severe burns and is harmful in contact with skin.

[d] Caution: SDS is harmful by inhalation and if swallowed. It may cause sensitization by inhalation. It is irritating to the eyes, respiratory system and skin. There is a risk of serious damage to eyes.

[e] Caution: dextran sulphate may cause harm to the unborn child. It poses a risk of serious damage to the eyes and is irritating to the respiratory system and skin.

[f] Caution: formamide may cause harm to the unborn child. It is irritating to the respiratory system and skin and may cause serious damage to the eyes.

[g] Caution: possible risk of irreversible effects.

[h] Caution: boric acid poses a possible risk of impaired fertility and there is a possible risk to the unborn child.

[i] Caution: paraformaldehyde may cause heritable genetic damage.

[j] Caution: irritating to eyes, respiratory system and skin. It can cause damage to liver and kidneys.

Protocol 1

Nick translation labelling

Equipment and reagents

A. Labelling

- Three water baths at 16°C, 37°C and 68°C
- Eppendorf tubes, sterile, 1.5 ml
- Agarose gel electrophoresis equipment
- Purified probe DNA
- UV transilluminator
- RNase A (Sigma R 4642)
- 25 nmol Cy3 dUTP, Cy5 dUTP (both from Amersham Pharmacia Biotech)
- 1 mM oestradiol-15-dUTP, biotin-16-dUTP, digoxigenin-11-dUTP (all from Boehringer Mannheim)[a]
- 10× nick translation buffer: 0.5 M Tris-HCl pH 8.0, 50 mM MgCl$_2$, 0.5 mg/ml nuclease-free BSA
- 10× dAGC[a] mix (no dTTP): 0.5 mM each dATP, dCTP, dGTP (Boehringer Mannheim)

- 0.1 M β-mercaptoethanol:[b] 0.1 ml β-mercaptoethanol in 14.4 ml distilled H$_2$O
- Spectrum Green dUTP (Vysis)
- DNase I stock solution: 20 000 U/ml (RNase free Grade 1 pure, Boehringer Mannheim)
- DNase I dilution buffer: 50% glycerol, 0.15 M NaCl, 20 mM sodium acetate, pH 5.0
- 10 U/μl DNA Polymerase I (New England BioLabs)
- 10× TBE: 108 g Tris base, 55 g boric acid,[c] 40 ml 0.5 M EDTA,[d] pH 8.0
- 0.5 M EDTA,[d]
- 2% TBE agarose gel
- PhiX174 HaeIII size marker

B. Purification of labelled probe

- Bench centrifuge
- Microcentrifuge
- Sephadex G-50 resin[e] for spin columns: 30 g in 400 ml column buffer. Hydrate at 95–100°C for 1.5 h, or 1 day at 37°C
- Column buffer: 10 mM Tris/HCl, pH 8.0, 1 mM EDTA,[d] 0.1% SDS[f]

- Fluorometer (e.g. Hoeffer DynaQuant, Amersham Pharmacia Biotech)
- Syringes, 1 ml
- Centrifuge tubes, 15 ml
- Eppendorf tubes, 1.5 ml

Methods

A. Labelling

1 First, RNase the DNA as follows: for each 1 μg DNA add 200 ng RNase A and incubate the DNA for 30 min at 37°C. Place the tube on ice.

2 Add the following (in order) to a 1.5 ml Eppendorf tube on ice: 1 μg probe DNA (RNA free); 1 μl (1 nmol) Cy3, Cy5 dUTP or 1 μl (1 mM) oestradiol-15-dUTP, biotin-16-dUTP, digoxigenin-11-dUTP, or 2.5 μl Spectrum Green dUTP (Vysis); 5 μl 10× nick translation buffer; 5 μl dAGC mix; 5 μl 0.1 M β-mercaptoethanol; sterile distilled water to make up to a final volume of 50 μl; 4 μl DNase I (dilute stock 1/2000 just before use: discard after use); 1 μl 10 U/ml DNA polymerase I. Mix well.

3 Incubate the tubes at 16°C for 2 h.

4 Stop the reaction by placing the tubes on ice.

5   Run a 5-μl aliquot on a 2% TBE agarose gel at 100 V for 1 h, with *PhiX174 HaeIII* as a size marker. The optimum size for labelled fragments is 100–500 bp (average 300). If the DNA is larger than this, reincubate with DNase for a further 30 min. If the DNA is smaller than 100 bp, it needs to be relabelled, using a lower concentration of DNase I.

6   When the DNA is the correct size, stop the reaction by adding 1.5 μl 0.5 M EDTA and incubating at 68°C for 10 min.

7   Store at −20°C until required.

B. Column purification of labelled probe

1   Prepare Sephadex G-50 spin columns as follows: plug 1 ml syringes with filter wool to the 0.1 ml mark and add Sephadex G-50 solution to the top of the syringe. Place the column in a 15 ml centrifuge tube and centrifuge at 200 **g** for 5 min. Discard the eluate, top up the column with more Sephadex and repeat the centrifugation. It is important to ensure that there are no air bubbles in the column.

2   Wash the column with 200 μl of column buffer and centrifuge at 200 **g** for 5 min. Repeat these washes five or six times.

3   Transfer the column to a new centrifuge tube with an Eppendorf tube at the bottom to catch the eluate from the column. Load a maximum of 150 μl of the labelled probe onto the centre of the column and centrifuge at 200 **g** for 5 min. The eluate contains the labelled probe.

4   Measure the probe concentration in a fluorometer. Store the purified, labelled probe at −20°C until required.

[a] Caution: nucleotide mixes are harmful to eyes, respiratory system and skin. Avoid contact and inhalation.

[b] Caution: mercaptoethanol is toxic in contact with skin and poses a risk of serious damage to eyes. It is harmful by inhalation and if swallowed.

[c] Caution: boric acid poses a possible risk of impaired fertility and poses a possible risk to the unborn child.

[d] Caution: EDTA is irritating to the eyes, respiratory system and skin.

[e] Caution: Sephadex is very toxic by inhalation, is harmful if swallowed and irritating to the eyes.

[f] Caution: SDS is harmful by inhalation and if swallowed. It poses a serious risk of damage to the eyes.

Protocol 2

Pre-treatment of slides

Equipment and reagents

- Fume hood
- Phase-contrast microscope
- Humid chamber[a]
- Coverslips, 24 × 50 mm

- 0.01 N HCl[b]
- RNase A (DNase free, Sigma)
- 1× PBS: 8 g NaCl, 0.2 g KCl, 1.44 g Na_2HPO_4, 0.24 KH_2PO_4 in 800 ml H_2O, pH to 7.4 with HCl. Add H_2O to 1 l
- PBS/50 mM $MgCl_2$: 50 ml 1 M $MgCl_2$ + 1 ml 1× PBS

- PBS/50 mM $MgCl_2$/1% formaldehyde[c]: 2.7 ml formaldehyde in 100 ml PBS/$MgCl_2$ (make up fresh each time in a fume hood)
- 100 mg/ml Pepsin[d] stock solution (Sigma)
- 30 µg/ml Pepsin: 150 µl of pepsin stock in 50 ml 0.01 N HCl (make up fresh before use)
- Shaking platform

Method

1 Place 100 µl RNase (100 µg/ml) on slides under a coverslip and incubate in a moist chamber at 37°C for 1 h at 37°C.

2 Wash twice (3 min each) in 2× SSC at room temperature (with agitation, on a shaking platform).

3 Incubate the slides in 30 µg/ml pepsin in 0.01 N HCl at 37°C for 2–5 min depending on the amount of cytoplasm present.

4 Wash twice (5 min each) in 1× PBS, with agitation.

5 Place the slides in PBS/50 mM $MgCl_2$ for 5 min.

6 Fix in PBS/50 mM $MgCl_2$/1% formaldehyde for 10 min.

7 Wash in PBS for 5 min (with agitation).

8 Dehydrate the slides through an alcohol series (70%, 95%, absolute) and allow to air dry. Check under phase-contrast at this stage to ensure that all the cytoplasm has been removed. Slides can be stored desiccated at 4°C for up to 1 month before use.

[a] The authors use a moist chamber consisting of a plastic microscope slide storage box with a lid (Raymond A. Lamb), floated in a water bath. In this case it is not necessary to put any moisture inside the chamber. However, if hybridizing in a dry oven, put some moist (not wet) tissue in the bottom of the box and suspend the slides above it on some sort of rack. Alternatively use immuno-slide staining trays (Raymond A. Lamb) placed in a water bath.

[b] Caution: HCl is corrosive and a poison. Avoid skin contact and inhalation.

[c] Caution: formaldehyde is toxic by inhalation, in contact with skin and if swallowed. It causes burns and poses a possible risk of irreversible effects. Handle in a fume hood.

[c] Caution: pepsin is irritating to the eyes, respiratory system and skin. It may cause sensitization by inhalation.

Protocol 3

Hybridization

Equipment and reagents

- Fume hood
- Hotblock, 95°C
- Parafilm
- Humid chamber (see *Protocol 2*)

- Ethanol, ice-cold 70%, 90% and 100%
- 70% Formamide[a] solution: 5 ml 20× SSC at pH 5.5, 35 ml Fluka formamide, 10 ml distilled H_2O. Check the pH with pH paper

- Waterbaths at 70°C (in a fume hood) and 37°C
- Vacuum dessicator
- Microcentrifuge
- Coverslips, 22 × 32 mm
- Labelled probe DNA (cosmid, YAC, PAC)
- 1 mg/ml *Cot-1* DNA (Gibco, BRL)

- 3 M Sodium acetate
- Hybridization buffer (warmed to room temperature): 50% formamide,[a] 10% dextran sulphate,[a] 2× SSC, pH 7.0
- Rubber solution (Cowgum or bicycle puncture repair solution)

Method

1 Heat 70% formamide in 2 × SSC at pH 7–8 to 70°C in a Coplin jar under a fume hood. Place the slides in the heated formamide for exactly 2 min.[b]

2 Transfer the slides to ice-cold 70% ethanol and leave for 4 min. Transfer to ice-cold 90%, then 100% ethanol for 4 min each and air dry.

3 Dry down the appropriate concentration of probe and competitor either in a vacuum dessicator (Speedivac) or by ethanol precipitation, e.g.: 100 ng labelled cosmid or 400 ng–1 μg YAC, PAC; 2.5 μg (2.5 μl) *Cot-1* DNA (for cosmids), or 5 μg (for YACs, PACs); 0.1 volumes 3 M sodium acetate; 2 volumes ice cold ethanol. Allow to precipitate for 1–2 h at −70°C.

4 Centrifuge and dry down the pellet as for labelled probes. Resuspend the pellet in 11 μl hybridization buffer.

5 Denature the probe mixture at 95°C on a hotblock for 10 min. Plunge the tubes in ice for a few minutes, then centrifuge briefly in a microcentrifuge.

6 Place the probe mixture in a waterbath at 37°C for 15 min to 1 h.

7 Centrifuge the probe mixture quickly to get the liquid to the bottom of the tube. Place this mixture on the previously treated slide containing denatured chromosomes and cover with a 22 × 32 mm coverslip (do not let the drop dry). Seal the coverslip with rubber solution and place the slides in a moist chamber at 37°C for 1–2 d.[c]

[a] Caution: See *Table 1* for risk information.

[b] If placing slides at room temperature into the formamide, the temperature of the formamide will decrease by 0.5°C for each slide used. The temperature should be adjusted accordingly, e.g. for three slides heat the formamide to 71.5–72°C. Alternatively, heat the slides in an oven or on a hotplate to 65–70°C for about 5–10 min before placing them in the denaturing solution.

[c] For repetitive probes, a few hours' hybridization is sufficient. Longer hybridization times are required for larger probes (e.g. YACs) or complex probe mixtures (e.g. M-FISH paints or CGH probe mixtures). For most FISH applications, overnight hybridization is sufficient.

Protocol 4

Post-hybridization washes and detection

Equipment and reagents

- Fume hood
- Coplin jars
- Water bath set at 42 °C in a fume hood
- Coverslips, 24 × 50 mm
- Parafilm
- 50% Formamide[a] solution: 15 ml 20× SSC at pH 5.5, 75 ml Fluka formamide, 60 ml distilled H_2O. Check the pH using pH paper
- 2× SSC, pH 7.0
- SSCT: 4 × SSC with 0.05% Tween 20[b]
- Blocking solution: 3% BSA in SSCT
- Detection solution: 1 volume of filtered blocking solution in 2 volumes SSCT

- Antibody solution (layer 1):[c] 1/300 avidin Cy3.5, 1/200 rabbit anti-estradiol, 1/100 sheep anti-dig, in detection solution
- Antibody solution (layer 2):[c] 1/500 donkey anti-rabbit Cy5.5, 1/100 donkey anti-sheep FITC in detection solution. Vortex the antibody solutions and incubate at 4 °C for at least 10 min, then centrifuge in a microcentrifuge for 15 min. Use the supernatant only
- Ethanol series (70%, 90% and 100%)
- Mountant: Vectashield[c] with DAPI (1 µl of 1 mg/ml DAPI stock solution in 1 ml of Vectashield (Vector Laboratories))

Method

1. Carry out the following post-hybridization washes (all at 42 °C): three washes (5 min each) in 50% formamide, 2 × SSC pH 7.0; three washes (5 min each) in 2 × SSC; one 5 min wash in SSCT.

For directly labelled probes, proceed directly to step 8.

2. Place the slides in blocking solution for 10–30 min at room temperature.

3. Wash the slides briefly in SSCT at room temperature

4. Briefly drain the slides (do not allow to dry out), then place 150 µl of antibody solution layer 1 on the slide. Cover with a coverslip (or 24 mm × 50 mm piece of Parafilm cut to size) and incubate at 37 °C for 20 min.

5. Wash in SSCT at room temperature for 5 min.

6. Briefly drain the slides (do not allow to dry out), then place 150 µl of antibody solution layer 2 on the slide. Cover with a coverslip (or 24 mm × 50 mm piece of Parafilm cut to size) and incubate at 37 °C for 20 min.

7. Wash in SSCT at RT for 5 min.

8. Wash twice in PBS for 5 min at RT.

9. Dehydrate the slides in 70%, 90% then 100% ethanol.

10. Mount the slides in Vectashield with DAPI and cover with 24 mm × 50 mm coverslip.

[a] See *Table 1* for risk information

[b] Caution: Tween 20 poses a possible risk of irreversible effects.

[c] Caution: antibody solutions and Vectashield are harmful to the respiratory system, eyes and skin.

3 Multicolour fluorescence *in situ* hybridization

3.1 Multiplex fluorescence *in situ* hybridization and spectral karyotyping

The availability of new fluorochromes and sensitive methods of imaging has enhanced one of the most attractive features of FISH, namely the ability to visualize several targets simultaneously in different colours. The basic protocols given above (*Protocols 1–4*), allow the detection of up to five colours simultaneously (using Digoxigenin-FITC, Cy3, Biotin-Cy3.5, Cy5, Oestradiol-Cy5.5). To increase the number of targets even further, the techniques of combinatorial or ratio-labelling can be used (3–5). Combinatorial labelling uses mixtures of unit amounts of fluorochromes such that no two probes have the same labelling combination. Ratio-labelling uses combinations of fluorochromes in different ratios, increasing the number of discernible targets even more. However, quantification of the varying ratios is more problematic than when the fluors are present in unit amounts. For this reason, combinatorial labelling is preferred. The theoretical number of targets which can be discriminated in this manner is 2^n-1, where n = number of fluorochromes available. Using only five fluorochromes allows painting of the entire chromosome complement in 24 colours, and provides the prospect of automated molecular karyotyping (6,7). Two methods have been used to discriminate the fluorochrome combinations.

The first, M-FISH, relies on capturing the separate fluorochrome images for each of the five fluorochromes using specifically selected narrow band pass filter sets (6). The second approach, SKY, uses a single exposure of the image and a combination of CCD imaging and Fourier transform spectrometry to analyse the spectral signature of the fluorochrome combinations (7). Both techniques use dedicated software to translate the unique labelling combination for each chromosome into a pseudocolour. Both of these techniques have already demonstrated hidden chromosome rearrangements in complex karyotypes in tumour cell lines and in haematological malignancies (6,8). However, the limitations of this technology are the reliance on metaphase analysis, and the imperfect coverage of painting probes. Preliminary studies indicate that the sensitivity of multicolour painting for the detection of translocations involving subtelomeric regions is approximately 2–3 Mb (L. Kearney, unpublished results). In addition, whole-chromosome painting will not detect deletions, duplications or inversions. Both M-FISH and SKY still require reference back to the G-banded karyotype and a combination of FISH approaches is still required to identify all abnormalities in complex karyotypes (9).

3.2 Colour 'bar codes'

To overcome the above limitations, chromosome arm painting probes (10) or chromosomal 'bar codes' have been developed. The concept of a colour bar code for each chromosome was first proposed by Lengauer *et al.* (11), using a series of region-specific YACs, labelled differentially and detected in different colours.

More recently, a set of painting probes from different gibbon species has been used to identify syntenic regions on human chromosomes, resulting in a colour-banded karyotype (12; reviewed in ref. 13). Other investigators have used amplified microdissected chromosome regions. The combination of ratio and combinatorial labelling (14) provides the promise of up to 96 colours. By conventional G-banding standards this would still produce low-resolution banding. However, the power of using even low resolution colour bar codes as a complementary technique to identify chromosomal inversions and insertions has been demonstrated (15).

3.3 Chromosome-specific subtelomeric probes

One of the remaining challenges for the new FISH techniques is to identify cryptic rearrangements in apparently normal karyotypes. A significant proportion (15–20%) of bone marrow karyotypes in leukaemia are reported as normal by conventional cytogenetic analysis. The t(12;21)(p13;q22), present in up to 25% of childhood B-cell ALL cases (16) is undetectable by conventional cytogenetic analysis. The difficulty in detecting chromosome abnormalities such as this lies in the fact that there is a reciprocal exchange of terminal, pale staining (G-band negative) regions of a similar size. It is likely that M-FISH and SKY will not be sufficiently sensitive to detect cryptic translocations in apparently normal karyotypes. The application of CGH to DNA microarrays promises sensitive detection of deletions and amplifications using clones approximately 1 Mb apart across the whole genome (2). However, this approach only detects unbalanced rearrangements, and will not detect balanced translocations. One approach to the sensitive detection of balanced rearrangements in normal karyotypes is to use a set of chromosome-specific subtelomeric probes (17). It has been shown that these probes can identify submicroscopic rearrangements in patients with mental retardation and apparently normal karyotypes (18). A 12-colour M-FISH assay using these probes has now been developed. This allows a full survey of all telomeres using only two hybridizations (see Plate 2), making this a feasible proposition for the screening of apparently normal leukaemic karyotypes.

3.4 Combinatorial labelling of probes for multiplex fluorescence *in situ* hybridization

The generation of combinatorially labelled probes for M-FISH or SKY is a complex procedure, beyond the scope of most diagnostic laboratories. Commercial versions of whole-chromosome painting sets are now available (Vysis, Metasystems, Appligene Orcor), which obviate the need to undertake such procedures. However, for those laboratories with the resources to undertake probe generation, some general principles will be outlined here. In order to produce a set of combinatorially labelled paints in 24 colours, five fluorochromes are needed. An example of the labelling scheme to produce a set of 24-colour whole-chromosome paints is given in Plate 3. Each chromosome is labelled with a unique fluorochrome combination, represented by a unique pseudocolour. A refinement of the labelling procedure has been described by Eils *et al.* (19), using fluorochrome pools. Pools for FITC, Cy3, biotin (detected with Cy3.5), Cy5 and digoxigenin (detected with Cy5.5) are prepared by adding equal amounts of each flow-sorted chromosome fraction to be labelled with a particular fluorochrome. Each fluorochrome pool is amplified by DOP-PCR (Protocol 5A) and an aliquot of this is labelled in the second-round PCR reaction (Protocol 5B). After labelling, it is necessary to test for homogeneity and equal intensity of the constituent chromosomes by hybridizing the individual pools to normal metaphase chromosomes. It may be necessary to adjust the concentration of some of the component chromosomes to generate balanced pools. This method has the added advantage that the pools can be re-amplified many times without visible loss of complexity (M. Speicher, personal communication).

The method in *Protocol 5* (20) can be used to label flow-sorted chromosomes or microdissected chromosomes for M-FISH

Protocol 5

DOP-PCR to generate whole-chromosome paints for M-FISH

Equipment and reagents

- Programmable thermal cycler capable of incorporating a ramp stage (e.g. Hybaid PCR Sprint or Express)
- Fluorometer (Hoeffer DyNAQuant, Amersham Pharmacia Biotech)
- Flow-sorted chromosomes (approximate concentration 500 chromosomes/μl)
- Microcentrifuge tubes, sterile 0.5 ml
- Mineral oil
- Agarose gel electrophoresis equipment
- Agarose gel, 1.2%
- Fluor-dNTPs for labelling:[a] biotin-16-dUTP, Digoxigenin-11-dUTP (Boehringer Mannheim); Cy3 dUTP, Cy5 dUTP, FluorX dCTP (all from Amersham Pharmacia Biotech)
- 10× PCR buffer (Gibco)
- Coverslips 22 × 22 mm

- 50 mM MgCl$_2$ (Gibco)
- dNTP mix:[a] 5 mM each of dATP, dCTP, dGTP and dTTP
- dAGC nucleotide mix:[a] 5 mM each of dATP, dCTP and dGTP
- dAGT nucleotide mix:[a] 5 mM each of dATP, dGTP, dTTP
- 100 μM 6-MW primer:[a] 5'-CCGACTCGAGNNNNNNATGTGG-3'
- *Taq* 1 polymerase[a] (Boehringer Mannheim)
- 1 mM biotin-16-dUTP[a] or 1 mM digoxigenin-11-dUTP (Boehringer-Mannheim)
- *Cot-1* DNA
- *Escherichia coli* tRNA
- Salmon sperm DNA
- Fluka formamide[b]
- 30% Dextran sulphate[b]
- 4 × SSC

Methods

A. First-round PCR

1 Combine in a sterile 0.5 ml microcentrifuge tube: 1 μl (= 500 flow sorted chromosomes), 2.5 μl 10× PCR buffer, 1 μl dNTP mix, 0.5 μl 100 μM 6-MW primer, 0.2 μl (1 U) *Taq* 1 polymerase and water to a final volume of 25 μl.

Protocol 5 continued

2 Overlay with 25 μl mineral oil and run the following program in a DNA thermal cycler: denature for 3 min at 94 °C; 5 cycles of 1 min at 94 °C, 1.5 min at 30 °C, 3 min at 30–72 °C transition and 3 min at 72 °C; 35 cycles of 1 min at 94 °C, 1 min at 62 °C, 3 min at 72 °C, with an additional 1 s/cycle and final extension time of 10 min.

3 Run a 3-μl aliquot of the amplified products on a 1.2% agarose gel with *Phi* X174 Hae III (see *Protocol 1A*) to check the success of the amplification. There should be no amplification in the negative control.

B. Second-round PCR and labelling

1 Add to a new sterile 0.5 ml microcentrifuge tube (final volume of 25 μl): 1 μl of amplified products from first round; 1 μl 50 mM $MgCl_2$; 2.5 μl 10× PCR buffer; 1 μl 5 mM dAGC nucleotide mix;[b] 0.75 μl 5 mM dTTP;[c] 0.5 μl 100 μM 6-MW primer; 1.25 μl 1 mM biotin-16-dUTP or Cy3 dUTP;[c] water to 25 μl.

2 Mix well, overlay with 25 μl mineral oil and run the following PCR program: denature for 3 min at 94 °C; 25 cycles of 1 min at 94 °C, 1 min at 62 °C, 3 min at 72 °C, with a final extension time of 10 min.

3 Remove the mineral oil. Run 3 μl of labelled products on a 1.2% agarose gel to check the size range. This should be in the range 200–600 bp. If the labelled fragments are too large, re-cut with 5 μl 3 μg/ml DNase 1 for 30–60 min.

4 Purify the labelled DNA through a Sephadex G50 column (see *Protocol 1B*). Measure the DNA concentration of the purified, labelled DNA in a fluorimeter (usually 20–50 ng/ml).

5 Prepare a hybridization mixture as follows: add 20 μl each of the FluorX, Cy3, biotin, Cy5 and digoxogenin-labelled pools to a tube and ethanol precipitate using 40 μg *Cot*1 DNA, 5 μg salmon sperm DNA, 15 μl 3M sodium acetate, 400 μl ice cold ethanol.

6 Place at −20°C overnight. Centrifuge, discard the supernatant, wash with 400 μl of 70% ethanol. Centrifuge, discard the supernatant and leave the pellet to dry at room temperature. Resuspend the pellet in 22 μl Fluka formamide and incubate at 37 °C until dissolved. Add 22 μl 30% dextran sulphate in 4 × SSC. Mix well. Use 10 μl of this hybridization mixture per 22 × 22 mm coverslip.

7 Carry out the hybridization as in *Protocol 3* and the washes and detection steps as in *Protocol 4* (without the oestradiol detection). Allow the hybridization to proceed at 37 °C for 2 nights.

[a] Caution: harmful to eyes, respiratory system and skin. Avoid contact and inhalation.

[b] For labelling with Fluor X-dCTP, substitute 1 μl of 5 mM AGT, 0.5 μl mM dCTP and 2.5 μl of label.

[c] For labelling with dig-11-dUTP or Cy5-dUTP, substitute 2.5 μl of label, and 0.5 μl of dTTP.

3.5 Multiplex fluorescence *in situ* hybridization imaging and analysis

The second most important requirement for M-FISH, after the generation of a good quality set of probes, is the requirement for multicolour microscopy and image analysis. There are a number of M-FISH imaging systems on the market, but experience with these is still limited. This section discusses the general principles of such systems. In choosing an epifluorescence microscope for M-FISH it is imperative to select filter sets for the optimum discrimination of the chosen fluorochromes. This requires the optimal combination of excitation, emission and dichroic beamsplitter filters. The specifications for one such filter set are given in *Table 2*. The requirements for up to six individual specific filter sets can be achieved using a combination of filter wheel (containing excitation filters only) and specific filter blocks in the microscope. However, most microscope manufacturers now supply a motorized filter turret to take up to eight individual filter blocks. The choice of light source also depends on the fluorochromes used. The authors use a microscope fitted with two light sources, a 75 W xenon arc lamp and a 100 W mercury lamp, and a switching mechanism to alternate between the two sources. The xenon lamp is superior at the red end of the spectrum, but requires longer exposure times in the blue and green ranges. The mercury lamp is superior in the green range. However, if only one lamp is used, the xenon lamp is preferable, at least for the fluorochrome combinations in *Table 2*. However, if SpectrumGold (Vysis) is used, a 100 W Mercury lamp is necessary for low-power scanning, as the xenon lamp is too weak. For image capture a Sensys cooled CCD camera with a Kodak KAF 1400 chip (Photometrics, Tucson, AZ, USA) is recommended.

There are two main approaches to the analysis of M-FISH images. The first relies on the calculation of intensity threshold levels for each fluorochrome (6). The second method relies on the calculation of feature vectors (19). For five fluorochromes, if we consider a two-dimensional image with each pixel having five-dimensional colour information, each of the specific combinations of fluorochromes for the 24 chromosome paints corresponds to a five-dimensional spectral feature vector. Most commercial M-FISH software packages incorporate one of these approaches to identify the unique spectral information, and apply an algorithm to assign a unique pseudocolour to each chromosome. The other essential requirements for M-FISH software are:

- some form of segmentation mask, based on either the DAPI or individual fluorochrome images

Table 2 M-FISH fluorescence filter sets for the Olympus AX-70 microscope (nm)

	DAPI	FITC	Cy3	Cy3.5	Cy5	Cy5.5
Excitation filter	360	470	546	581	630	682
Dichroic beamsplitter	400	497	557	593	649	697
Emission filter	470	522	567	617	667	721

- background removal
- pixel shift correction
- automated karyotyping based on colour classification.

Some form of built-in controls to check the colour classification are also desirable, for example the ability to view the individual fluorochrome channels and the pseudocoloured image in the same window. It is also important to be aware that spurious chromosome assignments can be given because of the overlap of fluorochromes at translocation borders. It is always wise to check the findings of multicolour karyotyping using single- or dual-colour FISH. An example of M-FISH analysis of a complex karyotype in a myeloid leukaemia derived cell line is given in Plate 4.

4 Interphase fluorescence *in situ* hybridization

One area which has contributed to the expansion in the use of FISH has been in the ability to use non-dividing cells as DNA targets, referred to as interphase FISH (21). This provides access to an almost unlimited variety of cells and confers considerable advantages particularly in cases where the proliferative activity is low, or the mitotic cells do not represent the neoplastic clone (e.g. in chronic lymphocytic leukaemia, Hodgkin's disease, multiple myeloma). However, it is important to realize that interphase FISH provides only limited information. There are also a number of pitfalls in the interpretation of FISH signals in interphase. As this technique is being increasingly relied upon, it is imperative that the limitations are fully understood. One important consideration is the choice of probe.

4.1 Types of probe for interphase fluorescence *in situ* hybridization

Whole-chromosome painting probes are generally not suitable for interphase FISH, as the extended chromosome domains are difficult to interpret in two dimensions. However, these have proved useful in the study of three dimensional chromosome structure in interphase nuclei (22). Chromosome-specific centromeric probes are perfectly suited to the detection of numerical abnormalities in interphase, as they exhibit strong, compact signals that are easy to evaluate. However, caution should be exercised in interpreting the number of signals from centromeric probes. These can only give information of the number of centromeres present, and are of limited use for the detection of structural rearrangements. It is also important to use suitably stringent hybridization conditions to avoid cross reaction with other centromeres. Certain tumour types may also exhibit decondensed heterochromatin, making interpretation difficult (23). Certain cell types may exhibit polymorphism in copy number, or pairing of centromeric regions (24). It is wise to test the usefulness of the chosen probe on the particular cell type under study.

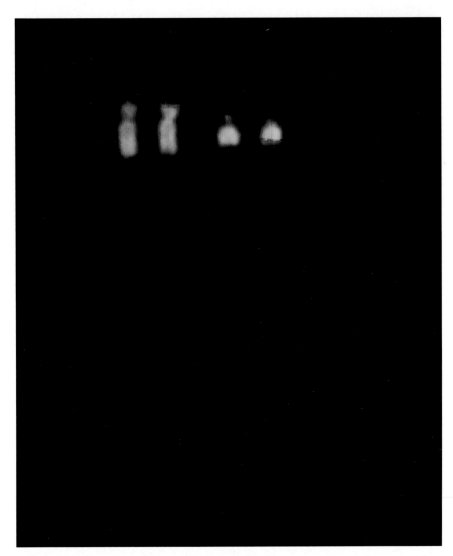

Plate 1 Partial karyotype of the t(12;21)(p12–13;q22) showing the cryptic nature of this translocation using FISH. The photograph of t(12;21) was kindly supplied by the LRF and UKCCG database in ALL, Royal Free Hospital, London, UK.

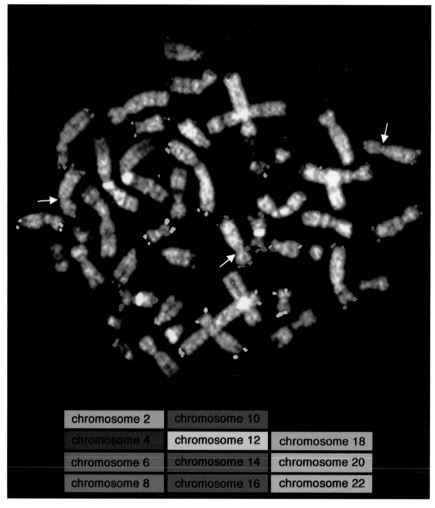

chromosome 2	chromosome 10	
chromosome 4	chromosome 12	chromosome 18
chromosome 6	chromosome 14	chromosome 20
chromosome 8	chromosome 16	chromosome 22

Plate 2 M-TEL assay for subtelomeric rearrangements. This allows the full survey of all telomeres in two hybridizations. Probes for the p and q arm subtelomeric regions of chromosomes 2, 4, 6, 8, 10, 12, 14, 16, 18, 20 and 22 were labelled with a unique combination of up to four fluorochromes and hybridized to a leukaemic bone marrow metaphase with trisomy 8. In each case the pa q arm probes for each chromosome have the same combination. The colour classification for each unique labelling is given at the bottom.

	FITC	Cy3	Cy3.5	Cy5	Cy5.5	
1	+					
2					+	
3		+				
4			+			
5		+			+	
6	+		+			
7	+	+	+			
8				+	+	
9	+	+		+		
10				+		
11			+	+		
12		+	+			
13	+	+			+	
14			+	+	+	
15	+		+		+	
16		+		+		
17	+				+	
18			+		+	
19		+	+	+		
20	+			+	+	
21	+		+	+		
22	+			+		
X		+	+			
Y	+	+				

Plate 3 Combinatorial labelling for M-FISH using whole-chromosome paints. The colour classification for each unique labelling combination is given on the right.

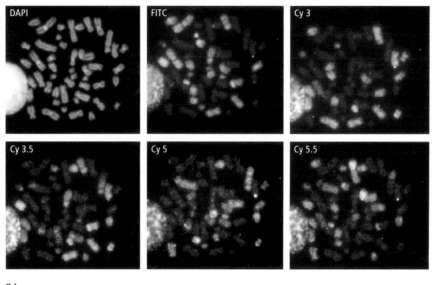

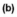

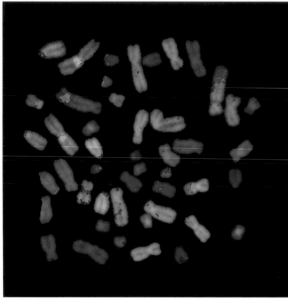

Plate 4 M-FISH analysis of the karyotype in the leukaemia-derived cell line GF-D8. (a) Individual fluorochrome greyscale images captured through specific narrow band pass filter sets for DAPI, FITC, Cy3, Cy3.5, Cy5, and Cy5.5 using a Sensys cooled CCD camera mounted on an Olympus AX-70 microscope fitted with an eight position filter turret. (b) Composite image of the fluorochrome channels shown in (a). All 24 chromosomes have been pseudocoloured according to their unique fluorochrome composition using Powergene M-FISH software (Perceptive Scientific International, Chester, UK). (See Plate 3 for classification colours).

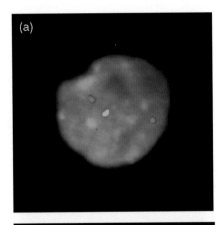

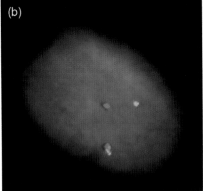

Plate 5 Interphase FISH on haemopoietic progenitor cells derived from colony assays. Cells in (a) were derived from the bone marrow of an AML patient with del(5q), whereas those in (b) were from a patient with Philadelphia translocation-positive acute leukaemia. In both cases, leukaemic blast cells were induced to differentiate into dendritic cells. (a) Using YAC 15DB10 (detected with FITC), which localizes to 5q31. A control probe, YAC13HH4, which localizes to 11q23, was co-hybridized (detected with Texas Red). Only one copy of the 15DB10 sequence is present (green signal), with of two copies of the control YAC13HH4 (red signal), confirming the del(5q) clonal marker. (b) Using a commercial *BCR–ABL* probe set (Appligene-Oncor). The presence of the Philadelphia translocation is shown by a red-green fusion as well as a single red and green signal.

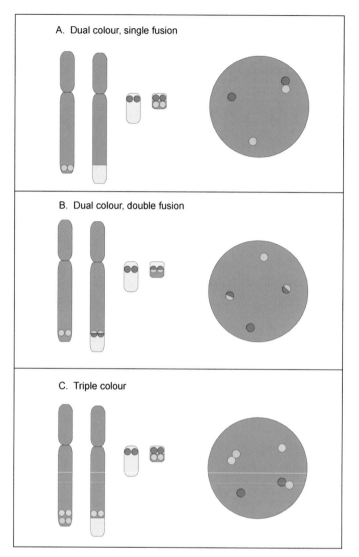

Plate 6 Schematic representation of different schemes to detect the Philadelphia translocation in interphase nuclei (reproduced from Kearney, L. (1999), *Br. J. Haematol.* **104**, 648, with permission). In each case, the left panel shows the location of the FISH signals on metaphase chromosomes (partial karyotype), and the right panel the interphase FISH signals. In (a), two probes from the flanking regions of the *BCR* and *ABL* genes are labelled and detected in different colours: *BCR* in red and *ABL* in green. The *BCR/ABL* fusion results in co-localization of the red and green signals on the der(22) (Ph) chromosomes, with a single red and green signal separated, corresponding to the normal chromosome 22 and 9 chromosomes, respectively. A *BCR–ABL*-negative cell would show two separate red and two green signals. The scheme in (b) uses two probes, this time spanning both the *BCR* and *ABL* breakpoint regions. In this case, two red/green fusion signals are formed: one corresponding to the der(9), and the second to the(22). A positive cell would therefore exhibit one red, one green and two red/green fusions (53). In (c), a third probe from the region just proximal to *ABL* on 9q34 is used, labelled in a different colour (represented here in yellow). A translocation-positive cell exhibits one green/yellow doublet, one red/green, and a single red and yellow signal.

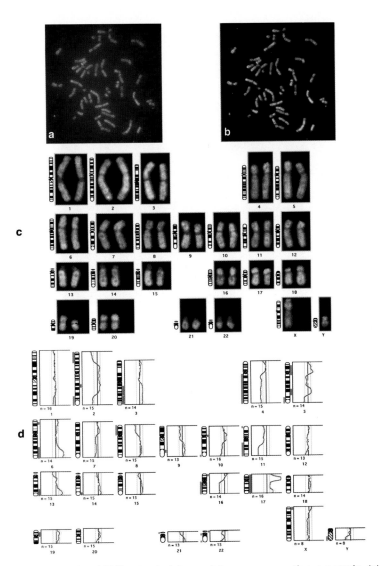

Plate 7 CGH analysis of DNA extracted from a leiomyosarcoma tissue sample. (a) Original captured digital image of one target metaphase from the experiment. Note the green colour cast; the green fluorescence (Spectrum Green) in the image was brighter than the red (Spectrum Red), although both showed a good signal to noise ratio. (b) Image from (a) after processing by CGH analysis software. (Quips, Vysis, UK). Background removal and normalization have dramatically enhanced the appearance of the chromosomes. (c) Target chromosones paired up by the program (on the basis of enhanced DAPI banding). Matching areas of amplification (in green) and/or deletion (in red) can be clearly seen on homologous chromosones. (d) Combined fluorescence ratio data from 8 target metaphases. Red and green bars to the left and right respectively of each chromosomes ideogram show regions of deletion and amplification. The red and green lines represent cut-off values of 0.8 and 1.2, and are derived from a normal vs. normal control slide which was included in the experiment. The blue graph lines represent mean values of each green/red fluorescence ratio. The orange lines represent the 95% confidence limits in each case.

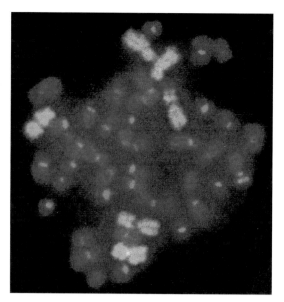

Plate 8 Translocation detected with whole chromosome paints.

For the reasons given above, it may be more prudent to choose locus specific probes to detect aneuploidy. Cosmid clones make ideal probes for interphase analysis as they usually hybridize with high efficiency (> 90% of cells have signal on all four chromatids), and produce signals which are easy to evaluate. Large cloned probes (e.g. YACs) can also be used, but these may detect regions which are decondensed in interphase, giving long, 'stringy' signals. Cosmid or YAC probes for the genes rearranged as a result of specific chromosome rearrangements can be used to detect these rearrangements in interphase. When labelled in two different fluorochromes, the fusion gene is identified by a red–green fusion signal representing the translocation, and a single red and green signal corresponding to the normal chromosome homologues. However, the random co-localization of fluorescent signals occurs in up to 5% of normal cells means that cut-off levels for false positives have to be established (see Section 4.5).

4.2 Types of target for interphase fluorescence *in situ* hybridization

Fluorescence *in situ* hybridization can be applied to a wide range of cellular targets, from standard methanol–acetic acid-fixed nuclei to previously intractable targets such as paraffin-embedded tumour tissue. These all need special treatment before hybridization to allow penetration of probe and detection reagents.

4.2.1 Bone marrow, peripheral blood smears

Protocol 6 can be used for unfixed, unstained bone marrow or peripheral blood smears. We have also found that this pretreatment is suitable for haemopoietic progenitor cells from colony assays (see Plate 5).

Protocol 6

Pretreatment of bone marrow or peripheral smears

Equipment and reagents

- Fume hood
- Phase-contrast microscope
- Water bath, 37 °C
- Humid chamber (see *Protocol 2*)
- Freshly prepared 3:1 methanol–glacial acetic acid[a]
- Ethanol: 70%, 90% and absolute
- 1× PBS
- Coverslips 24 × 50 mm

- 0.01 M HCl[b]
- PBS/50 mM MgCl$_2$: 50 ml 1 M MgCl2 + 1 ml 1× PBS
- PBS/50 mM MgCl$_2$/1% formaldehyde[b] (make up fresh each time): 2.7 ml formaldehyde in 100 ml PBS/MgCl$_2$.
- 100 µg/ml RNase A (DNase free, Sigma)
- 100 mg/ml Pepsin stock solution (Sigma)[b]
- 2 × SSC

Method

1 Fix the smears in methanol–acetic acid for 10 min.[c]
2 Put the slides through an ethanol series (10 min each in 70%, 90% and 100% ethanol) and air dry the slides.

3 Place 100 μl RNase (100 μg/ml) on the slides under a 24 × 50 mm coverslip and incubate in a moist chamber at 37 °C for 1 h at 37 °C.

4 Wash twice (3 min each) in 2× SSC at room temperature with agitation.

5 Incubate the slides in 50 μg/ml pepsin in 0.01 M HCl at 37 °C for 10 min.

6 Wash twice (5 min each) in 1× PBS, with agitation.

7 Place the slides in PBS/50 mM $MgCl_2$ for 5 min.

8 Fix in PBS/50 mM MgCl2/1% formaldehyde for 10 min.

9 Wash in PBS for 5 min, with agitation.

10 Dehydrate slides through an alcohol series (70%, 95%, absolute) and allow to air dry. Check under phase contrast at this stage to ensure that all the cytoplasm has been removed. Slides can be stored desiccated at 4 °C for up to 1 month before use.

[a] Caution: methanol is highly flammable and toxic by inhalation. Acetic acid causes severe burns and is harmful in contact with the skin.

[b] See Protocol 2 for risk information.

[c] For blood or bone marrow smears previously stained in May Grünwald–Giemsa or Wright's stain, incubate for 10 min in 10 mM Tris-HCl, pH 7.5, 1 mM EDTA for 5 min at 37 °C. For smears older than 2 weeks, this incubation should be extended to overnight.

4.2.2 Paraffin-embedded material

This type of target can present a range of difficulties. There is sometimes a marked degree of autofluoresence inherent in fixed tissues and probe penetration may also be a problem. Leaving preparations several days before viewing can reduce autofluoresence. The latter problem is addressed by slide pretreatments, initially described in detail by Hopman et al. (25). Protocol 7 should be used when it is important to visualize individual cells in the context of the surrounding tissue. Reasonable results have been obtained with this method, but individual cells can be difficult to image owing to unclear boundaries between nuclei and an overlap of cells within the section. Information may also be lost because of the inevitable presence of numbers of incomplete nuclei. Protocol 8, which utilizes whole nuclei extracted from thick paraffin sections, based on (26), is therefore recommended unless there is an overriding requirement to visualize the entire section.

Protocol 7

FISH on paraffin sections

Equipment and reagents

- Fume hood
- Coplin jars
- Waterbaths/incubators, 37 °C, 45 °C and 80 °C
- Waterbath at 73 °C (in a fume hood)
- Hotplate
- Coverslips, 22 × 22 mm
- Eppendorf tubes, 1.5 ml
- Paraffin sections
- Xylene[a]

Protocol 7 continued

- Methanol[b]
- Formaldehyde,[d] 10%
- Ethanol: 70%, 95% and absolute
- Pepsin (Sigma P7012):[d] 4 mg/ml in 0.9% NaCl, pH 1.5)
- Hybridization mix: 65% formamide,[e] 10% dextran sulphate,[e] 2 × SSC, pH 7.0
- Sodium thiocyanate 1 M

- 1× PBS
- Wash buffer 1: 0.4% SSC
- Wash buffer 2: 2× SSC, 0.1% NP-40
- Antifade AF1 solution (Citifluor UK) containing 200 ng/ml DAPI
- Rubber solution
- Nail varnish

Method

1 Dewax slides carrying 5 μm paraffin target sections with three 10-min washes in xylene followed by two 5-min washes in methanol.

2 Incubate the slides in 1 M sodium thiocyanate for 10 min in a water bath at 80 °C and wash twice for 3 min in water.

3 Incubate the slides in pepsin for 10 min at 37°C and then rinse twice in distilled water for 3 min and then in PBS twice for 3 min.

4 Fix the slides in 10% buffered formalin for 2 min then rinse twice in PBS for 3 min.

5 Dehydrate through 70%, 95% and 100% ethanol washes for 3 min each and then air dry the slides.

6 Prepare the labelled probe at an appropriate concentration (see *Protocol 3*) in 10 μl hybridization mix in an Eppendorf tube and heat in a water bath at 73 °C for 5 min. Allow the tubes to cool down to 45°C and incubate at this temperature for 30 min.

7 Denature the slides in 70% formamide, 2× SSC, pH 7.0, for 5 min at 73°C (in a water bath in a fume hood).

8 Dehydrate through 70%, 95% and 100% ethanol washes for 3 min each, air dry the slides and then prewarm each slide to 45–50 °C on a hotplate.

9 Add the warmed probe to the slide, cover with a coverslip, seal with rubber solution and incubate overnight at 37 °C in a humid chamber.

10 Carefully remove the coverslip, place the slide in wash buffer 1[f] at 73 °C, agitate the slide for 1–3 s and then leave for a further 2 min.

11 Transfer the slide to wash buffer 2 at room temperature for between 5 s and 2 min.[g]

12 Dehydrate the slide through a 70%, 95%, 100% ethanol series.

13 Air dry the slide, mount with 1 drop AF1 with DAPI and seal with nail varnish.

[a] Caution: xylene is highly flammable; the vapour/air mixture is explosive. Harmful by inhalation, in contact with skin and if swallowed. Irritating to skin and eyes, risk of blindness. Evidence of reproductive defects. Do not use uncovered on the open bench.

[b] See *Protocol 6* for risk information.

[c] Caution: sodium thiocyanate is irritating to eyes, respiratory system and skin. Contact with acids liberates very toxic gases. It is harmful if swallowed.

[d] See *Protocol 2* for risk information.

[e] See *Table 1* for risk information.

[f] If the probe(s) are not directly labelled then detection steps should be undertaken after this step, without allowing the slide to dry.

[g] Adding 0.1% NP40 to this buffer may reduce background.

Protocol 8

FISH on nuclei isolated from paraffin sections

Equipment and reagents

- Fume hood
- Coplin jars
- Water baths, 37°C, 75°C and 90°C
- Hotplate
- Vortex mixer
- Microcentrifuge
- Coverslips, 22 × 22 mm
- Vectabond or APES-treated slides
- 16–50 μm Paraffin sections on APES slides (1 × 16 μm section will work)
- Xylene[a]
- Ethanol series: 50%, 70%, 90% and 100%
- Metal mesh, 55 μm

- Carlsberg solution: 0.1% Sigma protease XXIV, 0.1 M Tris-HCl, pH 7.2, 0.07 M NaCl. Filter sterilize and store at −20°C
- RNase A solution: 100 μg/ml in 10 mM Tris-HCl, pH 7.5, 1 mM Na EDTA, 0.3% NP-40. Store at −20°C
- Proteinase K solution: 8 μg/ml final concentration in 20 mM Tris-HCl, 2 mM CaCl$_2$, pH 7.5
- Glycerol solution: 50% glycerol, 0.1× SSC, pH 7.5
- Denaturation solution: 70% formamide,[b] 2× SSC, pH 7.0
- 2× SSC

Method

1 Dewax the thick section by immersing the slide in xylene for 30 min. Transfer the slide into fresh xylene for 10 min.

2 Rehydrate through an ethanol series of 100%, 95%, 70% and 50% for 10 min each and then wash twice for 5 min in distilled water.

3 Keeping the slide wet, add 100–200 μl of Carlsberg solution to the section and scrape off the tissue with a syringe needle. Collect the material into an Eppendorf tube and wash the slide with sufficient additional Carlsberg solution to give a final digestion volume of 1 ml.

4 Vortex well and incubate the tube at 37°C for 1 h.

5 Vortex the tube thoroughly. Centrifuge at 4000 **g** in a microfuge for 4–5 s to produce a pellet and remove the supernatant.

6 Resuspend the pellet in 1 ml RNase A solution and incubate for 15 min at room temperature.

7 Filter the solution through a sterile 55 μM metal mesh and store at 4°C until the preparation of target slides is undertaken.

8 To prepare a target slide, pipette 10 μl of nuclear suspension onto a Vectabond or APES treated slide and spread out the liquid to approximately 22 × 22 mm with the pipette tip. Allow the slide to dry for at least 30 min and store at 4°C until use.

9 Prior to prehybridization treatment, equilibrate each slide at room temperature for 30–60 min.

Protocol 8 continued

10 Incubate the slide in glycerol solution for 3 min at 90°C and then cool to room temperature in 2× SSC for 30 min.

11 Incubate the slide in denaturation solution for 5 min at 74°C (in a water bath in a fume hood) and then dehydrate through 70%, 95% and 100% ethanol, chilled to −20°C for 3 min each.

12 Air dry the slide and then incubate it in proteinase K for 7.5 min at 37°C.

13 Wash the slide twice for 3 min in 2 × SSC at room temperature, dehydrate through a 70%, 95% and 100% ethanol series and air dry.

14 Hybridization is then carried out as for *Protocol 7*, step 6 onwards, apart from step 8, in which the slide is just warmed to 45–50°C.

[a] See *Protocol 7* for risk information.

[b] See *Table 1* for risk information. Handle in a fume cupboard.

4.3 Combined immunophenotyping and fluorescence *in situ* hybridization

The ability to identify the specific cell type in which clonal changes occur is desirable in a number of haematological disorders. In particular, there have been a number of conflicting reports on the cell lineages involved in the myelodysplastic syndromes (reviewed in ref. 27). One approach to this problem is the identification of clonal chromosome abnormalities linked to cell phenotype. The simultaneous detection of immunophenotype and chromosome abnormalities is possible using the APAAP immunophenotyping technique, followed by FISH (*Protocol 9*). The APAAP reaction product remains throughout the subsequent harsh FISH procedures and staining with Fast red produces auto-fluorescence visible through all filter sets, which can be viewed at the same time as the FISH signal (28).

Protocol 9

Combined immunophenotyping and FISH

Equipment and reagents

- Coplin jars
- Humid chamber (see *Protocol 2*)
- Thin bone marrow smears
- Acetone[a]–methanol,[b] 1:1
- First antibody layer:[c] choose the appropriate monoclonal antibody for the cell type under investigation, e.g. for haemopoietic cells, CD34 (early progenitor cell), CD3 (T lymphocytes), CD19 (B lymphocytes), all

from DAKO Ltd, Cambridge); CD13 (immature granulocytes and monocytes) from Prof. K. C. Gatter, John Radcliffe Hospital, Oxford; CD68 (monocytes), CD61 (megakaryocytes), glycophorin A (erythrocytes), all from Prof. D. Y. Mason, John Radcliffe Hospital, Oxford

- Second antibody layer:[c] rabbit anti-mouse antibody Z259 (DAKO Ltd)

Protocol 9 continued

- Monoclonal APAAP complex[c] (Boehringer Mannheim)
- Alkaline phosphatase substrate:[d] dissolve 2 mg of Naphthol[d] AS mix (Sigma) to 10 ml of 0.1 M Tris buffer, pH 8.2. To this add 10 mg of Fast Red TR[d] mix (Sigma) and

dissolve. Then add 0.1 M levamisole[d] (Sigma) to block endogenous alkaline phosphatase. Filter the solution before placing on the slides
- TBS: 1 M Tris, 0.5 M NaCl

Method

1 Store the bone marrow smears unfixed, wrapped in foil at −20 °C.

2 Allow the smears to reach room temperature, then unwrap.

3 Fix the slides in either acetone–methanol for 90 s or in acetone alone for 10 min, then transfer them immediately to TBS for 5 min at room temperature.

4 Add the appropriate primary monoclonal antibody and incubate the slides in a humid chamber at room temperature for 30 min.

5 Wash the slides in TBS for 5 min.

6 Add the second antibody layer to the slides and incubate for 30 min in a humid chamber.

7 Wash the slides in TBS for 5 min.

8 Add the monoclonal APAAP complex (1/500 dilution) to the slides and incubate for 30 min in a humid chamber at room temperature.

9 If necessary to enhance the staining, repeat the anti-mouse antibody and APAAP steps (steps 6–8), with reduced incubation times of 10 min.

10 Add alkaline phosphatase substrate to the slides and incubate for 10–20 min at room temperature.

11 Wash the slides in TBS, then distilled water and allow to air dry.

12 After immunostaining, FISH is carried out as described in *Protocol 7*, step 5 onwards.

[a] Caution: acetone is highly flammable and irritating to the eyes.

[b] See *Protocol 6* for risk information.

[c] See *Protocol 4* for risk information for risk information.

[d] Caution: harmful by inhalation, in contact with skin and if swallowed. Irritating to the eyes, respiratory system and skin and poses a possible risk of irreversible effects.

4.4 RNA-fluorescence *in situ* hybridization

There has been considerable interest in the *in situ* detection of mRNA, since this makes it possible to place the expression of specific genes in the context of the individual cell. The use of fluorescently labelled probes (29) has enabled more than one message to be targeted in cryostat sections (30) and in cultured cells (31). Paraffin-embedded material has been more difficult to work with, owing to auto-fluorescence, but it has recently proved possible to detect message in this material (32). *Protocol 10* describes a method for the simultaneous detection of multiple mRNAs in paraffin wax embedded sections using small oligonucleotides, thus permitting a wide variety of archival material to be investigated. This method also allows fluorescence immunocytochemistry to be applied in the same experiment and cell morphology may be ascertained on serial sections if required.

Protocol 10

Detection of multiple RNAs by FISH

Equipment and reagents

- Fume hood
- Coplin jars
- Hotplate, 70 °C
- Water bath, 37 °C
- Humid chamber (see *Protocol 2*)
- Coverslips, 22 × 50 mm
- 3 μm Paraffin-embedded sections on APES-treated microscope slides
- Xylene[a]
- 1× PBS
- 0.3% Triton X-100[b]
- 0.2% Glycine
- Hybridization mix: 50% formamide,[d] 10% dextran sulphate,[d] 0.5% SDS,[e] 1× Denhardts solution, 1 mM EDTA,[e] 240 μg/ml salmon sperm DNA, 240 μg/ml yeast tRNA
- Ethanol, 95%, 100%

- Paraformaldehyde[c] 4%
- Proteinase K (20 μg/ml in 50 mM Tris HCl, pH 7.6)
- Oligonucleotide probe cocktails: 5–8 probes each, 28–30 bp long, 5′-labelled with either FITC, rhodamine or digoxigenin
- 50 mM Tris, pH 7.6
- 4× SSC
- 2× SSC
- SSCTM: 4 × SSC, pH 7.0, 0.05% Tween 20,[f] 5% dried milk powder
- SSCT: 4 × SSC, pH 7.0, 0.05% Tween 20
- Anti-digoxigenin-AMCA, diluted 1:50 in SSCTM
- Antifade AF1 (Citifluor, UK)
- Rubber solution

Method

1 Dewax with xylene (2 × 5 min) and clean with 100% ethanol (2 × 5 min) and then 95% ethanol (2 × 5 min).[g] Wash slides sequentially in water (5 min), PBS (3 min) and 0.3% Triton X-100 (5 min).

2 Wash the slides with PBS for 5 min and 50 mM Tris for 5 min.

3 Incubate the slides with Proteinase K for 36 min at 37 °C.

4 Incubate for 1 min in 0.2% glycine and wash twice in PBS for 5 min each.

5 Fix the slides in 4% paraformaldehyde for 5 min and then wash the slides twice in PBS for 5 min each.

6 Prehybridize by covering each section with 300 μl of hybridization solution under a 22 × 50 mm coverslip and incubate the slides in a humid chamber for 1 h at room temperature.

7 After draining the slide, add oligonucleotide probes in the 100 μl hybridization solution (final concentration of 200 ng/ml) to the section under a 22 × 50 mm coverslip and seal with rubber solution.

8 Heat the slide for 10 min at 70 °C on a hotplate and then incubate overnight in a humid chamber at 37 °C.

9 After carefully removing the coverslips, wash the slides in 4× SSC (2 × 15 min), 2× SSC (15 min) and finally in distilled, deionized water (5 min).

10 Detect probes labelled with digoxigenin immediately as follows (do not allow the preparation to dry out): incubate the slides with SSCTM for 10 min at room temperature; incubate with SSCT for 3 min at room temperature; incubate the slides with anti-digoxigenin-AMCA at 37 °C for 30 min in a humid chamber

11 Wash the slides in SSCT (3 × 3 min) and PBS (2 × 5 min).

12 Air dry the slides and mount in AF1 antifade under a 24 × 50 mm coverslip.

[a] See *Protocol 7* for risk information.

[b] Caution: Triton X-100 is harmful if swallowed. It poses a risk of serious damage to the eyes.

[c] Caution: paraformaldehyde is very toxic by inhalation, in contact with the skin and if swallowed. It also causes burns, may cause sensitization by skin contact and poses a possible risk of irreversible effects.

[d] See *Table 1* for risk information.

[e] See *Protocol 1* for risk information.

[f] See *Protocol 4* for risk information.

[g] If immunocytochemistry is also required, this may be applied immediately after the ethanol washes, before probe hybridization.

4.5 Establishing cut-off levels

It is important to define 'in house' diagnostic cut-off levels for all interphase FISH analysis. This requires hybridization of the probes under test to a series of normal controls, to determine the mean. A useful cut-off level is the mean +3 standard deviations (33). Wherever possible, probes chosen for interphase analysis should have high hybridization efficiencies (> 90% of cells having signal on all four chromatids), particularly for assessing the presence of deletions. Incomplete hybridization or the overlap of two signals when viewing a three-dimensional nucleus in two dimensions will lead to the false assessment of monosomy. This type of false positive occurs more frequently than false trisomy (which is caused by counting artefactual fluorescent spots as true signals). Therefore, the cut-off levels for deletions are often higher. However, co-hybridization with a second control probe lowers the cut-off level considerably (34). The control probe should be of similar complexity to the target, and localized to a region not likely to be involved in a chromosome rearrangement in the particular malignancy under investigation.

4.6 Commercial probes for interphase fluorescence *in situ* hybridization

Commercial versions of virtually all probes diagnostic for recurrent transloca-tions and inversions in leukaemia are now available. The availability of a range of ready-labelled, quality controlled probes has been one of the main reasons for the widespread implementation of FISH. For the most part, these are of excellent quality, and save time and effort not only on labelling, but also on time-consuming detection protocols. However, it is important to be aware of the composition of commercial probes, particularly for interphase analysis. Commercial locus-specific probes are often a combination of cosmids or phage from the region of interest. These are not necessarily contiguous clones, and may give split signals in interphase nuclei. It is imperative that each probe is evaluated on a series of normal controls of the cell type under investigation. Below is a discussion of some of the commercial probes available for non-random rearrangements found in leukaemia. This is merely to illustrate the necessity for being informed and is not meant to be a criticism of the probes themselves.

4.6.1 *BCR–ABL* probes

There are a range of probes available for the detection of the *BCR–ABL* gene fusion (Vysis, Appligene-Oncor). These may be of the S-FISH or D-FISH type (see Plate 6). It is important to know whether the probe set will detect only the major breakpoint cluster region (M-BCR, the predominant type of rearrangement in CML), or the minor breakpoint cluster region (m-BCR, found in the majority of Ph positive ALLs) as well.

4.6.2 Breakpoint-spanning probes

Breakpoint-spanning probes give only limited information in interphase, and may be prone to misinterpretation owing to background signals. One such probe spans the 5.8 kb breakpoint cluster region of the *MLL* gene (Appligene-Oncor), resulting in three fluorescent signals in interphase cells if the *MLL* gene is rearranged. The advantage of this system is that it is independent of the translocation partner (at last count there were > 20 different partners for *MLL*). However, approximately 20% of cases with *MLL* rearrangements have a breakpoint 3′ of the breakpoint cluster region, which will not be detected by this probe. Furthermore, the finding of three signals in interphase does not always mean that *MLL* is rearranged. The other possible explanation is trisomy for chromosome 11. Since trisomy 11 is often associated with *MLL* self-fusion, molecular analysis by Southern blotting should be carried out (35) (see also Section 6.4). A newer dual colour FISH probe for *MLL* gene rearrangements which uses cosmids flanking the *MLL* gene (Vysis, UK) overcomes the above limitation.

4.6.3 *ETV6/AML1* probe

Vysis supply an *ETV6-AML1* probe set consisting of a probe for *AML1* that covers the *AML1* breakpoint, and 350 kb of *ETV6*, 5′ to the majority of breakpoints. This gives two red, one green and one fusion signal for *ETV6–AML1* positive cells, or 2 red, 1 fusion signal if the second *ETV6* allele is deleted. Deletion of the second *ETV6* allele is becoming recognized as an important factor in determining the outcome of t(12;21)-positive cases. In most cases, the whole of the *ETV6* gene is deleted. However, in a small proportion, the deletion is intragenic, involving one or two exons. In these cases, the commercial probe may not detect partial deletion, as only exons 1–4 are present.

5 Comparative genomic hybridization

5.1 Introduction

Comparative genomic hybridization is a novel approach to the global identification of chromosome copy number, which requires no previous knowledge of the tumour karyotype (36,37). The technique is carried out with DNA extracted from tumour cells and normal reference DNA. Tumour DNA is labelled by conventional nick translation (see below) with either biotin or a green fluorophore and normal DNA with either digoxigenin or a red fluorophore; after co-precipitation with unlabelled human *Cot-1* DNA, hybridization is carried out to normal human metaphase cells. Biotinylated probe is detected with avidin–FITC (green) and digoxigeninylated probe with anti-digoxigenin–rhodamine (red). Under normal circumstances, fragments from tumour and normal DNA have an equal chance of hybridizing to each appropriate locus on the target chromosomes. However, an increase in copy number in the tumour generates a relative increase in the green to red fluorescence ratio at the appropriate locus on the target metaphase, which will then appear green. Similarly, a deletion in the tumour will be indicated by an decrease in the green to red ratio, which will then appear red. Digital images of each target metaphase are captured and the red and green signals are quantified by a dedicated image analysis system, which generates a fluorescence ratio profile along the length of each target chromosome examined. Finally, data from several (5–10) metaphases are combined and a determination made as to which regions of the sample DNA contain amplifications or deletions.

The overwhelming advantage of CGH lies in its ability to give a picture of the genome with no prerequisite information. This is of course also true of conventional cytogenetics, but since only DNA is required for CGH, the number of situations in which it is applicable is considerably greater. However, balanced translocations are not detectable by this approach since they do not, in themselves, lead to a relative difference in DNA content between the tumour and the normal reference.

At present, the sensitivity of CGH is relatively low. The minimum amplification detectable, considered as amplicon size × copy number is about 2 Mb, which approaches the theoretical limit of the system (38,39). CGH is less sensitive when identifying deletions. The smallest region for which a reduction in copy number is detectable is approximately 10–12 Mb in length—about the size of a chromosome band (40,41).

Since CGH analysis averages the copy number changes in any particular DNA sample, contamination of the tumour by normal tissue is a potential problem. If this exceeds 50% of the test material, the results cannot be considered reliable (40). Another consequence of this effect is potential difficulties in detecting changes present only in minor clones. However, the technique may also be used in the analysis of archival material, since it has proved possible to use material from paraffin-embedded solid tumours for CGH experiments, in which DNA is extracted from tissue sections and amplified using DOP-PCR (20,42). Under these circumstances, microdissection may be used to secure a more homogenous population of cells (43,44).

Large numbers of both solid tumours and haematological malignancies have now been evaluated by CGH. For some recent reviews, see refs (45–47). In the overwhelming majority of cases, disease-associated changes have been identified and attempts are now being made to correlate these genotypic changes with phenotypic events such as disease progression (48).

Perhaps the aspect of CGH that would most benefit from improvement is resolution, as the current low level is determined by the reliance on metaphase chromosomes as targets. Efforts are currently being made to increase the sensitivity of the system by substituting microarrays for chromosomes, in which small spots of cloned DNA from specific regions of the genome are attached to a glass support. (2,49). These experiments have indicated a resolution of 40–130 kb and this is likely to improve in the future.

5.2 Preparation of targets

Good targets are critical for successful CGH but, unfortunately, it is difficult to predict the quality of any batch of slides in advance of the actual experiment. *Protocol 11* describes a screening procedure for potential CGH target slides. Phase-contrast microscopy enables chromosome morphology to be evaluated before hybridization. However, phase-contrast appearance does not predict how well chromosomes on a particular slide will hybridize. Karhu and colleagues (50) described a method of predicting the suitability of target metaphases by denaturing slides at a range of temperatures and then inspecting their morphology after DAPI staining. A modification of this approach is incorporated in *Protocol 11*, but does not provide sufficient information to replace a trial CGH experiment.

Protocol 11

Preparation and quality assessment of CGH target slides

Equipment and reagents

- Fume hood
- Phase-contrast microscope
- Denaturation solution 70% formamide,[a] 2× SSC, pH 7.0.
- Waterbath at 73 °C
- CGH capture and analysis system
- AF1 antifade (Citifluor, UK) containing 200 ng/ml DAPI
- Silica gel sachets

Method

1 Culture human lymphocytes from a range of male donors, harvesting and fixing metaphase cells by standard methods (see Chapter 1, *Protocol 7*).

Protocol 11 continued

2   Prepare one slide from each culture by dropping fixed cell suspension onto clean slides under humid conditions.

3   When the slides are dry inspect each slide carefully under phase-contrast microscopy. Reject any slides which demonstrate: cytoplasm surrounding the metaphases; many poorly spread, bent or overlapping chromosomes; a low mitotic index; chromosomes with a pale or glassy appearance; or a wide range of chromosome length between metaphases.

4   Use the whole of each acceptable culture to make slides and the following day, incubate one slide from each batch in denaturation solution at 73 °C for 3 min, air dry and then counterstain each slide with AF1 antifade containing DAPI. Capture an image of each slide and inspect the DAPI banding. Reject any slide at the extremes of chromosome quality, i.e. those that demonstrate either very good or very poor chromosome architecture and banding. Choose instead chromosomes with an 'average' morphology.

5   Subject a slide from each remaining batch of targets to CGH of normal male (labelled in green) versus normal female DNA (labelled in red) (Section 4.3), carrying out a full analysis and interpretation (Sections 4.4 and 4.5). A suitable CGH target slide should clearly demonstrate the sex difference ('amplification' of Y and 'deletion' of X), with no areas of false amplification or deletion.

6   Store the selected slide batches in an air tight container containing silica gel at −20 °C.

[a] See *Table 1* for risk information. Handle formamide in a fume hood.

CGH target slides are also available commercially and have the advantage of fulfilling most evaluation criteria. However, we have still found it necessary to test any new batch by CGH before committing valuable material.

5.3 Probe labelling

The importance of probe length was a key observation in the early development of CGH. Unlike most other FISH techniques which require labelled probe of 100–300 bp for effective hybridization, effective CGH requires longer probes (approximately 300–3000 bp). Most workers therefore label CGH probes by nick translation in order to control probe length: *Protocol 12* describes the method. Universal (DOP) PCR has also been used for labelling, particularly in cases with very small amounts of material (43) (see also *Protocol 5*).

Protocol 12

Nick translation of DNA for CGH

Equipment and reagents

- Water baths at 15 °C and 70 °C
- Microcentrifuge
- Vortex mixer
- Agarose gel electrophoresis equipment

Protocol 12 continued

- DNA polymerase I, 10 units/ml (Gibco-BRL, Cat. No. 18010–017)
- DNAse I (Gibco-BRL, Cat. No. 18162–016)
- Nick translation enzyme mix; 0.4 unit/ml DNA polymerase I, 40 pg/ml DNAse I
- Fluorescent labelled dUTP (Spectrum Red dUTP or Spectrum Green dUTP, Vysis)
- A4 mixture:[a] 0.2 mM dATP, 0.2 mM dCTP, 0.2 mM dGTP, 500 mM Tris-HCl (pH 7.8), 50 mM MgCl$_2$, 100 mM β-mercaptoethanol,[a] 100 mg/ml nuclease-free BSA
- Ultrapure water (18 Megaohm, Sigma)
- 1% Agarose gel
- dTTP 1 mM

Method

1 To an Eppendorf tube add 1 μl DNA, 5 μl A4 mixture, 1 μl 1 mM 1:1 mixture of dTTP fluorescent-labelled dUTP, 5 μl nick translation enzyme mix, 1 μl DNA polymerase I and sufficient ultrapure water to make the final volume up to 50 μl.

2 Vortex briefly, pulse in a microcentrifuge and then incubate at 15 °C for 45 min.

3 Incubate at 70 °C for 10 min.

4 Check the size of the DNA by running approximately 200 ng on an agarose gel.[b] The probe should be within the range 300–3000 bp. The amounts of enzymes used and time of reaction should be varied to give the required fragment range.

5 To decrease the fragment size increase the amount of enzyme mix; increase the reaction time or omit the DNA polymerase I. To increase the fragment size increase the amount of DNA polymerase I.

[a] See *Protocol 1* for risk information.

[b] For full details on preparing and running agarose gels, see ref. (51).

5.4 Hybridization

Hybridization for CGH is accomplished as in most other FISH techniques. Quite large amounts of probe are loaded by most workers, with an average of about 400 ng. *Protocol 13* is at the upper end of the range. Hybridization is carried out for several days; an overnight incubation will not give adequate results.

Protocol 13

Comparative genomic hybridization

Equipment and reagents

- Fume hood
- Water bath set at 73 °C (in a fume hood)
- Vacuum dessicator (e.g. Savant Speed Vac)
- Microcentrifuge
- Vortex mixer
- Humid chamber (see *Protocol 2*)
- Coverslips, 18 × 18 mm and 22 × 50 mm (No. 1 thickness)

Protocol 13 continued

- Diamond-tipped scribe
- CGH target slides (see *Protocol 11*)
- Spectrum Green-labelled test DNA (see *Protocol 12*)
- Spectrum Red-labelled test DNA
- *Cot-1* DNA (Gibco-BRL, Cat no. 15279–011)
- 3 M Sodium acetate
- Ethanol: 70%, 85% and 100%
- Hybridization buffer:[a] 50% formamide,[a] 10% dextran sulphate,[a] 2× SSC, pH 7.0
- Rubber solution

- Denaturation solution:[a] 70% formamide,[a] 2× SSC, pH 7.0. Prepare on day of use.
- Wash buffer 1: 0.4× SSC, 0.3% NP-40, pH 7.0. Filter through a 0.45 μm filter and store at room temperature. Discard after 6 months.
- Wash buffer 2: 2× SSC, 0.1% NP-40, pH 7.0. Filter through a 0.45 μm filter. Store at room temperature. Discard after 6 months.
- AF1 antifade (Citifluor, UK) with 200 ng/ml DAPI
- Clear nail varnish

Method

1   Combine 800 ng Spectrum Green-labelled test DNA with 800 ng Spectrum Red-labelled reference DNA and 60 μg Cot-1DNA.

2   Add 0.1 volumes of 3 M sodium acetate and 2.5 volumes of 100% ethanol, vortex briefly and then place at −80 °C for 30 min.

3   Centrifuge at 8000 **g** for 30 min at 4 °C to pellet the DNA.

4   Remove the supernatant, wash the pellet briefly with 70% ethanol and then dry in a vacuum dessicator.

5   Resuspend the pellet in 10 μl hybridization buffer. Store the tube on ice if any delay occurs but equilibrate it to room temperature prior to denaturing.

6   Remove a slide from the freezer and mark two hybridization areas with a diamond-tipped scribe. Immerse the slide in Coplin jar containing denaturation solution at 73 °C for 5 min.[b]

7   Just before the end of the denaturation period, denature the probe by incubating at 73 °C for 5 min.

8   Dehydrate the slide for 1 min in 70% ethanol, for 1 min in 85% ethanol and for 1 min in 100% ethanol.

9   Dry the slide by holding it upright and blotting the end on a paper towel. The probe denaturation will end while the slide is drying—allow the probe to self-anneal for up to 1 min before applying it to the target slide.

10   Apply the probe to the target area, apply an 18 × 18 mm coverslip, squeeze out any large bubbles and then seal with rubber cement.

11   Place in a sealed humid chamber and incubate at 37 °C for 4 days.

12   Remove the rubber solution and coverslip and place the slide in wash buffer 1 at 74 °C. Agitate the slide for 1–3 s and then leave for 2 min.

13 Transfer the slide(s) to wash buffer 2 at room temperature, agitate for 1–3 s and then leave for 1min.

14 Remove excess liquid from the slide by blotting the end on a paper towel and standing upright.

15 Add 25 μl AF1 antifade with DAPI in 2 drops (one over each hybridization area) and then cover with a 22 × 50 mm coverslip. Squeeze out any major bubbles, blot off any excess liquid around the coverslip with a tissue and then seal with clear nail varnish. Store the slides at 4 °C in the dark.

a See *Table 1* for risk information. Handle in a fume hood.

b The exact denaturation conditions depend on the batch and age of slides and can only be ascertained by trial and error. As slides age, the appropriate denaturation time will increase.

5.5 Analysis

5.5.1 System requirements

Unlike many FISH techniques, CGH requires a quantitative analysis of the fluorescence images obtained from each experiment. Thus, in addition to a capturing system, appropriate analysis software is essential. There are now a variety of systems available, and rather than attempt a full critique of each, only basic principles will be outlined here.

It was initially considered that a high-resolution camera was necessary for CGH. However, more recently it has become clear that even a video camera can capture images of sufficiently high quality and factors such as target slide characteristics play a more critical role (52). All adequate CGH software needs to carry out the functions of

- chromosome segmentation
- background removal
- normalization of fluorescence intensities
- chromosome axis location
- fluorescence ratio measurement
- summation of data within and between target metaphases.

Other preferable components are chromosome identification and statistical analysis of the combined data. (A fuller discussion of this topic may be found in refs. 39 and 53.)

5.5.2 Interpretation

When choosing which images to include in an analysis, preference should be given to metaphases demonstrating

- smooth hybridization
- high signal to background ratios
- a lack of extra-chromosomal signals.

However, high-quality hybridization does not necessarily predict a successful experiment. After analysing at least five metaphases, individual analysis files are combined into a single interpretation document. Prior analysis of the normal male versus female experiment that should be included in each run will enable cut-off values for amplification or deletion to be assigned. Good software will then enable the operator to assess the degree of deviation about the mean florescence ratios shown for each chromosome. If this is high, then any result should be treated with considerable caution. Heterochromatic and pericentric regions are generally excluded from analysis. Probe binding at these loci is low due to the hybridization of unlabelled *Cot-1* DNA and can result in spurious results. Care should also be taken when interpreting apparent amplifications or deletions in telomeric regions. A prudent approach should be taken to the interpretation of results on 1p34-pter, 16, 19 and 22, since artefactual CGH results have been reported at these GC-rich regions. (Extensive and helpful discussion of these topics may be found in refs. 40 and 50.) An example of CGH analysis of a leiomyosarcoma is given in Plate 7.

6 Guidelines for fluorescence *in situ* hybridization in diagnostic laboratories

The new molecular cytogenetic techniques, particularly CGH, M-FISH and SKY have created a lot of excitement among the cytogenetic and non-cytogenetic communities alike. However, in a diagnostic setting the desire to use FISH to identify all unknown chromosomes in a complex karyotype must be tempered by the lack of information on the diagnostic and prognostic significance of the findings. In addition, cost and time considerations are often paramount, limiting the number of special techniques which can be realistically applied. FISH is not a universal panacea, and it is important to use the technology to its best advantage. In some cases, conventional cytogenetics or molecular techniques may be more appropriate. The following is a discussion of the current thinking on the most appropriate use of available FISH technology in a diagnostic setting.

6.1 Chronic myeloid leukaemia

Conventional cytogenetics is still the method of choice for identifying the Philadelphia translocation (Ph) in CML at diagnosis. This applies not only to the standard Ph translocation, t(9;22), but also to the majority of simple variant and complex Ph translocations. However, in a small proportion ($\approx$ 5%) of definite CML cases, no Ph translocation is seen by G-banding, although the *BCR–ABL* fusion transcript can be detected by PCR. This may be due to submicroscopic rearrangements in a normal karyotype or to a masked translocation in a complex karyotype. In these cases, dual-colour metaphase FISH with differentially labelled probes for the *BCR* and *ABL* genes can be used to confirm the *BCR–ABL* fusion (see Plate 6). This has the added advantage of revealing the nature of the rearrangement. In the rare cases of failed cytogenetics on diagnostic CML cases, interphase FISH with *BCR* and *ABL* probes provides a rapid and accurate confirmation of the *BCR-ABL* fusion gene.

Cytogenetics also provides the best way to detect additional chromosome abnormalities in CML, which may provide the earliest indicator of the onset of blast crisis. It has also been suggested that interphase FISH may be suitable for monitoring regression of the Ph' chromosome in CML patients undergoing interferon treatment. However, because of the high incidence of false positives using the standard single fusion FISH probes, a number of alternative strategies have been employed (see Plate 6). These dual fusion and triple-colour, three-probe strategies all lower the false positive rate significantly (54,55). However, in the absence of reliable automated analysis techniques, they remain laborious and time consuming. The newer techniques of quantitative (56) and real-time PCR (57) are probably more suitable for the detection of small numbers of *BCR–ABL*-positive cells (i.e. for minimal residual disease detection) than either cytogenetics or interphase FISH, owing to their superior sensitivity and the speed with which they can be applied.

6.2 Acute myeloid leukaemia

The presence of certain specific chromosomal rearrangements in AML is associated with well defined risk categories. The t(15;17), t(8;21), and inv(16) are all identified as 'good risk' (58). Rapid identification of the t(15;17) is particularly important, as early treatment of t(15;17)-positive patients with retinoic acid is particularly beneficial. Conventional cytogenetic analysis of this translocation is not difficult, but does require 24 h cultures to enrich for t(15;17) positive metaphases. Interphase FISH with probes for *PML* and *RARα* provides the possibility of a rapid diagnosis. The t(8;21) is also readily identifiable by conventional banding. However, accurate identification of the inv(16) is difficult on poor cytogenetic preparations. Therefore, for cases of failed cytogenetics or poor chromosome morphology, FISH provides a valuable back-up. However, all of these rearrangements are readily detectable by RT-PCR. It has been recently shown that the presence of additional chromosome abnormalities have no detrimental effect on prognosis. Therefore, it may be more appropriate to carry out the initial screening by PCR for these good risk indicators, with cytogenetics and or FISH as a back-up procedure.

6.3 Myelodysplastic syndromes/myeloproliferative disease

Because of the diversity of possible abnormalities in MDS and MPD, FISH is not appropriate. Conventional cytogenetic analysis is the first line of investigation. Indeed, the identification of an abnormal karyotype is often required to confirm the diagnosis of leukaemia. Most FISH studies of MDS and AML fall into the category of research, e.g. defining the minimal region of deletion of 7q, 5q and 20q.

6.4 Childhood acute lymphoblastic leukaemia

Several specific rearrangements are associated with a well-defined prognosis in childhood ALL. The presence of the BCR–ABL fusion gene, rearrangements of the MLL gene, or near haploidy (≈ 23 chromosomes), are all associated with a poor outcome. In contrast, the presence of the ETV6–AML1 fusion, or the presence of a high hyperdiploid (50–65 chromosomes) karyotype are associated with a good prognosis. In ALL, cytogenetics often fails owing to poor-quality metaphases (which preclude the accurate identification of the Ph' translocation). The LRF and UKCCG ALL database at the Royal Free Hospital, London, reports approximately 18% of all childhood ALLs with a failed cytogenetic result, while a further 18% have a normal karyotype (Christine Harrison, personal communication). Interphase FISH may provide a valuable complementary technique for cases of failed cytogenetics.

Despite being present in up to 25% of childhood pre-B-cell ALL cases, the t(12;21) remained undetected until 1994, as it is cytogenetically invisible (16) (see also Chapter 3, Section 4.8). FISH with probes for ETV6 and AML1, or RT-PCR are the only reliable methods for detection. Deletions of the 'normal' ETV6 allele are often found and may be correlated with disease progression. Although generally considered to confer a good prognosis, this relationship has not been completely clarified. The presence of additional chromosome abnormalities, or of ETV6 deletions accompanying the translocation, have been reported to herald a poorer outcome. Cytogenetic analysis supplemented by metaphase FISH for the ETV6–AML1 fusion gene would seem to offer the method of choice to investigate the role of such additional changes.

High hyperdiploid karyotypes are found in approximately 30% of childhood ALLs. Interphase FISH with selected probes for the core additional chromosomes can provide a diagnosis in 'failed' ALL cases (see Chapter 3, Section 5.1). This is possible using the Multiprobe format. Indeed, one recent study has shown that 30% of failed or normal childhood ALL cases showed hyperdiploidy when screened using this method (35). The same approach can also be used to identify cases of near haploidy. All children entered into The MRC ALL'97 trial with a failed or normal karyotype are now routinely screened using this method (35).

Accurate identification of MLL rearrangements is crucial in infant leukaemias to ensure the correct treatment protocol, and to differentiate cases of transient abnormal myelopoiesis from true cases of infant leukaemias (see also Chapter 2, Section 6.1.8 and Chapter 3, Section 4.7). However, all of the available techniques for the detection of MLL rearrangements have their limitations. Some 11q23 translocations are subtle and may be missed by G-banding. The majority, but not all, MLL rearrangements can be detected by Southern blotting. Accurate detection of the fusion gene is possible by RT-PCR for those translocations in which the fusion partners have been cloned. However, multiplex PCR for all the known MLL translocations is laborious (59). Alternatively, interphase FISH with a commercially available breakpoint spanning probe (Appligene-Oncor) may give valuable information in cases of failed cytogenetics. However, it is necessary to be aware of the limitations of using this probe (see Section 4.2). Preliminary tests of a new dual colour probe set with cosmids from either side of the *MLL* breakpoint (Vysis) also show promising results (35). A sensible strategy is to apply all three techniques (Southern blotting, cytogenetics and FISH) in a complementary fashion for the accurate identification of these important translocations.

Acknowledgements

The authors wish to thank all of the members of their respective laboratories. In particular, Jill Brown, Sabrina Tosi and Rina Jaju (Institute of Molecular Medicine) for allowing us to use unpublished protocols and FISH pictures of their work, and to Helen Alcock, Jeannette Allen, Margaret Baird and Sarah Bottomley (Institute for Cancer Studies) for their contribution to protocol development. We also thank Roland Eils for the development of colour classification software for the M-FISH telomere assay (Plate 2), and Michael Speicher for expert advice on M-FISH techniques. We wish to acknowledge the Medical Research Council, UK, the Leukaemia Research Fund, UK and Yorkshire Cancer Research for financial support.

References

1. Forozan, F., Karhu, R., Kononen, J., Kallioniemi, A., and Kallioniemi, O.-P. (1997). *Trends Genet.* **13**, 405.
2. Solinas-Toldo, S., Lampel, S., Stilgenbauer, S., Nicolenko, J., Benner, A., Döhner, H., Cremer, T., and Lichter, P. (1997). *Genes, Chromosomes Cancer* **20**, 399.
3. Dauwerse, J. G., Wiegant, J., Raap, A. K., Breuning, M. H., and van Ommen, G. J. B. (1992). *Hum. Mol. Genet.* **1**, 593.
4. Nederlof, P. M., van, d. F. S., Wiegant, J., Raap, A. K., Tanke, H. J., and Ploem, J. S., van, d. P. M. (1990). *Cytometry* **11**, 126.
5. Ried, T., Landes, G., Dackowski, W., Klinger, K., and Ward, D. C. (1992b). *Hum. Mol. Genet.* **1**, 307.
6. Speicher, M. R., Ballard, S. G., and Ward, D. C. (1996). *Nature Genet.* **12**, 368.
7. Schröck, E., du Manoir, S., Veldman, T., Schoell, B., Wienberg, J., Ferguson-Smith, M. A. *et al.* (1996). *Science* **273**, 494.
8. Veldman, T., Vignon, C., Schröck, E., Rowley, J. D., and Ried, T. (1997). *Nature Genet.* **15**, 406.
9. Tosi, S., Giudici, G., Rambaldi, A., Scherer, S. W., Bray-Ward, P., Dirscherl, L. *et al.* (1999). *Genes Chromosomes Cancer* **24**, 213.
10. Guan, X.-Y., Zhang, H., Bittner, M., Jiang, Y., Meltzer, P., and Trent, J. (1996). *Nature Genet.* **12**, 10.
11. Lengauer, C., Green, E. D., and Cremer, T. (1992). *Genomics* **13**, 826.
12. Müller, S., Rocchi, M., Ferguson-Smith, M. A., and Wienberg, J. (1997). *Hum. Genet.* **100**, 271.
13. O'Brien, S. J., Wienberg, J., and Lyons, L. A. (1997). *Trends Genet.* **13**, 393.
14. Tanke, H. J., Wiegant, J., van Gijlswijk, R. P. M., Bezrookove, V., Pattenier, H., Heetebrij, R. J. *et al.* (1999). *Eur. J. Hum. Genet.* **7**, 2.

15. Uhrig, S., Schuffenhauer, S., Fauth, C., Wirtz, A., Daumer-Haas, C., Apacik, C. *et al.* (1999). *Am. J. Hum. Genet.* **65,** 442.

16. Romana, S. P., Le Coniat, M., and Berger, R. (1994). *Genes Chromosomes Cancer* **9**, 186.

17. National Institutes of Health and Institute of Molecule Medicine Collaboration (1996). *Nature Genet.* **13**, 86.

18. Knight, S. J. L., Regan, R., Horsley, S. W., Kearney, L., Homfray, T., Winter, R. M. *et al.* (1999). *Lancet*, **354**, 1676.

19. Eils, R., Uhrig, S., Saracoglu, K., Sätzler, K., Bolzer, A., Petersen, I. *et al.* (1998). *Cytogenet. Cell Genet.* **82**, 160.

20. Telenius, H., Pelmear, A. H., Tunnacliffe, A., Carter, N. P., Behmel, A., Ferguson-Smith, M. A. *et al.* (1992). *Genes Chromosomes Cancer* **4**, 257.

21. Cremer, T., Landegent, J., Bruckner, A., School, H. P., Schardin, M., Hager, H. D., and van der Ploeg, M. (1986). *Hum. Genet.* **74**, 346.

22. Lamond, A. I. and Earnshaw, W. C. (1998). *Science* **280**, 547.

23. Döhner, H., Pohl, S., Bulgay-Morschel, M., Stilgenbauer, S., Bentz, M., and Lichter, P. (1993). *Leukemia* **7**, 516.

24. Arnoldus, E. P., Peters, A. C., Bots, G. T., Raap, A. K., and van der Ploeg, M. (1989). *Hum. Genet.* **83**, 231.

25. Hopman, A. H. N., van Horren, E., van de Kaa, C. A., Vooijs, P. G. P., and Ramaekers, F. C. S. (1991). *Modern Pathol.* **4**, 503.

26. Hyytinen, E., Visakorpi, T., Kallioniemi, A., Kallioniemi, O. P., and Isola, J. J. (1994). *Cytometry* **16**, 93.

27. Knuutila, S. (1997). *Br. J. Haematol.* **96**, 2.

28. Price, C. M., Kanfer, E. J., Colman, S. M., Westwood, N., Barret, A. J., and Greaves, M. F. (1992). *Blood* **80**, 1033.

29. Lawrence, J. B., Singer, R. H., and Marselle, L. M. (1989). *Cell* **57**, 493.

30. Dirks, R. W., Vangijlswijk, R. P. M., Vooijs, M. A., Smit, A. B., Bogerd, J., van Minnen, J. *et al.* (1991). *Exp. Cell Res.* **194**, 310.

31. Raap, A. K., van Der Ijke, F. M., Dirks, R. W., Sol, C. J., Boom, R., and van der Ploeg, G. M. (1991). *Exp Cell Res*, **197**, 319.

32. Harper, S. J., Pringle, J. H., Gillies, A., Allen, A., Layward, L., Feehally, J., and Lauder, I. (1992). *J. Clin. Pathol.* **45**, 114.

33. Lichter, P., Bentz, M., and Joos, S. (1995). *Methods Enzymol.* **254**, 334.

34. Stilgenbauer, S., Dohner, H., Bulgay-Morschel, M., Weitz, S., Bentz, M., and Lichter, P. (1993). *Blood* **81**, 2118.

35. Harrison, C. J. (2000). *Br. J Haematol.* **108**, 19.

36. Kallioniemi, A., Kallioniemi, O. P., Sudar, D., Rutovitz, D., Gray, J. W., Waldman, F., and Pinkel, D. (1992). *Science* **258**, 818.

37. du Manoir, S., Speicher, M. R., Joos, S., Schrock, E., Popp, S., Dohner, H. *et al.* (1993). *Hum. Genet.* **90**, 590.

38. Joos, S., Scherthan, H., Speicher, M. R., Schelgel, J., Cremer, T., and Lichter, P. (1993). *Hum. Genet.* **90**, 584.

39. Piper, J., Rutovitz, D., Sudar, D., Kallioniemi, A., Kallioniemi, O.-P., Waldman, F. M. *et al.* (1995). *Cytometry* **19**, 10.

40. Kallioniemi, O.-P., Kallioniemi, A., Piper, J., Isola, J., Waldman, F. M., Gray, J. W., and Pinkel, D. (1994). *Genes, Chromosomes Cancer* **10**, 231.

41. Bentz, M., Plesch, A., Stilgenbauer, S., Döhner, H., and Lichter, P. (1998). *Genes Chromosomes Cancer* **21**, 172.

42. Speicher, M. R., du Manior, S., Schrock, E., Holtgreve-Grez, H., Schoell, B., Lengauer, C. *et al.* (1993). *Hum. Mol. Genet* **2**, 1907.

43. James, L. A., Mitchell, E. L. D., Menasce, L., and Varley, J. M. (1997). *Oncogene* **14**, 1059.

44. Alcock, H. E., Stephenson, T. J., Royds, J. A., and Hammond, D. W. (1999). *J. Clin. Pathol.* **52**, 160.

45. James, L. A. (1998). *J. Pathol.* **187**, 385.

46. Knuutila, S., Björkqvist, A.-M., Autio, K., Tarkkanen, M., Wolf, M., Monni, O. *et al.* (1998). *Am. J. Pathol.* **152**, 1107.

47. Rooney, P. H., Murray, G. I., Stevenson, D. A. J., Haites, N. E., Cassidy, J., and McLeod, H. L. (1999). *Br. J. Cancer* **80**, 862.

48. Ried, T., Heselmeyer-Haddad, K., Blegen, H., Schrock, E., and Auer, G. (1999). *Genes Chromosomes Cancer* **25**, 195.

49. Pinkel, D., Seagraves, R., Sudar, D., Clark, S., Poole, I., Kowbel, D. *et al.* (1998). *Nature Genet.* **20**, 207.

50. Karhu, R., Kahkonen, M., Kuukasjarvi, T., Pennanen, S., Tirkhonen, M., and Kallioniemi, O. (1997). *Cytometry* **28**, 198.

51 Ausubel F. M. (ed.) (1989). *Current protocols in molecular biology*. John Wiley and Sons, New York.

52. Tirkkonen, M., Karhu, R., Kallioniemi, O., and Isola, J. (1996). *Cytometry* **25**, 394.

53. du Manoir, S., Schrock, E., Bentz, M., Speicher, M. R., Joos, S., Ried, T. *et al.* (1995). *Cytometry*, **19**, 27.

54. Dewald, G. W., Wyatt, W. A., Juneau, A. L., Carlson, R. O., Zinsmeister, A. R., Jalal, S. M. *et al.* (1998). *Blood* **82,** 1929.

55. Sinclair, P. B., Green. A. R., Grace, C., and Nacheva, E. P. (1997). Blood **90**, 1395.

56. Cross, N. C. P., Feng, L., Chase, A., Bungey, J., Hughes, T. P., and Goldman, J. M. (1993). *Blood* **82**, 1929.

57. Heid, C. A., Stevens, J., Livak, K. J., and Williams, P. M. (1996). *Genome Res.* **6**, 986.

58. Grimwade, D., Walker, H., Oliver, F., Wheatley, K., Harrison, C. J., Harrison, G. *et al.*, and on behalf of the Medical Research Council Adult and Children's Leukaemia Working Parties. (1998). *Blood*, **92**, 2322.

59. Pallisgaard, N., Hokland, P., Riishoj, D. C., Pederson, B., and Jorgensen, B. (1998). *Blood* **92**, 574.

Chapter 7

Methods in solid tumour cytogenetics

N. Mandahl

Department of Clinical Genetics, University Hospital, S–22185 Lund, Sweden

1 Introduction

It has been demonstrated beyond doubt that the acquired chromosome abnormalities, which are a characteristic feature of human neoplastic cells, are non-randomly distributed throughout the genome and that certain aberrations are associated with specific histological tumour types (1,2). These chromosomal changes, including both structural and numerical aberrations, affect all chromosomes, autosomes as well as gonosomes, and may be found as sole changes, but, particularly in solid tumours, more often in a complex array of karyotypic changes. Some of the recurrent rearrangements are pathognomonic, whereas others are shared by a number of different tumour types. The number of neoplasms with cytogenetic aberrations investigated by chromosome banding techniques amounted, in December 2000, to almost 38 000 cases (3). Despite the fact that improved techniques for the cytogenetic study of solid tumours have been available since the mid-1980s, the solid tumours still represent only a minority (29%) of the data base, i.e., about 11 000 cases representing a large variety of subtypes. Thus, a lot of mapping work remains to be done on a research basis, and, at the same time, there are already sufficient data on some tumour types to make cytogenetic analysis an important tool to help improve the diagnostic work.

2 Logistics of tumour sampling

Cytogenetic analysis has been used for a long time to study genomic changes in neoplastic cells, but is, by no means, the only method that is available for such studies. Chromosome banding analysis has been challenged by a number of other methods, including a large variety of molecular genetic techniques and a number of FISH techniques (molecular cytogenetics). These methods may differ in resolution, precision, and sensitivity, they allow different questions to be asked and answers to be obtained, and the requirements on the handling of material differ. For example, molecular genetic analysis and CGH are not dependent on

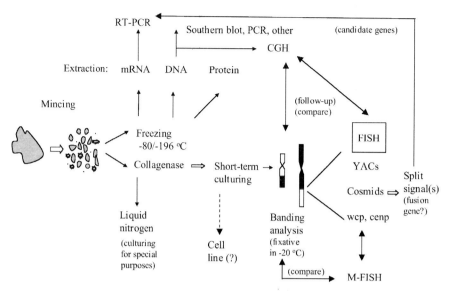

Figure 1 Tumour material should ideally be taken care of to allow multiple investigations (see Section 2). Embedding of tumour tissue for histopathological and related examinations and sampling for DNA flow cytometry are not included in the figure. Abbreviations: PCR, polymerase chain reaction; RT-PCR, reversed transcriptase PCR using cDNA obtained from mRNA; CGH, comparative genomic hybridization; FISH, fluorescence *in situ* hybridization; YAC, yeast artificial chromosome probes; M-FISH, multicolour FISH; wcp, whole-chromosome painting probes; cenp, centromere-specific probes.

the availability of viable tumour tissue and culturing procedures. In contrast, chromosome banding and most FISH analyses rely totally on the availability of dividing tumour cells. An exception to this is interphase FISH, which allows individual non-dividing tumour cells to be analysed. The prime screening procedures are chromosome banding, M-FISH, and CGH.

In the clinical setting, the choice of method(s) for analysis depends on factors such as the type of tumour to be analysed, necessity of rapid diagnosis, practical and economic aspects, and available expertise at the laboratory. For research purposes, however, it is obvious that multiple techniques need to be applied in a stepwise fashion; the results of one analysis enable educated questions to be asked for the next analysis. The cytogeneticist, surgeon, and/or pathologist should carefully consider the handling of tumour samples so as not to eliminate possibilities for further studies. Surplus tumour tissue should be stored in appropriate ways to enable a variety of additional studies to be carried out, taking advantage of the knowledge of chromosome aberrations and tumour heterogeneity as a starting point (*Figure 1*).

Although some genetic investigations can be made on paraffin embedded tissue, fresh frozen tissue is preferred and, in most cases, yields better results. DNA is fairly stable whereas mRNA usually is less so and sometimes quickly and easily degraded. To ensure that expression studies and RT-PCR analyses of chimeric mRNAs can be carried out, tumour tissue should be frozen as quickly as possible. Ideally, snap freezing in, for example, liquid nitrogen should be done in the operating theatre. Alternatively, the tissue could be placed in a $-20\,°C$ freezer or be kept on ice until transferred to low temperature storage. Freezing at later stages does not, however, exclude the possibilities of some RNA analyses. To allow repeated samplings from the frozen tissue, it is advantageous if the tissue is frozen in smaller pieces or in several tubes, so that aliquots can be withdrawn for analysis in an easy and safe way. Frozen tumour tissue should be stored in liquid nitrogen or in a deep-freezer at $-80\,°C$. Such material can be used for various DNA, RNA, and protein analyses as well as for CGH and DNA flow cytometric studies. The sample(s) to be frozen should preferably be adjacent to the sample(s) taken for cytogenetic and histopathological investigations. A sample of peripheral blood, or isolated lymphocytes, from the patient should also be frozen to allow for determination of the constitutional genotype and comparison with the tumour genotype.

After tissue disaggregation for tissue culturing (see Section 8.2), part of the rinsed cell suspension can be set aside and used for vital freezing in liquid nitrogen. This allows new cultures to be initiated in the future whenever new ideas, probes, techniques, larger series of a particular tumour type or several tumours with a specific aberration are available, or when there is a need to try to establish a cell line of a particular tumour. These cultures can be used for various molecular genetic studies and metaphase FISH analysis. Finally, every remaining suspension of abnormal cells in fixative and unstained slides should be kept frozen at $-20\,°C$ for future FISH analyses. Tubes for fixative suspensions should have especially tight caps to avoid, or at least minimize, evaporation of the fixative: dried out cell suspensions are useless for analysis and the evaporated fixative will destroy the interior of ordinary freezers. Any remaining unstained slides should be kept at $-20\,°C$ in closed boxes.

3 Application of cytogenetic analysis of human neoplasms

There are two major fields where the impact of cancer cytogenetics is highly significant. One is basic cancer research. The identification of chromosomal breakpoints involved in specific chromosome aberrations (primary as well as secondary changes) indicates the position of genes that through rearrangement, changed expression control, or inactivation are of importance in tumorigenesis. This is often the first step towards the identification of tumour-associated genes, and has to be followed by a search for split probe signals by FISH analysis, candidate gene approaches or positional cloning strategies.

The other major application is in clinical oncology. The type of aberrations found in individual cancer patients may be useful in reaching a diagnosis, in prognostication and in assessing the consequences of therapy (see Section 15). This is at present true primarily for the haematological disorders where abundant data are available and where the karyotypic changes are often simple. However, although solid tumours are frequently characterized by complex karyotypes, several consistent chromosome aberrations have been reported, some of which, particularly among the mesenchymal tumours, have diagnostic implications (1,2,4). In a few instances, differential diagnostic dilemmas may be resolved by cytogenetic analysis (5).

4 Techniques in solid tumour cytogenetics

Several different systems and techniques have been used to obtain chromosome preparations from solid tumours:

- xenografts of tumour cells to nude mice and rats
- long-term cultures and established cell lines
- direct preparations
- short-term cultures.

The descriptions that follow primarily deal with techniques for short-term culturing because it is the method of choice when the primary objective is to karyotype a tumour.

5 Xenografts

Subcutaneous injection of human malignant tumour cells into immuno-suppressed rodents gives rise to a proliferating solid tumour mass that may be propagated by serial transplantation to additional animals. Except for the advantage of getting rid of the human stromal cells, these tumours are no more suitable for cytogenetic analysis than the original tumour was. The major obstacle remains how to convert a solid tumour mass into a single-cell suspension, which is a prerequisite for making high-quality chromosome preparations. As with the primary tumour, tissue from the growing grafts can be used for direct preparations and short-term or long-term tissue cultures. However, a common problem is the contamination of rapidly proliferating host stromal cells that fairly soon may become the dominating population of cells. The system is laborious and expensive and is primarily suited to maintaining a tumour cell population *in vivo* for repeated sampling and experimentation.

6 Long-term cultures

When trying to establish cell lines from solid tumours, the stromal fibroblasts pose a major problem. Frequently, they outgrow the parenchyma cells in early *in vitro* passages. Some of the techniques for the development of cell lines take advantage of the fact that malignant tumour cells, but not fibroblasts, can grow in semisolid substrates. Given a suitable culture medium, tumour cells can proliferate in soft agar, soft agarose or methylcellulose and give rise to colonies that may be harvested or isolated under an inverted microscope and transferred to new culture flasks. Eventually, pure tumour cell cultures can be obtained, which may grow into established cell lines. Tumour cells may be transformed by trans-fection with plasmids including the early region of SV 40 (6). Frequently, at some stage the cultures end up in a period of crisis where there seems to be little hope for continued growth. These cultures should be given ample time as some recover and grow as permanent cell lines. Chromosome changes not seen in the primary tumour may be found in recovered cells, but most often specific aber-rations are retained. Cultures of permanent cell lines are most suitable for chromosome preparations, and stable cell lines are a practically unlimited source, in number and time, of identical or similar cells. A disadvantage is that it is not known which of the chromosome aberrations are acquired during the cells' *in vitro* life and which were present already *in vivo*, unless the primary tumour was cytogenetically characterized. Cell lines with known specific chromosome re-arrangements are quite useful as positive controls for molecular genetic investi-gations. Various tumour cell lines may be obtained from, for example, the American Type Culture Collection (http://www.atcc.org/atcc.html).

7 Direct chromosome preparations

Only tumours with a reasonably high spontaneous mitotic activity can be analysed in direct preparations, and for this reason most benign, slow-growing tumours are excluded. Most often, the mitotic index is lower and the chromo-some quality inferior to that which can be obtained from cultured cells. Direct preparations may be applied when quick cytogenetic diagnosis is required or when no successful short-term culture technique exists for that particular tumour type.

Protocol 1

Direct preparations, mechanical disaggregation

Equipment and reagents

- Class 2 microbiological safety cabinet
- Centrifuge with a swing-out rotor
- Incubator, 37 °C
- Centrifuge tube, conical-based
- Petri dish, plastic 35–60 mm
- Pasteur pipettes, plastic 3 ml
- Cleaned microscope slides[a]
- Disposable scalpels, steel blade shape 10 or 15, or a pair of curved scissors

- Complete culture medium: 100 ml standard culture medium (e.g. RPMI 1640), 15–20 ml FBS, 1 ml L-glutamine (200 mM) and 1 ml streptomycin/penicillin (10 000 µg/ml/10 000 U/ml)
- Colcemid[b] stock solution (10 µg/ml)
- Hypotonic solution: 0.075 M KCl
- Fixative: methanol[c]–glacial acetic acid[d] (Analar grade, BDH), 3:1

Method

1 Transport the tissue sample in isotonic saline or culture medium.

2 Place the tissue in a Petri dish containing 0.5–1 ml complete culture medium with 0.1 µg/ml colcemid, at room temperature.

3 Mince the tumour tissue as finely as possible with scalpels or scissors.

4 Add 2 ml of the same culture medium as above, but with only 0.01 μg/ml colcemid and transfer the suspension with a Pasteur pipette to a conical centrifuge tube. Add another 3 ml medium to the dish and transfer the remaining cells to the tube. Discard tissue fragments too large to pass into the pipette. Close the tube and incubate at 37 °C.

5 After 5 min, remove sedimented tissue fragments with a Pasteur pipette and discard. Continue the incubation for 2–4 h.

6 Centrifuge for 8–10 min at 200 **g**.

7 Discard all the medium and add 7–10 ml hypotonic solution. Resuspend the cells and let stand at room temperature for 10–15 min.

8 Centrifuge for 8–10 min at 200 **g**. Remove all but 0.5 ml of the hypotonic solution and resuspend the cells. Slowly add 2 ml fresh fixative.

9 Repeat centrifugation for 6–8 min at 200 **g** and fixation (freshly made fixative should be used every time) twice before the final cell suspension is prepared. The amount of fixative to be added depends on the number of cells.

10 Spread on to clean slides[a] and air-dry.

[a] Slides should not be used directly without any precleaning procedure, which can be cleaning in an ordinary dishwasher or treatment in 1 M HCl–absolute ethanol (1:1) followed by absolute ethanol.

[b] Caution: colcemid is toxic if swallowed and poses a possible risk of harm to the unborn child.

[c] Caution: methanol is highly flammable and toxic by inhalation.

[d] Caution: acetic acid causes severe burns and is harmful in contact with skin.

Protocol 2

Direct preparations, mechanical and enzymatic disaggregation

Equipment and reagents

As for *Protocol 1* and:

- Complete RPMI 1640 medium containing: 400 U/ml collagenase[a] (see Section 8.2.1), 0.5 μg/ml actinomycin D[b], 10 μg/ml ethidium bromide[c] and 0.05 μg/ml vinblastine[d]

Method

1 Mince the tissue as in *Protocol 1*, step 3 (but with a minimum of medium, just to prevent the tissue from drying out).

2 Cover the tissue fragments with complete RPMI 1640 medium.

Protocol 2 continued

3   Incubate at 37°C for 15–30 min.

4   Pipette vigorously to disperse cell clusters. Remove larger tissue fragments.

5   Proceed from step 6 of *Protocol 1*.

[a] Caution: collagenase may cause sensitization by inhalation and skin contact.

[b] Caution: actinomycin D may cause cancer, heritable genetic damage and harm to the unborn child and is very toxic by inhalation, in contact with skin and if swallowed.

[c] Caution: ethidium bromide may cause heritable genetic damage, is irritating to eyes, respiratory system and skin.

[d] Caution: vinblastine may cause harm to the unborn child, is harmful if swallowed, and irritating to the respiratory system and skin. There is a risk of serious damage to eyes.

An alternative protocol includes simultaneous enzymatic disaggregation (see Section 8.2.1), mitotic arrest, and condensation inhibition (see Section 9.1). This more complicated procedure may result in an inferior mitotic yield, but with less condensed chromosomes.

Disaggregated tumour cells may also be incubated in culture medium without colcemid overnight and then for 1–4 h with colcemid. Effusions and cells obtained by fine-needle aspiration from some tumour types are suitable for direct preparations or overnight culturing. To avoid cell aggregation, heparin (2 IU/ml) may be added. Effusions to be prepared directly are incubated for 1–2 h with 0.03–0.05 μg/ml colcemid in the fluid or in a 1:1 mixture of fluid and culture medium. After centrifugation, cells from effusions may be incubated overnight in supplemented medium. Suitable media for overnight effusion cultures and fine-needle aspirations are RPMI 1640, Ham's F12, and McCoy's 5A medium, supplemented as indicated in Section 8.3. Chromosome preparations are made according to *Protocol 1* from step 6.

8 Short-term cultures

Great efforts have been made to develop specialized tissue culture media in recent years. One trend has been to develop defined, serum-free media that may sustain the growth of particular types of normal, specialized cells. With such media, one gains control over different variables that influence cell proliferation and cellular metabolic activity. Attempts have also been made to develop defined media especially adapted for the growth of tumour cells. Sometimes these media have to be supplemented with a small amount (usually < 5%) of FBS. However, many tumour types do not need such complex media if the only aim is to keep the cells dividing for a short period of time, and some tumours can be grown in fairly simple media with few additives (see Section 8.3).

A problem common to the culturing of most tumour types is how to remove or reduce the number of stromal fibroblasts in the samples or how to counteract their growth in culture. If nothing is done, fibroblasts may, sometimes after a few days or a week, completely outgrow the tumour parenchyma cells.

A large variety of techniques applied in solid tumour cytogenetics have been reported. It is impossible to make a comprehensive summary here, and only a few references, adding to and completing the following presentation, are given (7–10). Anyone who is intending to work in this field has to try to develop routine procedures that balance a high success rate with simplicity. An experience shared by many is that success rate gradually improves with time, with seemingly negligible changes in the methods used, indicating the importance of systematic work, persistence, and experience.

8.1 Tissue samples

Saving of tumour material for future studies should be considered (see Section 2). For the purpose of cytogenetic analysis, large surgical specimens (several centimetres) may be kept dry in an operation cloth or a vial for up to 1 h. Smaller specimens should be immersed in culture medium or in sterile balanced salt solution; the most readily available is usually isotonic NaCl. Tissue can be transported in such solutions for 2–3 days and still retain good viability. After overnight transportation in liquid, the growth capacity of the tumour cells is not impaired compared with cells obtained from fresh specimens.

Tissue that is at risk of being contaminated with microorganisms (for example intestinal and head and neck tumours) should be exposed to antimicrobial agents, before and/or during disaggregation, to reduce the risk of infected cultures. The samples can be treated in a balanced salt solution containing benzylpenicillin and streptomycin (200 IU/ml and 400 μg/ml) or neomycin sulphate (50 μg/ml) against bacteria, and Amphotericin B (2.5 μg/ml) against yeasts and moulds for 30–60 min on a rotary shaker or a similar gentle agitation device. All antibiotic agents should be handled with caution (follow the instructions in the product information leaflets).

8.2 Preparing tumour samples for culturing

Before disaggregation of the biopsy, normal connective tissue, fat, clotted blood, and obvious necrotic tissue should be removed from the tumour tissue proper as carefully as possible. The quantity of material obtained may vary considerably, depending on the size of the tumour or on what could be spared by the pathologist. Almost no sample is so small that it is not worth a try. Many adipose tissue tumours contain fairly few cells per unit of volume, and therefore somewhat larger pieces of tissue should be used for culturing.

8.2.1 Tissue disaggregation

The tissue should always first be cut, in a Petri dish containing only the liquid that is already present on the sample, as finely as possible with scissors or scalpels. The minced tissue can then be treated in different ways.

- The tissue fragments may be used to initiate explant cultures. The pieces are distributed to culture flasks that are turned upside down after seeding and incubated with medium so as to obtain a humid atmosphere for 5-6 h or overnight. Thereafter, the flask is gently turned so that the tissue fragments are covered by medium (see *Protocol 12* in Chapter 3 of Human Cytogenetics: constitutional analysis for a detailed account of this technique). This method usually gives a slow outgrowth of cells and overgrowth of stromal fibroblasts may easily occur. The method is, therefore, not optimal for short-term culturing.

- In some tumours, a high proportion of the single cells released by mincing are tumour cells. These may be isolated by suspending the cut tissue in medium, after which the top fraction of the suspension, containing free cells, is transferred to a centrifuge tube, while the tissue fragments are left in the dish. After centrifugation and rinsing, cultures may be initiated. The fragments can be used for enzymatic disaggregation. The advantage is that few contaminating stromal cells are present in the first fraction of free cells but, unfortunately, the yield of viable tumour cells is usually fairly low.

- The tissue fragments obtained by cutting may be further dissociated by forcing them through a stainless steel sieve (1 mm^2) and then through a nylon screen (100 μm). The resulting suspension contains small cell aggregates and some free cells and can readily be plated.

- After cutting the tissue, a proteolytic enzyme may be added. The best results have been obtained with collagenase; trypsin frequently seems to cause more cell death. Collagenase II is commonly preferred, but other collagenases may be used in special cases. Crude collagenase attacks not only several types of collagen but also, owing to the presence of contaminating proteases, other intercellular substances. This may facilitate tissue disaggregation but may also cause cytotoxic effects. Pronase (0.05%) or hyaluronidase (100 U/ml) may be added to diluted (< 100 U/ml) collagenase solutions to enhance the breakdown of extracellular material.

Protocol 3

Preparation of standard collagenase II solution

Equipment and reagents

- Serum-free culture medium:[a] 100 ml standard culture medium (e.g. RPMI 1640), 1 ml L-glutamine (200 mM), 1 ml streptomycin/penicillin (10 000 μg/ml/10 000 U/ml) (add 2.5 μg/ml Amphotericin B if needed for samples at risk of being contaminated at source)[c]

- Membrane filter, 0.2 μm
- Syringes
- Collagenase II[b]

Method

1 Prepare a 1400 U/ml collagenase solution by dissolving the powder in medium.

2 Filter through one or more membrane filters.

3 Aliquot into required portion sizes, e.g. 1–4 ml.[d]

Protocol 4 continued

[a] Chelating agents should be avoided since collagenase activity depends on Ca^{2+} and Mg^{2+} ions.
[b] For risk information, see *Protocol 2*.
[c] e.g., intestinal, mouth, throat and lung tumours.
[d] Aliquots can be kept frozen at $-20\,^{\circ}C$ for several months.

The optimal concentration of collagenase, the time of treatment, and occasionally also the type of collagenase may vary among different tumour types. The activity of collagenase batches may differ by a factor of two or more and therefore concentrations should be given as U/ml. Two main protocols are applied: high concentration (1300–1500 U/ml) short-term (2–4 h) disaggregation or low concentration (200–400 U/ml) long-term (overnight or 15–24 h) disaggregation (see *Protocol 13* in Chapter 3 of Human Cytogenetics: constitutional analysis for a detailed account of a low concentration/long-term disaggregation method). To generalize, all tumour types may be subjected to the long-term treatment and most epithelial tumours should be treated this way, whereas most mesenchymal tumours are sufficiently well disaggregated by the short treatment. The tissue fragments should be covered by and dispersed in the collagenase solution in a Petri dish and then incubated at $37\,^{\circ}C$ in 5% CO_2 in humidified air. Although not necessary, a rotary shaker makes the digestion more efficient. Tiny biopsies, including core needle biopsies, usually need shorter treatment than pieces cut from larger specimens.

8.2.2 Sedimentation and rinsing

After the collagenase treatment, attempts may be made to fractionate fibroblasts from epithelial cells by sedimentation. Also, the cells need rinsing before they are plated.

Protocol 4

Rinsing of disaggregated tissue

Equipment and reagents

- Class 2 microbiological safety cabinet
- Centrifuge with a swing-out rotor
- Centrifuge tubes, sterile, plastic with a screw cap and conical-based
- Pipettes, sterile, plastic 5 or 10 ml
- Basic medium without supplements, or balanced salt solution

Method

1 Transfer the disaggregated tissue with a pipette to a centrifuge tube and add medium or balanced salt solution up to 10 ml.

2 Disperse by drawing the suspension up and down through the pipette several times.

3 Centrifuge for 10 min at 200–220 g.

4 Repeat the rinsing procedure once or twice.

Special problems may be experienced in sedimentation and rinsing:

(a) **Lipogenic tumours.** Large amounts of fat are released during the collagenase treatment and if not removed, this will interfere with the subsequent attachment of the cells in the flasks. The fat floats on top of the supernatant and should be removed carefully, which may be difficult if the rinsing is with cold solutions. The cells may be transferred to a clean tube after the second rinsing.

(b) **Bone tumours.** Fragments of bone or cartilage do not interfere with the culturing but may clog the pipette. Be careful not to draw these fragments into the pipette so as to avoid ending up with a completely clogged pipette containing part or all of the cell suspension.

(c) **Myxoid tumours.** In some cases it seems to be almost impossible to sediment the cells by centrifugation at **g** forces that are not harmful to the cells. It helps if the disaggregated cells are transferred to 50 ml centrifuge tubes filled with balanced salt solution. Be careful when removing the supernatant after the first centrifugation; there is often no distinct border between the pellet and the supernatant—all the material may suddenly get sucked into the pipette. Leave part of the solution, resuspend the cells, and add fresh solution. Gradually, after some changes of rinsing solution and centrifugation, the cells will sediment and can be resuspended for plating.

(d) **High viscosity.** When the viscosity of the suspension obtained after collagenase treatment is high, due to large quantities of released DNA, sedimentation of cells by centrifugation is difficult. This problem can be solved as indicated above in (c). When the tumour samples contain necrotic foci that cannot be removed by dissection, the problem can be circumvented by including DNase I, at concentrations of about 100 μg/ml, in the collagenase solution (this is done routinely by some researchers).

(e) **RBCs.** Large numbers of RBCs are sometimes present. Although they do not significantly impede either the attachment of tumour cells or their proliferation, they make it more difficult to determine an appropriate plating density and to monitor proliferation during the first days until they are lysed or washed off by medium changes. The RBCs may be lysed by buffer treatment before plating.

Protocol 5

Lysis of RBCs

Equipment and reagents

- Class 2 microbiological safety cabinet
- RBC lysing buffer: 8.29 g NH_4Cl, 1 g $KHCO_3$, 37.1 mg EDTA[a] and distilled water up to 1000 ml

- Centrifuge with swing-out rotor

Method

1   Resuspend the pelleted cells, rinsed according to *Protocol 4* in 3–5 ml RBC buffer.

Protocol 5 continued

  2   Let stand for 10 min at room temperature.

  3   Centrifuge for 10 min at 200 **g**.

  4   Rinse in medium or balanced salt solution.

  5   Centrifuge for 10 min at 200 **g**.

^{a} Caution: EDTA is irritating to eyes, respiratory system and skin.

Sedimentation by gravitation alone may be applied to reduce the fraction of fibroblasts in epithelial tumour samples (7). After mechanical and enzymatic disaggregation, clusters of epithelial cells may remain, whereas the connective tissue is more readily broken down to single cells. If left on the bench in a centrifuge tube for 5–15 minutes, the supernatant of the suspension becomes enriched in fibroblasts and the sediment in epithelial cells. The two fractions are rinsed and then cultured separately.

8.2.3 Choice and pretreatment of culture substrates

Different types of culture systems may be used, the most useful of which are:

- plastic flasks
- glass chamber slides
- plastic chamber slides.

Plastic flasks are convenient for the culture of a large number of cells. However, the cell density may be suboptimal when only small tumour samples are available. Another disadvantage is that during harvesting the cells have to be dislodged, which inevitably leads to loss of some cells. Chamber slides have a smaller surface and are suitable for *in situ* chromosome preparations with negligible loss of metaphase cells. Cells from epithelial tumours often grow in dense colonies. These cultures are not ideal for *in situ* preparations since only metaphase cells at the periphery of the colonies display well-spread chromosomes. Some cells, primarily from epithelial tumours, attach poorly to a glass surface. On the other hand, glass chamber slides are more resistant than plastic slides to treatments in the subsequent staining procedures and are also easier to mount.

Cell spreading and the ensuing proliferation require, in most cases, that cells adhere to a solid or semisolid substrate. Adhesion is dependent on the contact between the cells and attachment factors adsorbed to the growth surface. Since only some cells can synthesize the required factors, these must, in most cases, be supplied from an external source. One major attachment factor, fibronectin, is provided by the added serum. However, serum supplementation is not always sufficient for satisfactory cell attachment, in particular for epithelial cells, and additional factors may have to be added. This is even more important when serum-free or low-serum media are used. Fibronectin may be added to the culture medium at a concentration of 1–5 µg/cm^2. Culture flasks may also be pretreated by coating with collagen, fibronectin or Vitrogen 100 (Collagen Biomaterials) to improve cell attachment. A variety of flasks modified to sustain attachment and growth are commercially available such as flasks coated with extracellular matrix produced by cow endothelial cells, and Primaria flasks (Becton Dickinson). One advantage is that the surface in the Primaria flasks is more permanent and not degraded during cell growth as other coated surfaces may be.

Protocol 6

Collagen R coating

Equipment and reagents

- Incubator, 37 °C
- Tissue culture flasks, 25 cm^2
- Glass chamber slides, 10 cm^2
- Sterile rubber policeman or bent glass Pasteur pipette
- Distilled water, prewarmed (37 °C)
- Collagen R (2 mg/ml in 0.1% acetic acid)
- HBSS
- PBS

Method

1 Dilute one part of collagen R with three parts of HBSS.

2 Add 1 ml of the diluted collagen to flasks and 0.5 ml to chamber slides. Distribute evenly over the surface with a rubber policeman or a bent Pasteur pipette.

3 Incubate at 37 °C for 1 h.

4 Add 2 ml (flasks) or 1 ml (chamber slides) distilled water.

5 Incubate at 37 °C for 10 min.

6 Remove the water and add 4 ml and 2 ml, respectively, of PBS. Close the caps tightly.

7 Store in a refrigerator. The coated vessels may be kept for at least 1 month in this way. Remove the PBS before use.

Protocol 7

Collagen R and fibronectin coating

Equipment and reagents

Equipment as for *Protocol 6*

- Collagen R (2 mg/ml in 0.1% acetic acid)
- Fibronectin from bovine plasma (1 mg/ml in 0.5 M NaCl, 0.05 M Tris, pH 7.5)
- BSA, 10% w/v in PBS
- RPMI 1640 medium without additives
- Penicillin/streptomycin (10 000 U/ml/ 10 000 μg/ml)

Method

1 Mix the following: 200 μl fibronectin, 20 μl BSA, 300 μl collagen, 19 ml RPMI 1640, 400 μl penicillin/streptomycin.

Protocol 7 continued

2   Add 0.5–1 ml to flasks and 0.25–0.5 ml to chamber slides. Distribute evenly over the surface.

3   Incubate at 37°C for 30 min.

4. Remove carefully all remaining solution with a Pasteur pipette.

5. Put the culture vessels, with loosened caps, in an incubator at 37°C for at least 30 min.

6   Let the culture vessels stand at room temperature for 30 min.

7   Tighten the caps and store in a refrigerator. The coated vessels may be kept for 1 month. Inspect the flasks/chamber slides by the end of this period to avoid using those with crackled coating.

Protocol 8

Collagen I (Vitrogen) coating

Equipment and reagents

Equipment as for *Protocol 6*

- Vitrogen 100 (Collagen Biomaterials)
- PBS

Method

1   Dilute 1 ml Vitrogen in 44 ml PBS.

2   Add 3 ml of the Vitrogen solution to flasks and spread over the surface.

3   Keep the flasks in a refrigerator for 24 h.

4   Pour off the solution, add 3 ml PBS, and agitate gently.

5   Remove the salt solution and add another 3 ml PBS.

6   Store in a refrigerator. Remove the PBS before use.

8.2.4 Plating of cell suspensions

The balance between plating at too low and too high a cell density is difficult and can only be learned from experience. Low density may lead to slow growth accompanied, as a result of the prolonged culture time, by an increased risk of fibroblast overgrowth and the emergence of chromosome aberrations acquired *in vitro*. High cell density reduces the number of cultures that can be initiated and may make subcultivation necessary before chromosome preparations can be made, thereby again increasing the culture time. Five millilitres of culture medium are added to 25-cm^2 flasks and 3 ml to chamber slides. Cells from fine-needle aspirates, and in some cases even detached cells concentrated from transport medium, may be plated directly. Aspirates from some tumours, for example Ewing family tumours, may be grown in suspension in overnight cultures.

8.3 Culture media and additives

Culturing of cells from some tumour types can be made in simple standard media (e.g. RPMI 1640, Eagle's MEM, Ham's F12, TC 199, and McCoy's 5A medium) whereas others require complex media with multiple additives. Attempts are being made to develop defined media but most of those presently available have to be supplemented with serum, preferentially FBS, as an unspecific growth-promoting agent and as a source of adhesion factors and protease inhibitors. A variety of growth factors, hormones, vitamins, and detoxification reagents have been tested for substitution of the serum. One advantage with serum-free media is that growth of normal fibroblasts is counteracted. However, attachment of cells may be poor, proliferation of tumour cells may be slow and there is a risk that some normal differentiated cells are also stimulated. For these reasons small amounts of serum may be needed for the first day(s) after plating or throughout culturing. Some media intended to facilitate the growth of non-neoplastic, highly differentiated cells are not necessarily optimal for culturing the corresponding neoplastic cells.

A large variety of culture media and supplements used for short-term culturing of solid tumours have been reported. These include both simple and complex media, and it is impossible to list them all. A good rule, when starting to culture a new tumour type, is to confront the literature on that particular tumour type and try to make it as simple as possible while still obtaining good results. Some media with multiple additives are commercially available, for example the Pandis medium (Irvine Scientific), Keratinocyte-SFM (Gibco BRL), and Chang medium D (Irvine Scientific). Below are listed a few examples of media, simple as well as complex (*Table 1*), known to be suitable for cytogenetic studies of some types of solid tumours. All are supplemented with L-glutamine and penicillin/streptomycin as in *Protocol 3*; hence these constituents are not included in the lists.

(a) Benign and malignant soft tissue tumours, brain tumours:
  - RPMI 1640 medium with HEPES buffer
  - 17% FBS
  - Good results have also been obtained by adding 5 µl/ml Mito+ serum extender (Collaborative Biomedical Products).

(b) Chondrosarcoma, Ewing sarcoma, soft tissue sarcoma that do not grow well in (a):
  - Ham's F12 medium
  - 12% FBS
  - 10 µl/ml ITS (Collaborative Biomedical Products)
  - 1 µl/ml Mito+ serum extender.

(c) Simple medium for some epithelial tumours, for example renal tumours:
  - RPMI 1640 medium with HEPES buffer
  - 17% FBS
  - 5 µg/ml insulin
  - 1 ng/ml epidermal growth factor.

Table 1 Complex media used for various epithelial tumours

Component[a,b]	Brt	Pt	Lit	Blt	Ot	Lut	Git	Vt
Dulbecco MEM: Ham's F12, 1:1	X	X	X	X				X
RPMI 1640, HEPES					X	X	X	
FBS (%)	(20)	10	10	5	17	10	10	(10)
Ascorbic acid (μg/ml)	10	10		10				50
BSA (mg/ml)	0.1						1.25	
Catalase (U/ml)								50
Cholera toxin (μg/ml)	0.1–0.5	0.5		0.5	0.1			
Dibutyryl cAMP (nM)	10	10	10	10				
EGF (ng/ml)	20–100	20		100	1	1	10	4
Estradiol (nM)	0.1							
Fetuin (μg/ml)	20	20		20				
Fibronectin (ng/ml)	100	100		100				
Glucagon (μg/ml)								0.2
Hydrocortisone (μg/ml)	0.5	0.5	0.5	0.5		0.36		0.004
Insulin (μg/ml)	3	3		3	5	5	6.25	10
ITS (%)		1						
Linoleic acid (μg/ml)							5.35	
Non-essential amino acids (%)								1
Phosphoethanol amine (nM)	0.1	0.1		0.1				
Pituitary gland extract (μg/ml)				80				
Selenious acid (ng/ml)							6.25	
Sodium selenite (ng/ml)	2.6	2.6				4		
Trace element mix	1:100	1:100						
Transferrin (μg/ml)	25	25		25			0.006	
Triiodothyronine	10 nM	10 nM					0.6 ng/ml	

[a] Tumours of: Brt, breast, FBS may be present for the initial 1 or 2 days of culture; Pt, pancreas; Lit, liver; Blt, bladder; Ot, ovary; Lut, lung; Git, gastrointestinal tract; Vt, various benign and malignant tumours, FBS is added after about 5 days of culture.

[b] Several of the additives to culture media are bioactive agents and hazardous or potentially hazardous. See information leaflets or product catalogues for further details.

(d) Prostatic tumours:
- PFMR-4 medium (Peehl and Stamey (16))
- 15% FBS
- 10 ng/ml epidermal growth factor
- 0.36 μg/ml hydrocortisone
- 20 ng/ml dihydrotestosterone
- 1 μg/ml sodium selenite

(e) Head and neck tumours:
- Keratinocyte-SFM (Life Technologies)
- add accompanying solutions of pituitary extract and epidermal growth factor
- 3–5% FBS may improve attachment and growth

8.4 Maintenance of cultures

During culturing, glass chamber slides must be loosely capped or they may start to leak. They must also be incubated in a humidified atmosphere containing 5% CO_2. The cultures should be inspected regularly under the inverted microscope, preferably once every day. It is important to monitor the attachment, flattening, and proliferation of tumour cells. The appearance of mitotic activity may be seen as cells rounding up into spheres in some tumours or even by the identification of various mitotic stages at high magnification (*Figure 2*). The cultures should also be monitored for outgrowth of normal-looking fibroblasts (*Figure 3*) and should be harvested if these tend to take over completely. In some cases, in particular benign mesenchymal tumours, the tumour cells and stromal fibroblasts are morphologically indistinguishable and a variety of other cell types may also be present (*Figure 4*).

8.4.1 Feeding of cultures

The medium should be exchanged the day after or, if few cells have attached, 2 days after the plating. Sometimes, it may be difficult to see the attached cells because of the presence of large quantities of blood cells and cell debris. However, these are only loosely attached and may easily be suspended by gently tilting the cultures a few times. If viable tumour cells are suspected to remain floating in the medium, which is often the case, they can be transferred to additional flasks,

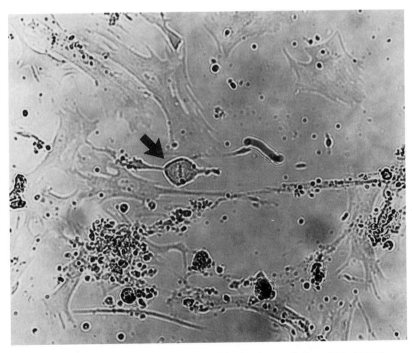

Figure 2 Haemangioma. A metaphase cell in side view is seen in the middle (arrow).

(a)

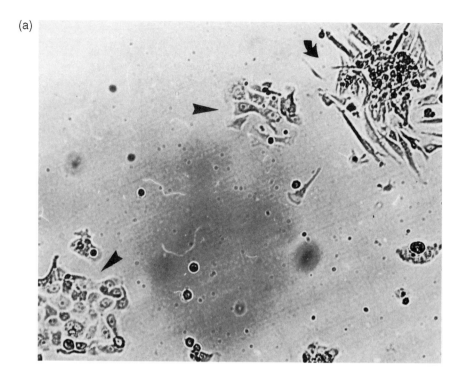

(b)

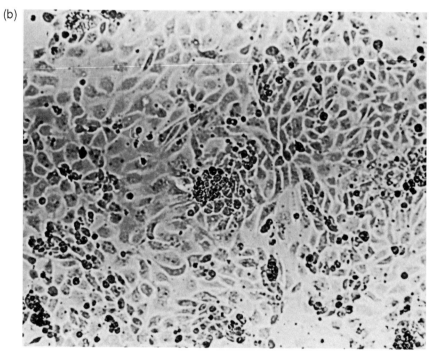

Figure 3 Colon adenocarcinoma. (a) Early culture (3 days) showing two colonies with epithelial cells (arrowheads) and one with fibroblasts (arrow). (b) Almost pure colony of epithelial cells.

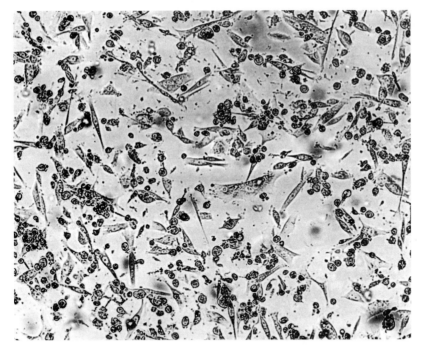

Figure 4 Leiomyosarcoma. Several morphologically different cell types are present.

either directly or after centrifugation and rinsing. Alternatively, unattached cells can be used for making chromosome preparations (see Section 9) after transfer to a centrifuge tube for colcemid treatment. If few cells have attached after 1 day of culturing in uncoated flasks, the cell suspension could be transferred to coated flasks. The cells are fed with fresh medium after another 2 or 3 days, or depending on their growth capacity, which may be estimated from the shift of colour of the pH indicator in the medium.

8.4.2 Subcultivation

Ideally, cells should be plated at a density that allows harvest of subconfluent primary cultures. It may happen, however, that the cultures are already confluent or even multilayered the day after plating. These cultures have to be subcultured, at least if *in situ* preparations are going to be made. This eliminates the possibility of making chromosome preparations from primary cultures and delays the time span before the first harvest can be made. Another reason why subculturing should be avoided is that some tumour cells have low plating efficiency. Trypsin, commonly used to detach cells, may cause unacceptable cell death of cells grown in serum-free media because of the lack of protease inhibitors. This adverse effect may be overcome by spinning down the cells and then rinsing them before replating or by adding soya bean trypsin inhibitor. Descriptions of the handling of cultures should follow accepted terminology (11).

Protocol 9

Subcultivation

Equipment and reagents

- Class 2 microbiological safety cabinet
- Tissue culture flasks, 25 cm²/glass chamber slides, 10 cm²
- Pasteur pipettes, sterile, glass or plastic, 1.5–3 ml
- Inverted microscope with ×2.5 and ×6.3 objectives and ×10 eyepieces

- Incubator, 37°C
- Trisodium citrate[a] solution (2.5% w/v)
- Complete culture medium (see Section 8.3)
- Trypsin[b] solution (0.25% w/v)

Method

1 Remove the medium.

2 Add 3 ml (flasks) or 2 ml (chamber slides) trisodium citrate solution.

3 After 2–3 min, remove all but 0.3–0.5 ml of the citrate solution.

4 Add 0.5–0.7 ml (flasks) or 0.3–0.5 ml (chamber slides) trypsin solution. Incubate at 37°C for 2–5 min and inspect under an inverted microscope. If cells have not detached, shake and incubate for another 2–5 min.

5 Add supplemented medium and disperse the cells carefully.

6 Distribute the cell suspension to two or more new flasks and incubate at 37°C.

[a] Commercially available trypsin-EDTA solution is as effective as citrate/trypsin.

[b] Caution: trypsin is irritating to eyes, respiratory system and skin and may cause sensitization by inhalation.

9 Harvest of cultures

The first harvest should be made as soon as possible after plating. If multiple cultures have been initiated, these can be harvested consecutively over several days, which is especially useful when the mitotic activity is difficult to estimate. In most cases, no mitoses are found until the second or third day. Most often, cells grown in serum-supplemented media can be harvested within 3–7 days, whereas cells in serum-free media often need 1–2 weeks. Exposure of cells to enzymes (including disaggregation and subcultivation procedures) cause a lag in cell proliferation. Cultures initiated from fine-needle aspirations and only mechanically disaggregated tissue may be harvested after 1 day. In these situations, cells that have not attached after overnight incubation can be harvested, whereas those that have attached can be used for continued culturing. Not all tumours can be analysed in this way and the mitotic yield is usually very low, but such a quick harvest may still be useful in diagnosis. Very dense cultures and cultures with scattered but dense colonies can be used for partial harvest. After colcemid treatment of the culture, metaphase cells can be shaken off or removed by a short (less than 1 min), mild trypsin treatment. The remaining attached cells are fed fresh medium and allowed to continue to grow. One advantage with the use of chamber slides is that they can be harvested at very low cell densities because practically no cells are lost during the preparation procedure. However, only one slide is obtained per culture, reducing the chances of applying both banding and FISH analyses.

9.1 Pretreatment of cultures for long chromosomes

Techniques for obtaining prometaphase chromosomes should be applied with moderation for short-term cultured tumours. Cultures with a low mitotic activity are not suitable because the procedures frequently reduce the mitotic index. Excessively long chromosomes often make it more difficult to interpret the rearrangements in karyotypes with very complex aberrations when G-band analysis is applied, but may be quite useful for addressing specific questions, such as breakpoint localization, using FISH analysis. Only two of many available techniques will be outlined here. In both, subconfluent, actively proliferating cultures should be used.

Protocol 10

Methotrexate synchronization

Equipment and reagents

- Class 2 microbiological safety cabinet
- Incubator, 37°C
- Micropipette, 10 or 20 μl, and sterile tips
- Methotrexate[a] stock solution, 5×10^{-5} M
- Thymidine stock solution, 5×10^{-3} M
- Colcemid[b] stock solution, 10 μg/ml
- Complete culture medium[c] (see Section 8.3)

Method

1 Add methotrexate (final concentration 10^{-7} M) to the cultures and incubate at 37°C.

2 Discard the medium after 16–17 h. Rinse with prewarmed medium and add fresh medium.

3 Add thymidine (final concentration 10^{-5} M) and incubate at 37°C for 6–7 h.

4 Add colcemid (final concentration 0.02 μg/ml) and incubate at 37°C for 2–3 h.

5 Harvest according to *Protocols 12* or *13*.

[a] Caution: methotrexate may cause harm to the unborn child, heritable genetic damage and may impair fertility. It is toxic if swallowed, irritating to eyes, respiratory system and skin.

[b] For risk information, see *Protocol 1*.

[c] Media containing thymidine should not be used.

Protocol 11

Condensation inhibition

Equipment and reagents

- Class 2 microbiological safety cabinet
- Incubator, 37°C
- Micropipettes, 10 and 100 µl, and sterile tips
- BrdU[a] stock solution:[b] 1.6 mg/ml, dissolved in complete culture medium and sterile filtered

- FdU[c] stock solution:[b] 3.76 µg/ml, dissolved in complete culture medium and sterile filtered)
- Ethidium bromide[d] stock solution:[b] 10 mg/ml, dissolved in sterile distilled water
- Colcemid[e] stock solution, 10 µg/ml

Method

1 Add BrdU (final concentration 40 µg/ml) and FdU (final concentration 9.4×10^{-2} µg/ml) to cultures and incubate at 37°C for 16–17 h.

2 Add ethidium bromide (final concentration 5 µg/ml) and incubate at 37°C for 1 h.

3 Add colcemid (final concentration 0.04 µg/ml) and incubate at 37°C for 30 min.

4 Harvest according to *Protocol 12* or *13*.

[a] Caution: BrdU may cause heritable genetic damage and harm to the unborn child. It is harmful by inhalation, in contact with skin and if swallowed.

[b] Can be kept frozen at −20°C in aliquots of 0.5–1 ml.

[c] Caution: FdU is harmful by inhalation, in contact with skin and if swallowed and poses possible risks of irreversible effects.

[d] For risk information, see *Protocol 2*.

[e] For risk information, see *Protocol 1*.

9.2 Mitotic arrest

Different mitotic arrest protocols can be chosen, e.g., those that give a reasonably large number of metaphase cells, some of which contain fairly condensed chromosomes, and those that yield chromosomes that are relatively long, but also fewer metaphase cells. The two important variables in the treatment with colcemid are time and concentration. Some short-term cultures of solid tumours have a fairly low mitotic activity and should be treated with low concentrations (0.01–0.02 µg/ml) overnight; too low concentrations may allow cells to escape mitotic arrest and re-enter cycling. The chromosomes in cells arrested in metaphase continue to condense until the cells are harvested. Low concentrations can also be used for 3–4 h treatment, but more often actively proliferating cultures are exposed to 0.03–0.1 µg/ml for 0.5–2 h.

9.3 Hypotonic treatment

A variety of hypotonic solutions have been used (*Table 2*). The most frequently used hypotonic solution for chromosome banding analysis is KCl, but different tumours may have different requirements to obtain good results. There is a

Table 2 Solutions used for hypotonic treatment of tumour cells

- Culture medium and distilled water, 1:4
- FBS and 0.052 M KCl, 1:4
- 0.060–0.075 M KCl
- 0.075 M KCl and 1% (w/v) trisodium citrate, 1:1
- 0.21–0.30% (w/v) NaCl
- 3 g/l KCl, 0.2 g/l EGTA and 4.8 g/l HEPES
- Equimolar solution of 0.055 M KCl, NaNO$_3$ and sodium acetate, 10:5:2

(a)

(b)

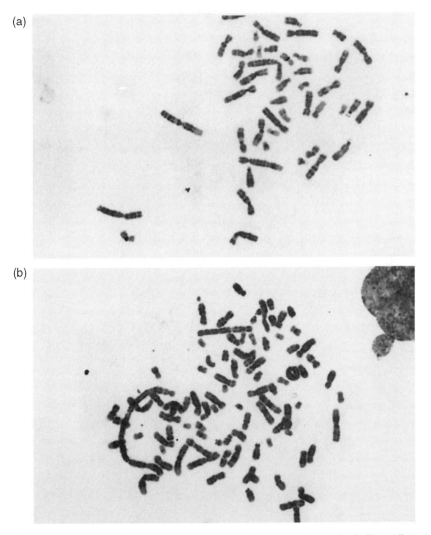

Figure 5 *In situ* preparations showing metaphase cells from benign and borderline malignant tumours. (a) Lipoma with loss of chromosome 1 and five structural aberrations. (b) Atypical lipomatous tumour; metaphase cell at the tetraploid level with a clonal, supernumerary ring chromosome, telomeric associations, and some non-clonal markers.

balance between obtaining an optimal swelling of the cells without losing cells that burst before they stick to the slide. When making *in situ* preparations from chamber slides, a short rinsing of the slides in a solution with a very low salt concentration, to remove remaining medium, gives good results (see *Protocol 13*).

9.4 Chromosome preparations

Chromosome preparations from cells grown in flasks are made by an air-drying procedure of detached, suspended cells. From cells grown on chamber slides *in situ* preparations are made (*Figures 5* and *6*). Essentially, both techniques are standard

(a)

(b)

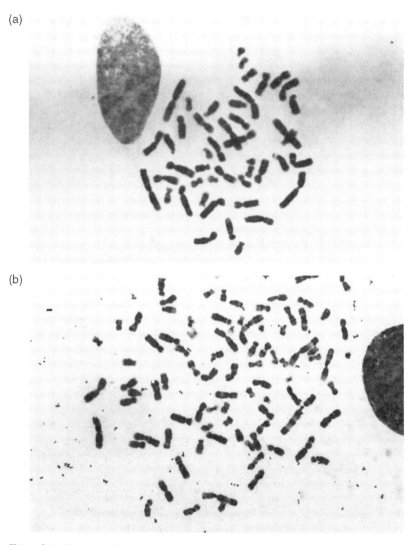

Figure 6 *In situ* preparations showing metaphase cells from highly malignant tumours. (a) Synovial sarcoma with a t(X;18) as the sole anomaly. (b) Part of metaphase cell from a malignant fibrous histiocytoma with multiple aberrations.

procedures that do not need to be modified depending on the type of tumour. The major variation experienced is the ease and the time it takes to detach the cells by enzymatic treatment (the solutions described in *Protocol 9* are usually quite effective). The final step of spreading may also be varied extensively, and depend partly on the relative humidity in the preparation room. For banding analysis, the cells are usually spread all over the slide, whereas the cells are often concentrated to one or two spots on the slide for FISH analysis, to reduce probe consumption.

9.4.1 Preparations from suspended cells

The advantage of this type of preparation is that multiple slides can be obtained from a single culture, and that cells can be concentrated to a small area for FISH analysis. It is less suitable for cultures with few cells and low mitotic activity.

Protocol 12

Chromosome preparations from flasks (25 cm^2)

Equipment and reagents

- Class 1 or 2 microbiological safety cabinet
- Centrifuge with a swing-out rotor
- Centrifuge tubes, conical-based, plastic 15 ml
- Pasteur pipettes, plastic 3 ml
- Pipettes, plastic 1 and 5 ml
- Incubator, 37°C
- Inverted microscope with ×2.5 objective and ×10 eyepieces
- Cleaned microscope slides (as in *Protocol 1*)
- Trisodium citrate solution (2.5% w/v)
- Trypsin[a] solution (0.25% w/v)
- Hypotonic solution: 0.06 M KCl
- Fixative I: methanol[b]–glacial acetic acid[b], 4:1, freshly prepared
- Fixative II: methanol–glacial acetic acid, 3:1, freshly prepared at each fixation

Method

1 Remove all medium from the flask and save in a centrifuge tube.

2 Add 3 ml trisodium citrate. Shake the flask gently and let stand for 2–4 min at room temperature.

3 Transfer the citrate solution to the tube and add 0.5–1 ml trypsin solution (or trypsin-EDTA if cells attach firmly) to the flask. Incubate at 37°C for 3–5 min. Check under an inverted microscope that all cells are detached. If needed, suspend cells detached in aggregates with a Pasteur pipette. Transfer to the centrifuge tube.

4 Centrifuge for 8–10 min at 200 **g**. Remove all medium, resuspend the cells in 7–10 ml KCl and stand for 10–15 min at room temperature.

5 Centrifuge for 8 min at 200 **g**. Remove all but 0.5 ml of the hypotonic solution, resuspend and slowly add 4–6 ml Fixative I.

6 Centrifuge for 6–8 min at 200 **g**. Exchange the fixative with 5–7 ml Fixative II. Repeat this procedure once or twice.

Protocol 12 continued

7 Add Fixative II after the last centrifugation. The volume depends on the number of cells; the resulting suspension should be slightly opalescent.

8 Spread on to clean slides and air-dry.

[a] For risk information, see *Protocol 9*.

[b] For risk information, see *Protocol 1*.

9.4.2 *In situ* preparations

In situ preparations are illustrated in *Figure 5*. The advantage of this type of preparation is that few metaphase cells are lost and that it can easily be automated by robotic harvest. It is not suitable for confluent cultures or cultures with dense colonies.

Protocol 13

Chromosome preparations from chamber slides

Equipment and reagents

- Class 1 or 2 microbiological safety cabinet
- Coplin jar
- Pipette, 50 ml
- NaCl solution (0.1% w/v)
- NaCl solution (0.21% w/v)
- Fixative: methanol[a]–glacial acetic acid[a], 3:1, freshly prepared before each fixation step

Method

1 Remove the chamber from the slide and discard the medium. Rinse briefly in 0.1% NaCl.

2 Submerge the slides into 100 ml 0.21% NaCl in a Coplin jar. Let them stand for 30 min at room temperature.

3 Add 20 ml fixative. Let stand for 5 min.

4 Remove 30 ml of the hypotonic/fixative mixture, add 30 ml fixative and let stand for 5 min.

5 Remove 50 ml of the mixture, add 50 ml fixative and let stand for 5 min.

6 Remove all of the mixture, add 100 ml fixative and let stand for 10 min.

7 Exchange the fixative and let stand for 30 min. Repeat once.

8 Withdraw the slides and let them air-dry.

[a] For risk information, see *Protocol 1*.

9.5 Treatment of slides prior to banding

Pretreatment of chromosome preparations prior to banding is done to 'age' the slides and/or to remove remaining cytoplasm covering the chromosomes. Without pretreatment, fresh chromosome preparations may easily result in poorly banded, fuzzy-looking chromosomes. Too much remaining cytoplasm interferes with the banding procedure and also takes up some stain, resulting in chromosomes with few bands and poor contrast between dark and light bands. 'Ageing' of chromosomes can be obtained by incubating the preparations dry in an oven at 60°C overnight or at 90°C for 30 min. Preparations, in particular *in situ* slides, may routinely be pretreated according to *Protocol 14*.

Protocol 14
Pretreatment of chromosome preparations

Equipment and reagents
- Oven, 60°C
- Distilled water
- 2× SSC (0.3 M NaCl and 0.03 M trisodium citrate)

Method
1   Incubate the slides dry in an oven at 60°C overnight.
2   Incubate the slides in 2 × SSC at 60°C for 2–3 h.
3   Rinse carefully in tap water and finally in distilled water.
4   Dry the slides and wait for 1–2 h before banding.

---

10 Chromosome staining

A variety of chromosome banding techniques may be used to characterize the chromosome aberrations. Most G-, Q-, or R-banding techniques will be suitable (see Human Cytogenetics: constitutional analysis, Chapter 4). Only one technique that has proven quite useful for solid tumours will be presented in detail.

Protocol 15
Preparation of Wright's stain solution

Equipment and reagents
- Fume hood
- Flask or beaker, glass 250–400 ml
- Aluminium foil
- Magnetic stirrer
- Flasks, glass with screw cap, 25 ml
- Filter paper (filter speed, medium fast; retention, medium crystalline)
- Incubator, 37°C
- Wright's stain[a]
- Methanol[b]

Method
1   Dissolve 0.5 g Wright's stain in 200 ml methanol in a flask covered with aluminium foil on a magnetic stirrer for 30 min.
2   Let the solution drain through a filter paper into 25 ml foil covered flasks.
3   Incubate the tightly capped flasks at 37°C for 3–4 days.
4   The stain solution can be kept at room temperature for 1–2 months.

[a] Caution: Wright's stain is harmful if swallowed. It poses a risk of serious damage to eyes.
[b] For risk information, see *Protocol 1*.

Protocol 16

G-banding with Wright's stain

Equipment and reagents

- Test tubes, plastic
- Pasteur pipettes, plastic 3 ml
- Light microscope with ×10, ×25 or ×40, and ×100 objectives
- Coverslips, 24 × 60 mm
- Stock A solution: 0.06 M Na_2HPO_4
- Stock B solution: 0.06 M KH_2PO_4
- Wright's stain solution (see *Protocol 15*)
- Distilled water
- Standard mounting medium[a] for microscope slides, e.g. Eukitt, Euparal, or Pertex (Histolab Products)

Method

1. Prepare a buffer by mixing 49 ml of stock A with 51 ml of stock B.
2. Cover the slide with buffer for 10 s to 3 min.
3. Pour off the buffer and cover the slide with a mixture of 1.5 ml buffer and 0.5 ml Wright's stain solution, prepared immediately before use. Stain for 2–4 min.
4. Discard the staining solution and rinse in tap water and then briefly in distilled water.
5. Inspect the stained slide with the microscope.
6. Dry the slide, add mounting medium and put on a coverslip. Keep the slide horizontal until the mounting medium has polymerized.

[a] Caution: mounting medium is flammable and harmful by inhalation; see product information.

If, at inspection with the microscope (preferably with a ×40 objective), the chromosomes are overstained, the slide may be rinsed in tap water until the differentiation is optimal. For older slides, G-banding with Wright's stain may be superior to trypsin-Giemsa banding. If it is known that the slides are subsequently going to be used for FISH analysis, mounting in permanent mounting media should be avoided. However, it should be noted that slides that are not mounted are vulnerable to mechanical damage and dust, and one should be aware that some immersion oils destain Wright- and Giemsa-stained chromosomes. G-banding can be followed by C-banding or FISH analysis of the same metaphase cells. Slides that have been mounted for some days to some weeks can usually be demounted and reused.

Protocol 17

Demounting and destaining of chromosome slides

Equipment and reagents

- Fume hood
- Coplin jars
- Xylene[a]
- Absolute ethanol
- Methanol[b]
- Glacial acetic acid[b]

Method

1 Remove the immersion oil from the slide and immerse in xylene.

2 Leave the slide until the coverslip falls off or can be removed easily with a scalpel or razor blade. If the slide has been mounted for a long time, this may take 1–3 days.

3 Take the slide through a series of Coplin jars (5 min in each) containing: (i) xylene, (ii) xylene–absolute ethanol, 1:1; (iii) absolute ethanol; (iv) methanol–acetic acid, 3:1.

4 Air-dry and wait for at least 1 h before starting the next staining procedure.

[a] Caution: xylene is highly flammable, toxic by inhalation and if swallowed. Keep the Coplin jars in a fume hood.

[b] For risk information, see *Protocol 1*.

11 Analysis of chromosome preparations

Frequently, multiple cultures are harvested at different intervals from plating, and the slides may show very different mitotic indexes and fractions of metaphase cells with chromosome abnormalities. The slides have to be analysed carefully; only in exceptional cases do all metaphase cells originate from the tumour parenchyma. Mostly, there is a mixture of dividing cells displaying normal and abnormal chromosome complements, and the latter, which are sometimes in the minority, may have clonal or non-clonal chromosome aberrations. Benign tumours in particular, but also some malignant tumours (*Figure 6*), may have pseudodiploid karyotypes with subtle aberrations. If metaphase cells from the tumour parenchyma constitute a small proportion of all dividing cells, these may escape detection unless many cells are karyotyped under the microscope. Tumour cells with more extensive aberrations, structural and especially numerical changes, are more easily detected (*figures 5b* and *6b*). There may be a distinct difference between chromosomes from stromal cells and tumour cells in banding quality, condensation, and/or spreading. Hence, poor-looking metaphase cells should not be disregarded when screening at low magnification, since a large fraction of these may represent tumour cells.

The number of abnormal metaphase cells that should be analysed depends on the type of aberrations found and on the purpose of the analysis, whether clinical-diagnostic or research, but is sometimes self-limiting. If, in tumours with simple karyotypic changes and little heterogeneity, a total of 20–25 metaphase cells are routinely analysed, the risk of missing a subclone is negligible. A few cells with a specific translocation may be sufficient for diagnosis. In tumours with complex aberrations the heterogeneity is frequently extensive and, in some cases with a basic set of clonal aberrations, no two cells have identical chromosome complements. In epithelial tumours in particular, cytogenetically unrelated clones may be found (12). Although important, the task of identifying subclones and the events of clonal evolution may become overwhelming. Hence, the number of analysed metaphase cells becomes a cost-benefit consideration.

12 Karyotyping, interpretation and description

It may be useful not only to make chromosome images (whether photographic or digitized on an image analysis system) from abnormal metaphase cells but also to include a few with a normal chromosome complement. This will help to determine whether certain abnormal-looking chromosome segments, especially the short arms of acrocentric chromosomes and the centromeric regions, represent acquired aberrations or constitutional extreme variants of polymorphisms. Moreover, for FISH analysis, normal cells may be quite useful as a control of hybridization efficiency.

Occasionally, only metaphase cells with chromosome abnormalities are found. Simple aberrations such as balanced reciprocal and Robertsonian translocations, small deletions, numerical and structural sex chromosome aberrations, trisomy 21, and small supernumerary markers, may represent either constitutional or acquired aberrations. In these situations a cytogenetic analysis of lymphocytes from the patient is required to establish the constitutional karyotype.

Large-scale gene amplification manifests cytogenetically as double minutes (dmin, *Figure 7a*), homogeneously staining regions (hsr, *Figure 7b*), or sometimes as ring chromosomes or other chromosomal structures with an abnormal repetitious or diffuse banding pattern (*Figure 5b*). Although more common in established cell lines, these structures may also be found in primary untreated tumours.

The number of dmin may vary between tumours from a few to more than 100. Although less extensive, there is also a variation in number between metaphase cells from the same tumour, because at mitosis these acentric chromatin bodies are unequally distributed to the daughter cells. The size of dmin may vary from about the width of a chromatid to barely detectable. Small, acentric sister chromatid fragments should be distinguished from true dmin by virtue of their sporadic occurrence. Occasionally, dmin may appear as single bodies because of the spreading forces at preparation. Since dmin are usually G-band negative the presence of few and small dmin may escape detection, in particular in 'overbanded' metaphase cells with very light stained negative G-bands. Suspected presence of dmin in banded preparations can be verified or rejected by staining a slide without banding pretreatment (7–8 min in 2–3% Giemsa in phosphate buffer). The same slide can then be destained and used for banding or FISH.

The majority of hsr appear as G-band and C-band negative, fairly uniformly stained chromosome segments, although a weak, diffuse banding may occur; it is usually only seen in one or a few chromosomes. Because of the similarity between hsr and distal 1p and 12q the involvement of these segments in rearrangements have to be considered. Simultaneous presence of hsr and dmin is seldom found in the same tumour.

Ring chromosomes frequently vary in number and size because they are more prone than rod-shaped monocentric chromosomes to anaphase malsegregation. Size variation seems to be particularly common when the essential outcome of ring formation is gene amplification. Thus, uniform size, or for that matter an

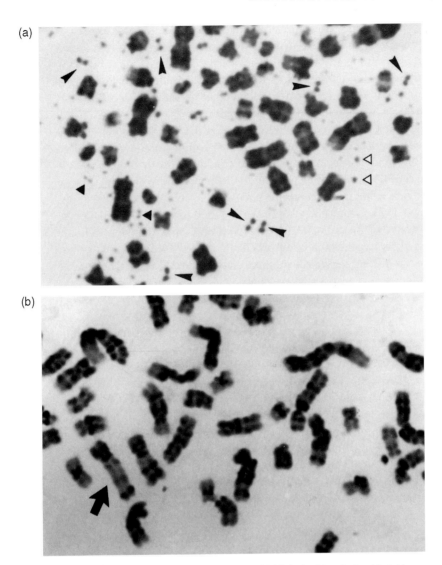

Figure 7 Cytogenetic signs of gene amplification. (a) Multiple double minutes (dmin) in a malignant fibrous histiocytoma. Note the size variation (large indicated by arrowheads and intermediate by solid triangles) and the occasional separation of chromatids (open triangles). Several dmin are not indicated. (b) Squamous cell carcinoma with a large homogeneously staining region (hsr) in a derivative chromosome 11.

identical banding pattern, is not a requirement to describe the presence of a ring as a clonal aberration.

The amplicon, i.e., the amplified chromosome segment, typically comprises a number of genes and the identification of the essential target gene in the amplicon may be difficult. The amplicon may even be discontinuous, with some linked genes being amplified and intervening genes lacking, and amplified genes may be present in different copy numbers. The position of hsr does not necessarily disclose the chromosomal origin of amplified genes and in some cases the amplified sequences may originate from two or more chromosomes. Amplified chimeric genes resulting from translocations have also been identified (13). Banding analysis can only demonstrate the presence of amplification but further characterization has to be performed using other techniques such as FISH (including M-FISH), CGH, or Southern blot analysis.

The finding of a normal karyotype is inconclusive. The result may represent a false negative (an effect of technical failure) so that only stromal cells entered mitosis, or the tumour specimen may have contained no or too few viable parenchyma cells. This will not be possible to distinguish from dividing tumour parenchyma cells with microscopically undetectable mutations. Preparations containing non-dividing tumour cells can be used for interphase FISH analysis to detect particular fusion genes and numerical chromosome changes. Tumours with a normal karyotype should be recorded and reported since it may be that they represent a distinct biological subgroup, possibly with a more favourable prognosis than tumours with rearrangements.

Small clones of two or three metaphase cells could represent *in vivo* clones but the fear is that they may sometimes be *in vitro* artefacts. If the same aberration, at least the same structural aberration, is found in different preparations from primary cultures, it is highly probable that the abnormality was present *in vivo*. It may also be reasonable to accept a structural aberration as clonal when it is found in metaphase cells at a large distance from each other on the same *in situ* preparation. Chamber slides also offer another advantage. Colonies of cells displaying different morphology are found frequently in different areas of the slides. This can be documented by photography and if the stage of the inverted microscope is equipped with a fixed position holder allowing a particular colony to be localized using an England finder, the same colony can be found again after the chromosome preparations have been made. Thus, the cytogenetic findings can be correlated with cell and colony morphology.

13 Nomenclature

It is essential for communication without misunderstanding that the cytogenetic findings are described in accordance with the international standard, ISCN (1995) (14). In most cases, even for complex chromosome aberrations, the short system is adequate and to be preferred. Detailed descriptions, explanations and multiple examples make the ISCN recommendations self-explanatory. The banding nomenclature is well established, whereas the first attempts of a FISH nomenclature may be seen as provisional. There is also an accepted terminology that should be used when describing the handling and status of cultures (11). The cytogeneticist is often referring to genes when discussing the molecular genetic consequences of chromosome aberrations and should be aware of the existing recommendations of the Human Gene Nomenclature Committee (http://www.gene.ucl.ac.uk/nomenclature).

14 Chromosome aberrations in solid tumours

In general, simple karyotypic changes characterize benign and low-malignant solid tumours while complex changes are found in most highly malignant tumours. However, several exceptions are known (*Figures 5* and *6*). For example, multiple aberrations are occasionally found in lipoma, uterine leiomyoma, and pleomorphic adenoma of the salivary gland, whereas the highly malignant Ewing sarcoma and synovial sarcoma may have reciprocal, balanced translocations as the sole aberrations. No comprehensive overview of chromosome rearrangements in solid tumours will be presented here; such data can be found in (1–4,15). A quite useful internet address to obtain up-dated information on recurrent chromosome and gene aberrations is: http://www.ncbi.nlm.nih.gov/CCAP/mitelsum.cgi. A short list of some recurrent chromosome changes and their molecular genetic consequences is provided in *Table 3*, and some of these aberrations are shown in *Figure 8*. The frequent involvement of the two related genes, *EWS* and *FUS*, in human neoplasms is illustrated in *Figure 9*.

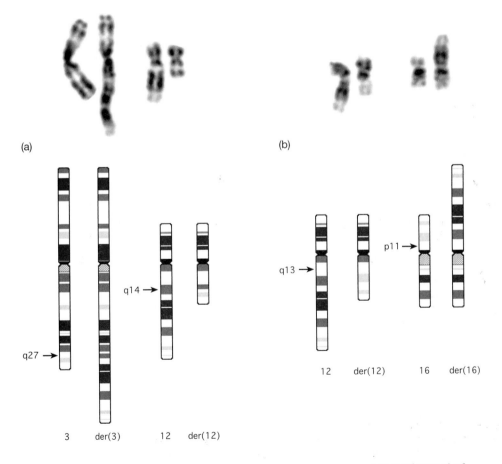

(a)

(b)

See caption overleaf.

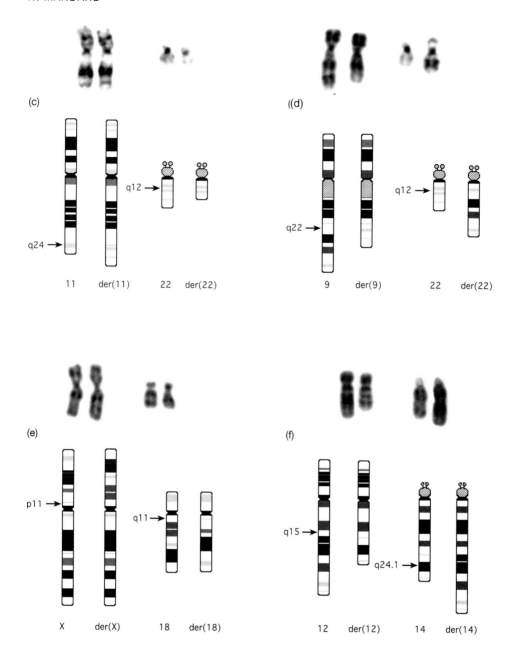

Figure 8 Some characteristic structural chromosome aberrations (arrows indicate breakpoints). (a) Lipoma: t(3;12)(q27–28;q14–15). (b) Myxoid liposarcoma: t(12;16) (q13;p11). (c) Ewing sarcoma: t(11;22)(q24;q12). (d) Extraskeletal myxoid chondrosarcoma: t(9;22)(q22;q12). (e) Synovial sarcoma: t(X;18)(p11;q11). (f) and (g) Uterine leiomyoma:

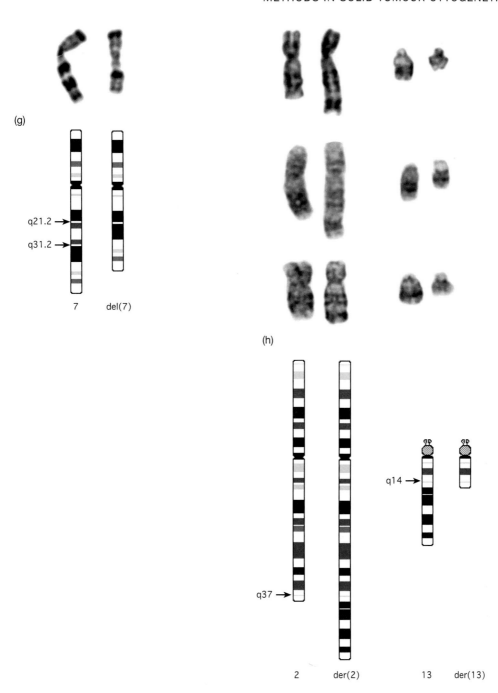

(g)

q21.2 →
q31.2 →

7   del(7)

(h)

q14 →

q37 →

2   der(2)   13   der(13)

t(12;14)(q15;q24) and del(7)(q2lq31). (h) Alveolar rhabdomyosarcoma: t(2;13)(q35;q14). The t(2;13) photographs were kindly supplied by B. Gibbons, ICRF, Department of Medical Oncology, St Bartholomew's Hospital, London, UK.

Table 3 Short list of some characteristic chromosome and gene aberrations in solid tumours[a]

Tumour	Cytogenetic aberration	Molecular genetic aberration
Lipoma	Various changes of 12q13–15 common: t(3;12)(q27–28;q14–15)	*HMGIC* rearrangements *LPP/HMGIC* fusion
Hibernoma	Various changes of 11q13	Gene losses (e.g. *MEN1*)
Lipoblastoma	Various changes of 8q11–13	*PLAG1* activation
Atypical lipomatous tumour	Ring or giant marker chromosomes	12q amplification (e.g. *MDM2*)
Myxoid liposarcoma	t(12;16)(q13;p11) t(12;22)(q13;q12)	*FUS/CHOP* fusion *EWS/CHOP* fusion
Uterine leiomyoma	Various changes of 12q14–15 common: t(12;14)(q14–15; q23–24)	*HMGIC* and *RAD51B* changes
Fibromatosis/desmoid	+8,+20 or changes of 5q	
Neurilemoma	−22 or del(22q)	Loss of *SCH*
Dermatofibrosarcoma protuberans	r(17;22) or t(17;22)(q22;q13)	*COL1A1/PDGFB* fusion
Clear cell sarcoma	t(12;22)(q13;q12)	*EWS/ATF1* fusion
Desmoplastic small cell, round cell tumour	t(11;22)(p13;q12)	*EWS/WT1* fusion
Fibrosarcoma, juvenile	+8,+11,+17,+20,t(12;15) (p13;q25-26)	*ETV6/NTRK3* fusion
Synovial sarcoma	t(X;18)(p11;q11)	*SYT/SSX1* fusion *SYT/SSX2* fusion *SYT/SSXY* fusion
Rhabdomyosarcoma, alveolar	t(2;13)(q35;q14) t(1;13)(p36;q14)	*FKHR/PAX3* fusion *FKHR/PAX7* fusion
Alveolar soft part sarcoma	Changes of 17q25	
Osteocartilaginous exostosis	del(8)(q24)	Loss of *EXT1*
Giant cell tumour of bone	Telomeric associations	
Parosteal osteosarcoma	Ring chromosomes	12q amplification
Myxoid chondrosarcoma	t(9;22)(q22;q12) t(9;17)(q22;q11)	*EWS/CHN* fusion *RBP56/CHN* fusion
Ewing tumours	t(11;22)(q24;q12) t(21;22)(q22;q12) t(7;22)(p22;q12) t(2;22)(q33;q12) t(17;22)(q12;q12)	*EWS/FLI1* fusion *EWS/ERG* fusion *EWS/ETV1* fusion *EWS/FEV* fusion *EWS/EIAF* fusion
Pleomorphic adenoma of the salivary gland	t(3;8)(p21;q12)	*CTNNB1/PLAG1* fusion
Papillary renal cell carcinoma	t(X;1)(p11;q21)	*TFE3/PRCC* fusion
Papillary thyroid carcinoma	inv(10)(q11q21)	*RET/PTC* fusion

[a] For more extensive information, see Mitelman *et al.* (2).

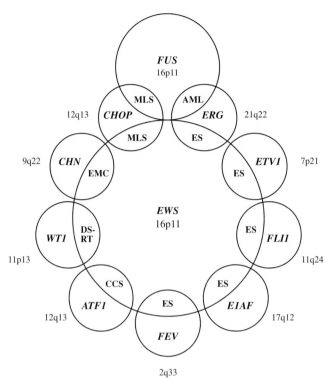

Figure 9 Overview of translocations resulting in chimeric genes involving *EWS* and *FUS*. Gene symbols are shown in italics and the chromosome bands indicated represent the translocation breakpoints and localization of the genes. Abbreviations (indicating the tumour type associated with particular gene fusions): MLS, myxoid liposarcoma; AML, acute myeloid leukaemia; ES, Ewing tumour family (including Ewing sarcoma); CCS, clear-cell sarcoma of tendons and aponeuroses; DSRT, desmoplastic small cell, round cell tumour; EMC, extraskeletal myxoid chondrosarcoma.

15 Significance of the study of genetic changes

As indicated (Section 1, *Table 3*), cytogenetic analysis is becoming more and more important in diagnostic work because of the identification of an increasing number of specific or characteristic chromosome aberrations associated with particular tumour subtypes. In some situations where there are difficult differential diagnostic dilemmas, cytogenetic analysis can be an important adjunct to clinical data and histopathological and cytological examinations (5). Cytogenetic analysis may lend support to a particular diagnosis, help distinguish between two or more suspected diagnoses, or even provide an alternative diagnosis. The precision or lack of precision of cytogenetic analysis can be illustrated by a few examples. The t(X;18) (p11;q11) seems to be pathognomonic for synovial sarcomas, and among the small, blue cell childhood tumours, causing great diagnostic problems, all differential diagnoses have different karyotypic profiles. Conversely, the t(12;22)(q13;q12) found as characteristic changes in clear cell sarcomas and a minor subset of myxoid liposarcomas are cytogenetically indistinguishable. Yet these aberrations are not only associated with different tumour types but have also different consequences at the gene level. Furthermore, cytogenetic analysis may help distinguish neoplasia from non-neoplastic lesions and benign from malignant tumours (5). However, acquired chromosome aberrations, in particular trisomy 7 as the sole anomaly, have been found in normal tissues, and should be interpreted with caution. Although chromosome studies in solid tumours play a role in diagnosis, the impact on prognostication is, in contrast to the situation in haematological malignancies, less significant, although a few examples are known (5).

Another important role of cytogenetic analysis is to identify chromosome aberrations and chromosomal breakpoints for further studies with molecular techniques. Thus, cytogenetics is an integrated part of a set of genetic techniques (see Section 2) used both for the search for better prognostic factors and attempts to reach a deeper understanding of basic tumour biology and tumorigenesis. Access to multiple techniques may be quite useful, not only in basic research but also in the diagnostic setting, once the affected genes have been identified (17). As an example, the diagnosis of a case of suspected Ewing sarcoma could be considered. Cytogenetic analysis, being an excellent screening procedure, will reveal any of the variant translocations as well as secondary aberrations (which may turn out to be of prognostic importance). The rare cases with cytogenetically cryptic Ewing sarcoma-associated chimeric genes will be missed. The finding of chromosome aberrations other than those seen in Ewing tumours may suggest an alternative diagnosis. The failure rate, however, appears to be as high as 25–40%. RT-PCR analysis is accurate and sensitive. Not all variant translocations can be analysed in one reaction, but can cover the two most common gene fusions comprising almost 95% of the cases. A negative result will not provide any alternative diagnosis. Identification of the type of fusion transcript may be of prognostic importance (18,19). Finally, interphase FISH analysis with 3′and 5′ *EWS* probes in different colours can be used. This will detect all variant translocations, but cannot distinguish the Ewing sarcoma-associated translocations from rearrangements in other tumours characterized by a split *EWS* gene (*Figure 8*). Another example is synovial sarcoma in which cytogenetics readily can detect the t(X;18) but is unable to discriminate between the involvement of *SSX1* or *SSX2*. This can be done by RT-PCR, and there are indications that this may be prognostically important; patients with *SYT/SSX1* seem to have a worse prognosis (20).

Acknowledgements

Colleagues at the Department of Clinical Genetics, Lund University Hospital are greatly acknowledged for all discussions and for sharing with me their knowledge and experience on the culturing and analysis of solid tumours.

References

1. Heim, S. and Mitelman, F. (1995). *Cancer cytogenetics*, 2nd edn. Wiley-Liss, New York.
2. Mitelman, F., Mertens, F., and Johansson, B. (1997). *Nature Genetics* **15**, 417.
3. Mitelman Database of Chromosome Aberations in Cancer (2000). Mitelman, F., Johansson, B., and Mertens, F. (Eds.), http://cgap.nci.nih.gov/chromosomes/mitelman
4. Mandahl, N. (1996). *Adv. Cancer Res.* **69,** 63.
5. Mitelman, F., Johansson, B., Mandahl N., and Mertens F. (1997). *Cancer Genet. Cytogenet.* **95**, 1.
6. Kazmierczak, B., Bartnitzke, S., Hartl, M., and Bullerdiek, J. (1990). *Cytogenet. Cell Genet.* **53**, 37.
7. Limon, J., Dal Cin, P., and Sandberg, A. A. (1986). *Cancer Genet. Cytogenet.* **23**, 305.
8. Freshney, R. I. (1987). *Culture of animal cells. A manual of basic technique.* Alan R. Liss, New York.
9. Thompson, F. H. (1991). In *The ACT cytogenetics laboratory manual* (ed. Barch, M. J.), pp. 451–488. Raven Press, New York.
10. Lawce, H. (1997). *Applied Cytogenet.* **23**, 167.
11. Schaeffer, W. I. (1990). *In Vitro Cell. Dev. Biol.* **26**, 97.
12. Gorunova, L. (1998). *Genes Chromosomes Cancer* **23**, 81.
13. Barr, F. G., Nauta, L. E., Davis, R. J., Schäfer, B. W., Nycum, L. M., and Biegel, J. A. (1996). *Hum. Mol. Genet.* **5**, 15.
14. ISCN (1995). *An international system for human cytogenetic nomenclature* (ed. F. Mitelman). S. Karger, Basel.
15. Carey, T. and Mertens, F. (2001). In *Clinical laboratory medicine* (ed. K. McClatehey), 2nd edn. Lippincott/Williams & Wilkins, Philadelphia.
16. Peehl, D. M., and Stamey, T. A. (1986). *In Vitro Cell Dev. Biol.* **22**, 82.
17. Sreekantaiah, C. (1998). *Cytogenet. Cell Genet.* **82**, 13.
18. Zoubek, A., Dockhorn-Dworniczak, B., Delattre, O., Christiansen, H., Niggli, F., Gatterer-Menz, I. *et al.* (1996). *J. Clin. Oncol.* **14**, 1245.
19. De Alava, E., Kawai, A., Healey, J.H., Fligman, I., Meyers, P.A., Huvos, A.G. *et al.* (1998). *J. Clin. Oncol.* **16**, 1248.
20. Kawai, A., Woodruff, J., Healey, J. H., Brennan, M. F., Antonescu, C. R., and Ladanyi, M. (1998). *N. Engl. J. Med.* **338**, 153.

Chapter 8

In vivo mutagen-induced chromosome damage in human lymphocytes

E. J. Tawn and C. A. Whitehouse

Genetics Unit, Westlakes Research Institute, Westlakes Science and Technology Park, Moor Row, Cumbria CA24 3JY, UK

1 Introduction

The study of induced chromosome changes in human lymphocytes is well established for monitoring the genotoxic effects of *in vivo* exposure to radiation and chemicals. Cytogenetic studies can be used to monitor populations for a range of environmental and occupational clastogens and mutagens (1–3) and, for radiation, can provide an estimate of individual dose (4,5). Various endpoints can be studied. These include structural chromosome aberrations, SCE and micronuclei. All require short-term cultures of peripheral blood lymphocytes with modifications to allow the manifestation of the different types of genetic changes.

2 Principles of lymphocyte culture for aberration and sister chromatid exchange analysis

Chromosome aberrations are usually scored in cells undergoing their first metaphase in culture for individuals exposed *in vivo*, and SCE are observed in cells that have undergone two cycles in the presence of BrdU which permits differential labelling of the chromatids. Certain media appear to encourage faster growth than others and it is important that the rate of cell progression through the cell cycle be established and appropriate culture medium and harvest times chosen. BrdU labelling is therefore also applicable to aberration analysis since it allows differentiation of cells in their first and subsequent divisions. For convenience, it is useful to establish a protocol for aberration analysis which minimizes the number of cells in second metaphase at 48–50 h and to culture for 72 h for SCE analysis.

2.1 Lymphocyte culture

Precautions must be taken in any process which involves the handling of potentially toxic or infective materials. Suitable protective clothing and the use of a safety cabinet conforming to appropriate standards is essential.

BrdU-substituted DNA is degraded by natural and artificial light. These cultures should therefore be kept in the dark for as much of the time as is reasonably practicable, and certainly throughout the incubation period. If lighting is unavoidable, use an orange or yellow light source.

Protocol 1

Lymphocyte culture, harvesting and slide preparation

Equipment and reagents

- Class 2 biological safety cabinet
- Incubator, 37 °C
- Fume hood
- Gilson pipette, 20 μl
- Pressmatic 2000 pipette dispenser (Bibby Sterilin Ltd)
- Plastic syringes with quills (1 ml, 2 ml and 10 ml)
- Syringe needles (essential use only)
- Universal containers, plastic 25 ml, sterile
- Centrifuge tubes, plastic 10 ml
- Pasteur pipettes, plastic
- Glass microscope slides, pre-cleaned
- RPMI 1640 medium with L-glutamine stored at 4 °C

- BrdU[a] final concentration 3.074 mg/ml (Sigma) stored at −20 °C
- 5000 IU/ml Penicillin and 5000 μg/ml Streptomycin stored at −20 °C
- FCS stored at −20 °C
- PHA[b] M-form dehydrated, rehydrated in sterile water and stored at 4 °C for up to 1 month once reconstituted
- KaryoMax colcemid[c] solution in HBSS final concentration 0.1 μg/ml (Gibco BRL)
- Hypotonic solution: dissolve 5.595 g of KCl in 1 l of distilled water
- Fixative: methanol[d]–glacial acetic acid[e], 3:1

Method

1 Dispense 0.1 ml of BrdU into 100 ml RPMI and mix well.

2 Measure into 25 ml plastic universal containers: 8.5 ml RPMI plus BrdU, 1.5 ml FCS, 0.2 ml penicillin and streptomycin, 0.2 ml PHA.

3 Inoculate the culture medium with 0.8 ml of heparinized whole peripheral blood and incubate at 37 °C for 48–50 h or 72 h.

4 Four hours before the end of culturing, add 0.1 ml colcemid.

5 At 48–50/72 h transfer to a 10 ml plastic centrifuge tube and centrifuge at 200 **g** for 10 min at room temperature. Discard the supernatant.

6 Resuspend the pellet in 10 ml hypotonic solution, mix well and allow to stand for 10 min (times will vary between laboratories).

7 Centrifuge at 200 **g** for 10 min. Discard the supernatant.

Protocol 1 continued

8 Resuspend the pellet and add freshly prepared fixative, drop-wise at first, to a final volume of 10 ml.

9 Repeat steps 7 and 8 until the cells have been fixed a total of six times. Store the sample at −20 °C overnight, at least, before making slides.

10 For slide making, centrifuge the fixed suspension, discard the supernatant and resuspend the cell pellet in a small amount of fresh fixative.

11 Using a Pasteur pipette, drop the cell suspension onto clean, grease-free polished slides. Alternatively pipette 2 drops of 20 μl of fixed suspension onto the slide.[f]

[a] Caution: BrdU may cause heritable genetic damage and harm to the unborn child. It is harmful by inhalation, in contact with skin and if swallowed.

[b] Caution: PHA may cause serious systemic effects.

[c] Caution: colcemid is toxic by skin contact and by inhalation and may cause irreversible effects. It poses a possible risk of harm to the unborn child.

[d] Caution: methanol is highly flammable and toxic by inhalation.

[e] Caution: glacial acetic acid causes severe burns and is harmful in contact with skin.

[f] This latter method alleviates the need to drop the suspension from a height onto the slide. Aim to produce slides having the highest density of metaphases commensurate with cytoplasm-free cells. Thinly spread preparations are more time-consuming to analyse.

2.2 Staining techniques

2.2.1 Fluorescence-plus-Giemsa

Fluorescence-plus-Giemsa staining of cells cultured in the presence of BrdU will allow the identification of cells in their first, second and subsequent divisions in culture, and enable differentiation of SCE in cells undergoing their second division cycle. Occasionally, FPG staining on 48 h cultures results in poor-quality first division cells that are difficult to score. In these cases, it is advisable to use the FPG-stained slides to establish the proportion of metaphases in first division but to perform the analysis on conventional Giemsa slides.

Protocol 2

FPG staining

Equipment and reagents

- Slide staining rack and glass trough
- Hoechst 33258 (bisbenzimide)[a] (Sigma) stock solution: 0.5 mg/ml sterile water, this can be stored for up to 1 month in the dark at 4 °C
- PBS (Unipath Ltd): dissolve eight tablets of PBS buffer in 1 l of distilled water and store at 4 °C

- UV light source (365 nm)
- Glass Coplin jars
- Coverslips (22 × 50 mm)
- Giemsa improved R66 stain[b] (Merck)
- Gurr's Buffer tablets pH 6.8 (Merck): dissolve one Gurr's Buffer tablet in 1 l of distilled water and store at 4 °C
- DPX mountant[c] (Merck)

Protocol 2 continued

Method

1 Dilute Hoechst 33258 1:100 with PBS.

2 Arrange the slides in a staining rack and immerse in the Hoechst solution for $\approx$ 25 min.

3 Wash the slides twice with PBS and blot dry carefully.

4 Place 12 drops of PBS onto each slide and cover with a 22 × 50 mm coverslip.

5 Expose the slides to UV light (365 nm) at a distance of $\approx$ 10 cm for 2–5 h.[d]

6 Remove the coverslips by washing in PBS.

7 Stain the slides for 5 min in Giemsa diluted 1:9 with Gurr's buffer.[e]

8 Leave to air dry and mount on a coverslip with DPX mountant.

[a] Caution: Hoechst 33258 is a possible mutagen.

[b] Caution: contains methanol which is highly flammable and toxic by inhalation.

[c] Caution: contains xylene which is flammable and harmful by inhalation.

[d] Alternative UV sources can be used but some trial and error will be needed to establish the time of exposure and distance from the slides.

[e] It is advisable initially to Giemsa stain just one slide from each batch. If this shows unsatisfactory differential staining apply more UV light to the remainder.

2.2.2 Fluorescence *in situ* hybridization

Fluorescence *in situ* hybridization chromosome analysis using a cocktail of whole chromosome probes (also called paints) to a number of pairs of chromosomes is based on the detection of exchanges between painted and unpainted chromosomes. The addition of a centromeric probe allows the different types of aberrations to be distinguished.

The whole chromosome and centromeric paints may be either biotinylated or directly labelled with, for example, FITC or Cy3. Single-colour labelling with one fluorochrome or multicolour labelling with more than one fluorochrome are both possible. All chromosomes are additionally counterstained with either DAPI or propidium iodide. In the authors' laboratory a cocktail of biotinylated paints for chromosomes 1, 3 and 4, detected with FITC, and a centromeric probe directly labelled with Cy3 are routinely used.

Protocol 3

FISH using whole-chromosome paints and a pancentromeric probe

Equipment and reagents

- Glass Coplin jars
- Water baths at 42 °C and 65 °C
- Ovens at 37 °C and 42 °C
- Gilson pipettes (all sizes)
- Fume hood (for steps involving formamide)
- Microcentrifuge

Protocol 3 continued

- Moist chamber (e.g. wet tissues in a plastic box)
- Eppendorf tubes
- Coverslips, 22 × 50 mm
- Ethanol series: 70%, 90% and 100%
- Ethanol: 70%, ice cold
- Biotinylated concentrated chromosome paints (Cambio)
- Hybridization solution[a] (Cambio)
- Genomic DNA (Cambio)
- Vulcanizing rubber solution
- 4× SSC: 0.06 M sodium citrate (Merck), 0.6 M sodium chloride (Merck)
- 2× SSC: 0.03 M sodium citrate, 0.3 M sodium chloride

- 1× SSC: 0.015 M sodium citrate, 0.15 M sodium chloride
- 70% formamide[a] (Merck)/2× SSC
- 50% formamide/1× SSC
- 50% formamide/2× SSC
- Cy3 pancentromeric probe (Cambio)
- Wash solution: 4× SSC, 0.05% Nonidet P-40 (Sigma)
- Blocking solution: 15% blocking protein (Cambio)/wash solution
- Fluorescein avidin (Vector Labs)
- Biotinylated goat anti-avidin (Vector Labs)
- DAPI (Sigma), 0.1 mg/ml
- Vectashield Mountant (Vector Labs)
- Coverslips, 22 × 50 mm

Method

1 Prepare fresh slides from fixed preparations (*Protocol 1*) and leave at room temperature for 2–3 days or age at 65°C for 1.5 h. Dehydrate the slides through an ethanol series, (70%, 90%, 100%) and air dry. Denature the slides by incubating in 70% formamide/2× SSC at 65°C for 2 min then quench in ice-cold 70% ethanol, dehydrate in ethanol as above and air dry.

2 To prepare the chromosome probe, warm the three biotinylated paints to 42°C for ≈ 10 min and mix well. Pipette 6 μl per slide of each probe into an Eppendorf tube, add 1 μl per slide of genomic DNA and 11 μl per slide of hybridization buffer, then denature the paints by incubating at 65°C in a water bath for 10 min and pre-hybridize at 37°C for 60 min.

3 Pipette 30 μl of probe onto each slide, cover with a coverslip, seal the edges with rubber solution and incubate at 42°C overnight.

4 Post hybridization wash: prewarm to 42°C three Coplin jars of 2× SSC and two jars of 50% formamide/1× SSC; remove the rubber solution and wash off the coverslip and excess paint by incubating the slides in 2× SSC at 42°C for 5 min, then wash the slides twice in 50% formamide/1× SSC at 42°C for 5 min in each jar, and then twice in 2× SSC at 42°C for 5 min in each jar; dehydrate the slides in ethanol as above and air dry.

5 For pancentromeric probe preparation, warm the probe to 37°C for 5 min, mix well, then pipette 30 μl per slide of probe into an Eppendorf tube and denature the probe at 85°C for 10 min. Immediately chill on ice until required.

6 Pipette 30 μl of probe onto the slide, cover with a 22 × 50 mm coverslip, seal with rubber solution and hybridize for 16 h at 37°C.

7 Post-hybridization wash: pre-warm to 42°C three Coplin jars of 2× SSC and two jars

Protocol 3 continued

50% formamide/2× SSC; remove the rubber solution and wash off the coverslip and excess paint by incubating the slides in 2× SSC at 42°C for 5 min, then wash the slides twice in 50% formamide/2× SSC at 42°C for 5 min in each jar and then twice in 2× SSC at 42°C for 5 min in each jar.

8 To prepare the detection reagents, prewarm to 42°C seven Coplin jars of wash solution. Make up enough blocking solution to incubate the slides and dilute the detection reagents. Rinse the slides briefly in wash solution and incubate the slides in 100 μl blocking solution in a moist chamber at 37°C for 30 min. Dilute fluorescein avidin 1:500 in blocking solution and biotinylated goat anti-avidin 1:100 in blocking solution, then incubate the detection reagents at room temperature in the dark for at least 10 min and microfuge at 11 000 **g** for 10 min.

9 For detection, pipette 100 μl fluorescein avidin onto each slide, cover with a coverslip (but do not seal) and incubate at 37°C in a moist chamber for 20–30 min, then wash slides three times in fresh wash solution at 42°C for 5 min in each jar. Then pipette 100 μl biotinylated goat anti-avidin onto each slide, cover with a 22 × 50 mm coverslip (but do not seal) and incubate in the dark at room temperature for 15–30 min. Wash slides twice in fresh wash solution at 42°C for 5 min in each jar, then pipette 100 μl fluorescein avidin onto each slide, cover with a 22 × 50 mm coverslip (but do not seal) and incubate at room temperature for 15–30 min. Wash slides twice in fresh wash solution at 42°C for 5 min in each jar. Dehydrate slides in an ethanol series as above.

10 To mount slides, mix 2 μl DAPI per 200 μl Vectashield mountant and pipette 40 μl of DAPI/mountant onto each slide, cover with a coverslip and seal the edges with nail varnish. Allow to harden at 4°C before observing under a fluorescence microscope.

[a] Caution: formamide may cause harm to the unborn child. It may cause serious damage to the eyes and is irritating to the respiratory tract.

3 Structural chromosome aberrations

Structural chromosome aberrations arise as a result of discontinuities or breaks in the DNA. Failure to rejoin such breaks leads to deletions, whereas aberrant rejoining results in exchanges. Aberrations are usually divided into chromosome-type, involving both chromatids at identical loci and chromatid-type involving one chromatid. A detailed classification is provided by Savage (6). Chromosome analysis for genotoxic studies has traditionally been restricted to scoring aberrations that can easily be identified using a conventional block staining technique. For the chromosome-type these are the asymmetrical aberrations e.g. dicentrics, rings, fragments (*Figures 1* and *2*). Symmetrical (or stable) chromosome aberrations, e.g. translocations, insertions and inversions, can be detected using a G-banding technique (see Human Cytogenetics: constitutional analysis,

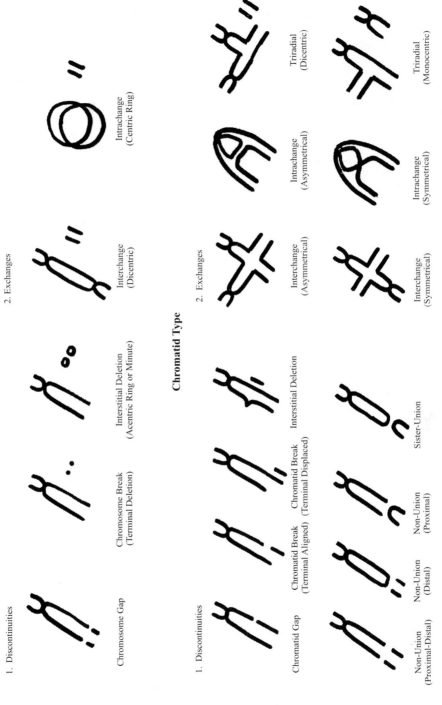

Figure 1 The main types of chromosome aberrations observed with block staining. Derived from the classification of Savage (6).

211

(a)　　　　　　　　　　　　　　　　(b)

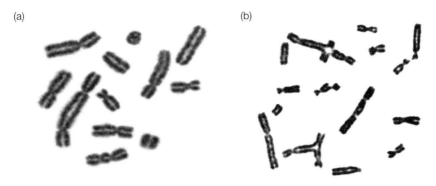

Figure 2 (a) Chromosome-type aberrations; (b) chromatid-type aberrations (*Figure 2b* kindly provided by Dr J. R. K. Savage, MRC Radiation and Genome Stability Unit, Chilton, Oxon, UK).

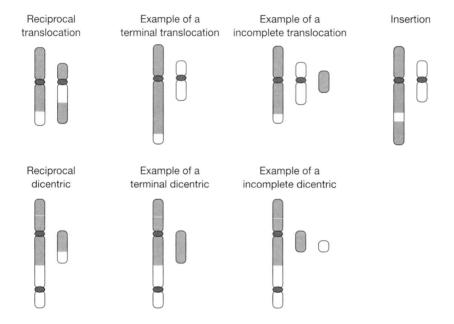

Figure 3 The main types of chromosome aberrations observed with FISH chromosome painting.

Chapter 4) but this is very time consuming. More recently, FISH techniques have been applied allowing the rapid detection of both symmetrical and asymmetrical chromosome aberrations (*Figure 3* and Plate 8). For chromatid-type aberrations the configurations produced allow most types of both asymmetrical and symmetrical aberrations to be detected with block staining (*Figures 1* and *2*).

3.1 Lymphocyte culture for aberration analysis

It is essential that the population of cells scored does not include cells in their second post-exposure division since this will result in an underestimate of aberration yield due to loss of damaged cells. This can be avoided by the choice of a suitable culture time which should be checked with BrdU labelling and FPG staining (see Section 2 and *Protocols 1* and *2*).

3.2 Aberration analysis with block staining

Analysis should only be undertaken by an experienced observer who has knowledge of the human karyotype, and has undergone a period of training in the identification and classification of aberrations. This training should include working through test slides with known aberration frequencies. In order to avoid observer bias in the selection of cells, rigid criteria should be adopted. It is important that the slides are randomly coded so that the scorer is unaware of the identity of the sample. The slide should be scanned systematically using a low-power objective (×10) and cells that appear suitable analysed at high magnification (×100). Computer-aided metaphase finding can speed up this process. Having moved to high power, the observer should ignore the presence of any abnormalities and make a snap judgement on whether the chromosomes are of sufficient quality to allow the cell to be scored. Once a cell is observed at high magnification it should only be rejected if the quality is poor, e.g. inadequate spreading, dirt on the slide preventing full analysis, or if the cell is incomplete. Some laboratories will analyse cells with 46 ± 2 centromeres, whereas others will only accept cells with 46 centromeres. Similarly, some will accept only those cells that are chromosomally balanced, e.g. a dicentric must have an accompanying fragment, whereas others will accept the cell with the fragment missing. The important thing is to set the criteria and apply them consistently. In the authors' laboratory, cells are only accepted if they have 46 centromeres and appear chromosomally complete. Other aberrant cells are noted and although not included in frequency calculations may provide useful information if the results are inconclusive.

On finding a suitable cell, the number of chromosome pieces should be counted and the aberrations noted. Exchanges which include the formation of an acentric fragment, e.g. dicentrics, are classed as one aberration and the acentric is not scored separately. Additional acentrics are placed in a separate category. Occasionally, cells are seen with multiple aberrations and an attempt should be made to analyse these in detail. If this proves impossible, they should be placed in a complex aberration category.

Data are usually recorded on a score sheet. This can be done manually or electronically, in which case there needs to be a provision for producing a paper printout. The precise design of the score sheet is not critical and will to some extent depend on the main type of aberration induced. An example is provided in *Figure 4*. Some provision should be made for a full description of every aberration, although for statistical analysis of the data it is legitimate to combine them into general classes.

In order to identify any scorer bias and to enable the study of intra-laboratory variation, it is advisable that the analysis be carried out by more than one individual.

213

Study Name .... Subject ID Number.............................. Slide ID...................

Analysed By .... Microscope Used............................... Date.......................

Cell No.	Verniers	2N	N	dic	cr	ace	chtg	chtb	chte	chsg	Comments
1	20.3 x 132.0	46	1								
2	20.6 x 132.3	46		1						1	
3	19.6 x 131.6	47			1			1			
4	19.8 x 128.3	48				2	1				minute and fragment
5	19.4 x 124.8	46	1								
6	19.9 x 118.3	46		2							tricentric
7	19.3 x 116.9	46					1				
8	19.4 x 108.1	48			1	1					fragment
9	18.2 x 109.6	47				1					acentric ring
10	18.5 x 112.8	45							1		quadradial

Figure 4 Score sheet used for chromosome- and chromatid-type aberration analysis using block staining.

3.3 Aberration analysis using fluorescence *in situ* hybridization

General analysis criteria have been described in Section 3.2. As with block staining, a period of training needs to be undertaken to ensure proficient identification and classification of aberrations. This should include the analysis and written description of a number of aberrant cells. FISH is usually confined to the analysis of chromosome-type aberrations.

A system of speed scoring is applied in the authors' laboratory. The slides are scanned at ×40 magnification using a filter relevant for the counterstain and suitable cells analysed at ×100 magnification. It is not necessary to count all the chromosomes and centromeres but only apparently intact metaphases with all the painted material present should be included. Damaged cells or those where some painted material is missing must be rejected. The cells should be observed using both the correct filter for the counterstaining and a filter for the painted chromosomes to enable all aberrations to be identified as fully as possible.

Using combinations of whole chromosome paints, aberration analysis is based upon the recognition of altered colour patterns. A normal cell with chromosomes 1, 3 and 4 painted will have 6 painted objects. A cell containing a rearrangement between a painted and a counterstained chromosome will usually have 7 or more painted objects. FISH analysis only allows a proportion of aberrations to be identified and it is therefore essential that a scorer has a full understanding of the derivation of the possible painting patterns (7). Two principle methods of classification have been proposed. S&S has been designed to allow a mechanistic interpretation of the origin of an aberration by considering each exchange in all its parts as an entity (8), and PAINT has been derived to allow a rapid description of each resulting rearranged chromosome (9). In the authors' laboratory each aberration is fully described so that either nomenclature can be applied as appropriate.

The aberrations most commonly seen are translocations and dicentrics. Although reciprocal exchanges form the majority, a number of incomplete patterns can sometimes be observed (*Figure 3*). It is also possible to find more complicated aberrations, defined as three or more breaks in two or more chromosomes. However, these cannot always be separated into simple rearrangements because only a proportion of aberrations are detected using chromosome painting. All abnormal cells should either be drawn on paper or captured using a computerized image analysis capture system. In the authors' laboratory a Perceptive Scientific International plc (PSI) computer with a black and white camera is used to capture and analyse all aberrant cells.

Data are recorded on a score sheet, an example of which is shown in *Figure 5*. It is not necessary to record the verniers of all cells, only those containing chromosome rearrangements. All aberrations should be recorded even if they will not be used in the final analysis. These may include rearrangements between two painted chromosomes or between two counterstained chromosomes. As with solid-stained scoring, where possible, the analysis be carried out by more than one individual to prevent scorer bias.

Because only a proportion of the total genome is being 'painted' it is usual to convert the aberration frequency detected to a whole genome equivalent by applying the formula $Fp = 2.05fp(1 - fp)F_G$ (10) where Fp is the frequency of translocations (or dicentrics) detected by fluorescence *in situ* hybridization, *fp* is

Study Name .... Subject ID Number.............................. Slide ID....................

Analysed By .... Microscope Used................................ Date.......................

Normal cells
╫╫ ╠╬ ╫╫ ╫╫ ╫╫

Abnormal Cells			
Cell No.	Vernier	Rearrangements	Comments
1	34.3 x 96.2	reciprocal translocation involving chromosome 1	
2	38.5 x 90.1	terminal translocation involving chromosome 3	
3	40.8 x 88.4	reciprocal dicentric involving chromosome 4	
4	41.5 x 86.7	incomplete translocation involving chromosome 1	blue acentric fragment
5	42.3 x 93.6	complex rearrangement involving chromosome 3	
6	42.9 x 89.3	normal cell	translocation between chromosomes 1 and 4

Figure 5 Score sheet used for chromosome-type aberration analysis using FISH

the fraction of the genome painted (11) and F_G is the genomic aberration frequency. This assumes that breaks occur randomly throughout the genome, there is no preference for breaks between particular pairs of chromosomes and therefore that the number of aberrations seen involving a particular chromosome is proportional to its length.

4 Sister chromatid exchange

Sister chromatid exchanges are reciprocal exchanges between sister chromatids. They do not result in a change in chromosome morphology and the exchange occurs, as far as is known, at homologous loci. Although DNA breakage and reunion is presumably involved, the exact molecular mechanism remains unknown. SCE are most efficiently induced by substances that form covalent adducts with the DNA, or interfere with DNA precursor metabolism or repair. They are produced during DNA replication. SCE induction is maximal at the start of DNA synthesis but falls to zero at the end of S phase, implying that SCE arise at the replication point. SCE appear to be unrelated to other cytogenetic phenomena. The poor SCE inducing ability of potent clastogens such as bleomycin and ionizing radiation shows that SCE are unrelated to structural chromosome aberrations and the mechanisms involved in the two types of lesion are obviously dissimilar.

4.1 Culture factors influencing sister chromatid exchange frequency

Sister chromatid exchanges can be observed in cells that have undergone two division cycles in the presence of BrdU thus allowing differential labelling of the chromatids (*Protocols 1* and *2*) (*Figure 6*). A number of culture factors can influence SCE frequency (for reviews, see refs. 12 and 13). These include BrdU concentration, time of harvest, culture medium, serum, antibiotics and temperature. BrdU will itself cause SCE and its concentration should be kept to the minimum required for good differential labelling of the chromatids. The influence of harvest time reflects the presence of different populations of lymphocytes with different cell progression times and different SCE levels. It has been suggested that the more slowly cycling cells have a higher SCE frequency in control individuals. Media components and temperature may simply exert an influence on cell cycle time, although there are suggestions that they have a more direct effect on SCE frequency. In order to minimize variation and maximize sensitivity the use of standardized procedures is essential. Some laboratories recommend performing a total white cell count so that the number of cells per culture can be controlled.

4.2 Sister chromatid exchange scoring

General scoring criteria have been described in Section 3.2. Only cells with clear harlequin staining should be scored. Each exchange (i.e. switch in colour) is

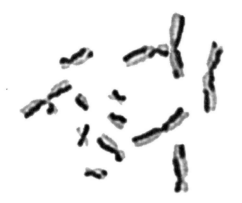

Figure 6 Sister chromatid exchanges.

scored as one SCE. Care should be taken to avoid confusing a twist about the centromere with a chromatid exchange. It is conventional to report frequencies as SCE per chromosome and SCE per cell.

5 Micronuclei

Micronuclei are discrete round bodies, of nuclear origin, found in the cytoplasm outside the main nucleus. They resemble nuclei in shape, structure and staining properties, and can vary widely in size. They arise from acentric fragments which have been excluded from the daughter nuclei during cell division. Micronuclei can also be formed by entire chromosomes that lag behind during mitosis due to a failure of the mitotic spindle or to complex configurations that pose problems at anaphase. The formation of micronuclei can therefore be induced by both clastogenic agents and mitotic inhibitors. The earliest appearance of micronuclei is at the end of the first post-treatment mitotic division, but additional micronuclei can be formed in the next few divisions. Their usefulness for mutagenicity testing was first established with rodent bone marrow smears and later extended to human lymphocytes. In principle, the lymphocyte micronucleus assay is also applicable to a wide range of occupational and environmental monitoring programmes but, until recently, quantification was difficult.

5.1 Lymphocyte culture for micronucleus determination

Micronuclei can be seen in cells that have undergone a complete post-treatment division cycle. However, both dividing and non-dividing interphase nuclei will be scored using conventional Giemsa stain. Changes in mitotic rate will therefore result in different observed frequencies of micronuclei. A technique has recently been developed which enables the dividing cell population to be differentiated from the unstimulated remainder (14). This employs a cytokinesis block which results in the formation of binucleated cells, i.e. cells which have undergone nuclear division but where the cytoplasm has been prevented from dividing (*Figure 7*). To achieve this, Cyt B is added to the culture medium towards

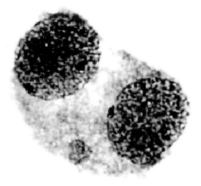

Figure 7 Binucleate cell with micronucleus from cultures treated with cytochalasin B.

the end of the first division cycle to catch the first wave of cells as they complete mitosis. Cells which have divided once will have two nuclei and can therefore be easily distinguished from non-dividing cells.

A prerequisite of the micronucleus assay is preservation of the cytoplasm of the cell. This allows a micronucleus to be assigned to a main nucleus and eliminates the scoring of blobs and spots on the slide. This is facilitated by eliminating the hypotonic treatment and minimizing the fixation. To avoid problems with red blood cells in the final lymphocyte suspension, the use of a buffy coat preparation for culture initiation is recommended.

Protocol 4

Lymphocyte culture, harvesting and slide making for micronucleus determination

Equipment and reagents

Equipment as for *Protocol 1*

- Coplin jars
- RPMI medium (see *Protocol 1*)
- FCS (see *Protocol 1*)
- PHA[a] (see *Protocol 1*)
- Penicillin and streptomycin (see *Protocol 1*)
- DMSO (Merck)
- Cyt B[b] (Sigma): 1 mg/ml in DMSO and store at −20 °C

- Phosphate buffer solution (Unipath Ltd): 10 tablets dissolved in 1 l of distilled water and store at 4 °C
- Fixative (see *Protocol 1*)[a]
- Giemsa staining solution[c] (Merck)
- Gurr's buffer (Merck Limited): one tablet dissolved in 1 l of distilled water

Method

1 Prepare the culture medium as for *Protocol 1* excluding the BrdU.

2 Centrifuge the whole peripheral blood at 800 **g** for 15 min. Carefully remove the

Protocol 4 continued

buffy coat from the interface between the red blood cells and plasma using a sterile Pasteur pipette.

3 Inoculate 10 ml of medium with 0.2 ml of buffy coat preparation and incubate at 37 °C for 44 h.

4 After 44 h add Cyt B to a final concentration of 3 μg/ml and continue incubation to 72 h.

5 Transfer the cells to a 10 ml plastic centrifuge tube and centrifuge at 200 **g** for 10 min. Discard the supernatant.

6 Resuspend the cells in PBS and centrifuge at 200 **g** for 10 min. Discard the supernatant.

7 Resuspend the cells in 1 ml fixative and centrifuge at 200 **g** for 10 min. Discard the supernatant.

8 Resuspend the cells in a few drops of fixative. Store at −20 °C until required.[d]

9 Spread the slides according to *Protocol 1*.

10 Stain the slides with Giemsa diluted 1:9 with Gurr's buffer for 5 min.

[a] Caution: see *Protocol 1* for risk information.

[b] Caution: Cyt B is very toxic by inhalation, in contact with the skin and if swallowed. It poses a possible risk of irreversible effects and is a possible risk to the unborn child.

[c] Caution: see *Protocol 2* for risk information.

[d] The minimal fix protocol is designed to avoid the disruption of the cytoplasm. Use of as little height as is commensurate with satisfactory spreading will assist in this.

5.2 Scoring of micronuclei

Compared with conventional chromosome analysis, the scoring of micronuclei does not require highly trained personnel and is much faster. The following criteria for identifying micronuclei should be applied:

(1) Score only binucleate cells with well-preserved cytoplasm;

(2) In groups of cells, individual cellular boundaries must be distinct;

(3) A micronucleus must have the same structure and staining properties as the main nucleus;

(4) a micronucleus must be a discrete round body visibly separated from the main nucleus;

(5) a micronucleus must have a diameter no greater than half that of the main nucleus.

The slide should be systematically scanned. Since it is intended that this should be a rapid technique, it is not recommended that cell locations are recorded unless this can be done electronically. However, provision should be made for noting the numbers of cells with one, two, three, etc., micronuclei.

Image analysis and flow cytometric methods for micronucleus detection are currently being developed and offer the potential for scoring large numbers of cells.

6 Radiation dosimetry

Ionizing radiation produces aberrations at all stages of the cell cycle and therefore irradiation prior to chromosome replication will result in the observation of chromosome-type aberrations at the following metaphase. Since peripheral blood lymphocytes are essentially non-cycling cells in the G_0 stage of the cell cycle, they provide a fairly synchronous population of cells with uniform sensitivity. If sampled at the first metaphase *in vitro* it is possible to make a quantitative assessment of any chromosome damage. The aberration used for dose estimation in cases of recent acute exposure is the dicentric and this is determined by block staining analysis. It is easily scored and has the advantage of having a low background frequency in the general population (1 in 1000–2000 cells).

6.1 The dose response

The dose response for dicentrics is the same *in vitro* as *in vivo*, thus allowing *in vitro* curves to be produced and used in the *in vivo* situation where an acute exposure to radiation is suspected (4,5). The production of dicentrics depends on both the dose and the radiation quality. The data are usually fitted to a linear quadratic model (*Figure 8*). Ideally a laboratory should generate its own calibration curves, including background data, although this involves the analysis of many thousands of cells. If published dose–response curves (5) are used, the same laboratory criteria for culturing and aberration scoring employed in the production of the curves should be followed.

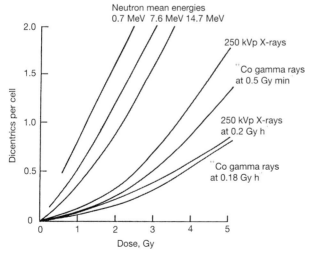

Figure 8 *In vitro* dose–response curves for the production of dicentrics by radiation (kindly provided by Dr D. C. Lloyd, NRPB, Chilton, Oxon, UK).

6.2 Blood sampling, culturing and slide preparation

It is advisable, particularly in the case of partial body or non-uniform exposures, to wait 24 h after the radiation exposure before taking the blood sample. This will allow the lymphocytes in the circulating and vascular pools to reach equilibrium and ensure that the sample contains a representative proportion of irradiated cells. Ideally, sampling should occur within 1 month of the exposure. After this time, the aberration yield will fall thus increasing the uncertainty in the dose estimate. In serious cases, where there is the likelihood of a severe drop in the white cell count, there may only be a few days after the accident when a viable blood specimen can be taken. In such cases, medical treatment may include blood transfusion and it is essential that a sample is obtained before this occurs.

Replicate cultures should be set up for 48–50 h (see *Protocol 1*) and the slides stained according to the FPG method (see *Protocol 2*).

6.3 Aberration scoring and dose estimation for acute recent exposures

All observable aberrations are scored, although only the dicentric frequency is used to estimate the radiation dose. At low frequencies there are considerable statistical uncertainties on the dose estimates. These are usually expressed as 95% confidence limits based on Poisson statistics. The confidence limits can be narrowed by increasing the number of cells scored. The decision on how many cells to score is usually a compromise based on the importance of the case, the time available, the quality of the preparations and the radiation dose. For a low or zero dicentric yield, 500 cells are routinely scored and this provides dose estimates of sufficient accuracy for most purposes. High doses can be detected by analysing comparatively few cells. Thus, following a major accident, cytogenetic analysis of just a few tens of cells can be invaluable for initially sorting patients into broad dose groups.

The lower limits of detection are usually based on finding 1 dicentric in 500 cells. At this level, which is approaching background, a number of other factors may confound and it is essential to identify age and anything in the individual's lifestyle (e.g. smoking) or working environment which could result in such a dicentric frequency. It is sometimes possible to consider previous exposure to radiation by assuming that lymphocytes carrying dicentrics have a half-life in the peripheral blood of 3 years. If detailed radiation records are available, then the recorded doses can be weighted appropriately and an estimate of the frequency of dicentrics expected from previous exposure established. Any increase over this can then be attributed to a new exposure.

The dose estimate is expressed as an equivalent whole body dose although in certain cases this may mask a partial body exposure. For a uniform whole-body exposure, the aberrations will be distributed amongst the cells according to Poisson expectations but with partial exposures there will be over-dispersion, with the aberrations contained in fewer cells. This is because a proportion of the lymphocytes will have been outside the radiation field. From the degree of over-dispersion, and making certain assumptions, it is sometimes possible to calculate the proportion of the body that has been irradiated, although in most cases, where the number of damaged cells is small, this is impractical.

Protocol 5

Determination of dose from dicentric frequency

Method

1   Score 500 first division metaphases from 48 to 50 h lymphocyte cultures recording all aberrations.

2   Using standard statistical tables for Poisson distributions determine the upper and lower 95% limits of the dicentric count.

3   Calculate the dicentric frequencies for the observed count and for the upper and lower limits.

4   Refer to the appropriate dose response curve for dose estimate and upper and lower confidence limits. (N.B. if the curve itself has wide errors, then these also will have to be taken into account, but in practice the variance due to the curve is usually small compared with the variance of the observed yield from the subject.)

6.4 Retrospective dosimetry

The development of FISH chromosome painting for the analysis of stable aberrations, e.g. translocations, offers potential for evaluating historical and chronic exposures, since translocation frequencies in peripheral blood lymphocytes have been shown to remain at steady levels for many years following exposure. Although a number of attempts have been made to assess individual dose in cases of past exposure using genomic translocation frequencies derived from analysis of 1000–2000 painted cells, considerable variation in translocation frequencies has been reported between apparently normal individuals and the use of FISH for individual biodosimetry is currently the subject of considerable debate (15). Translocation frequency is likely to be a measure of cumulative lifetime clastogenic exposure. Thus, while the effects of radiation exposure may be detectable in young people, the interpretation of translocation frequency in any one individual of an older age group may be difficult owing to the variability resulting from the increased influence of a range of confounding lifestyle factors.

7 Population monitoring

The incorporation of cytogenetic biomarkers in carcinogenicity/mutagenicity monitoring is becoming an increasingly important aspect of epidemiological studies assessing environmental health risks (1–3). However, while their use as markers of exposure is well established, the relevance of any particular endpoint and its method of induction needs to be evaluated in relation to any health out-come before the results of such studies can be directly applied to risk assessment (16,17). The nature and persistence of DNA damage induced by genotoxic agents will determine the type and degree of cytogenetic damage seen. Radiation-induced aberrations arise within a short time of exposure as a consequence of mis-repair and can remain in the circulating lymphocytes for a considerable time. In contrast, most chemicals produce aberrations exclusively during S phase irrespective of the cell cycle stage treated. Chemically induced DNA damage in non-cycling lymphocytes will not generally be converted into aberrations until the cells are stimulated to divide *in vitro* and chromatid-type aberrations will therefore predominate at the first mitosis. The time between exposure and sampling will allow cellular repair of lesions and only those that remain can be expressed as aberrations. Therefore, the quantitative approach used for radia-tion exposure, in which observed aberration frequencies can be directly related to exposure, must be applied with caution to chemical exposures. If an increase in aberrations is observed in a population suspected of being exposed to a chemical agent it is reasonable to assume that there has been some clastogenic exposure. However, no estimate of exposure level or of subsequent adverse health effects can safely be made. Conversely the absence of aberrations does not rule out an exposure. SCE are also replication dependent and their production will therefore be similarly influenced by post-exposure repair prior to sampling.

Although this Chapter deals only with cytogenetic endpoints in peripheral blood lymphocytes, assays for other genetic effects should also be considered and the choice of an appropriate genetic endpoint made with reference to the type and timing of the exposure. Extensive reviews are available (1–3) and only the key points which must be addressed will be described here. These include:

(1) Some idea of the nature of the clastogen and/or its source;

(2) Means of identifying the exposed population;

(3) Availability of a similar unexposed group to act as control;

(4) Some measure of exposure, i.e.
   (i) length of time exposed
   (ii) direct measurement of the agent either in the environment or patho-logically
   (iii) measurement of metabolites;

(5) Separation into different dose levels;

(6) Identification of confounding variables.

7.1 Setting up the study

Population monitoring is time consuming and expensive and it is advisable to know if the suspected mutagen has proved positive in short-term tests. Exposure should be quantified since the establishment of a dose–response relationship will support any suggestion that the association is causal. However, if resources are limited, initial studies can be restricted to a high-dose group. A statistical evaluation of the amount of work required to produce a reliable conclusion should be undertaken based on knowledge of expected background frequencies and the nature of the suspected exposure. Following identification of individuals in the exposed group, controls should be matched for confounding variables. As well as occupational and medical exposures to potential mutagens it should be appreciated that age and smoking have been found to have important influences on background frequencies of a range of cytogenetic endpoints (2,12,18,19). A questionnaire designed to provide relevant information on occupation, lifestyle and medical history (2) should be completed by each participant in the study.

7.2 Blood sampling, culturing and slide preparation

The exposed and the control groups should be sampled concurrently, randomly coded, and replicate cultures set up and stained for chromosome aberration analysis and SCE analysis (*Protocols 1, 2* and *3*) and micronucleus determination (*Protocol 4*), as appropriate. Culture conditions must be standardized particularly for the study of SCE.

7.3 Chromosome aberration analysis

It is usual to score 100–200 cells per individual using block staining for popula tions where exposure is expected to have been of recent occurrence. For populations with chronic or historical exposures FISH analysis for stable aberrations is more appropriate. Stable aberrations are likely to represent a lifetime's exposure to a wide range of genotoxins and it is therefore very important when using FISH for aberration analysis to match controls as closely as possible, in particular for age and smoking habits (15,18,19). A number of statistical tests are available for data analysis but there is no unified agreement on a proper statistical method. The choice will depend to some extent on the design of the study and the nature of the data collected. One approach is to use Poisson expectations to estimate standard errors and to perform a simple difference test (e.g. χ^2) on the means. In some studies distribution-free methods may be more appropriate.

7.4 Sister chromatid exchange analysis

A total of 50 cells, 25 from two replicate cultures should be scored for SCE analysis. A Student's *t*-test is most commonly used for data analysis.

7.5 Micronucleus analysis

At present, there is little quantitative data on background frequencies of micronuclei in human lymphocytes, and the technique has not been widely applied to exposed populations. However, recent technical advances have improved the reliability and sensitivity of the technique, and the simplicity of the endpoint and the potential for automation is likely to make it attractive for large-scale screening programs. For visual analysis, 1000 binucleate cells per sample should be examined for the presence of micronuclei and the group means can be compared by Student's *t*-test.

References

1. WHO (1985). *Guidelines for the study of genetic effects in human populations. Environmental health criteria 46.* WHO, Geneva.
2. Carrano, A. V. and Natarajan, A. T. (1988). *Mutat. Res.* **204**, 379.
3. WHO (1993). *Biomarkers and risk assessment: concepts and principles. Environmental health criteria 155.* WHO, Geneva.
4. IAEA (1986). *Biological dosimetry: chromosome aberration analysis for dose assessment. Technical report no. 260.* IAEA, Vienna.
5. Edwards, A. A. (1997). *Radiat. Res.* **148**, 539.
6. Savage, J. R. K. (1975). *J. Med. Genet.* **13**, 103.
7. Savage, J. R. K. and Simpson, P. J. (1994). *Mutat. Res.* **312**, 51.
8. Savage, J. R. K. and Simpson, P. J. (1994). *Mutat. Res.* **307**, 345.
9. Tucker, J. D., Morgan, W. F., Awa, A. A., Bauchinger, M., Blakey, D., Cornforth, M. N. *et al.* (1995). *Cytogenet. Cell Genet.* **68**, 211.
10. Lucas, J. N., Awa, A. A., Straume, T., Poggensee, M., Kodama, Y., Nakano, M. *et al.* (1992). *Int. J. Radiat. Biol.* **62**, 1, 53.
11. Morton, N. E. (1991). *Proc. Natl. Acad. Sci.* **88**, 7474.
12. Perry, P. E. and Thomson, E. J. (1984). In *Handbook of mutagenicity test procedures*, (ed. Kilbey, B. J., Legator, M., Nichols, W., and Rauel, C.), p. 495. Elselvier Science Publ., New York.
13. Tawn, E. J. and Earl, R. (1988). *J. Med. Genet.* **25**, 419.
14. Fenech, M. and Morley, A. A. (1985). *Mutat. Res.* **147**, 29.
15. Fluorescence *in situ* hybridization (FISH) biological dosimetry (2000) (ed. Edwards A. A.) *Radiat. Prot. Dosim.*, **88**, (1).
16. Tucker, J. D. and Preston, R. J. (1996). *Mutat. Res.* **365**, 147.
17. Albertini, R. J., Nicklas, J. A. and O'Neill, J. P. (1996). *Environ. Health Perspect.* **140** (Suppl. 3), 503.
18. Tucker, J. D. and Moore II, D. H. (1996). *Environ. Health Perspect.* **140**, 489.
19. Bolognesi, C., Abbondandolo, A., Barale, R., Casalone, R., Dalpra, L., De Ferrari, M. *et al.* (1997). *Cancer Epidemiol. Biomarkers Prevent.* **6**, 249.

Chapter 9

Chromosome instability syndromes

R.T. Howell

SW Regional Cytogenetics Centre, Southmead Hospital, Westbury on Trym, Bristol, BS10 5NB, UK

1 Introduction

A number of clinically diverse inherited human diseases, unified by the abnormal behaviour of their chromosomes, are sometimes grouped together under the heading of chromosome instability syndromes. Depending on the syndrome, the abnormal chromosome behaviour may take the form of:

- an elevated spontaneous aberration frequency
- an elevated level of SCE
- hypersensitivity to chromosome-damaging agents, manifesting as high levels of aberrations or SCE
- clonal or recurrent stable chromosome rearrangements.

As a part of normal cellular processes, the genetic material is under the management of a wide variety of proteins responsible for replication, repair, recombination, generation of novel immunoglobulin genes, sister chromatid exchange, cell cycling and chromosomal division. It is clear that a mutation responsible for a protein defect disrupting any one of these systems might have a serious effect. Recent advances in molecular methodology confirm the involvement of just such mutations in at least some of the disorders.

These single gene disorders mostly have an autosomal recessive mode of inheritance. The pleiotropic effect of the mutation results in a syndrome embracing a variety of clinical features, the abnormal chromosome behaviour being but a single manifestation. Despite their clinical diversity, some of the syndromes have important features in common, including tumour predisposition, immune deficiency, growth retardation and premature ageing—probably a direct consequence of the effect of genetic instability on normal patterns of cell proliferation. Identification of the genes involved, and the mechanism of activity of their protein products, is currently having an important impact on the understanding of cellular mechanisms, particularly with regard to tumourigenesis.

Ataxia telangiectasia, Fanconi anaemia and Bloom syndrome are the conditions originally grouped together in the 1960s as the classic 'chromosome breakage syndromes'. Analysis of chromosome instability still provides an important aid to the clinical diagnosis of these three syndromes, despite recent advances in molecular methodology and unravelling of the underlying molecular defects. There are a variety of reasons for discussing the other conditions included in the chapter: some are of diagnostic importance, whereas some are included simply for their interest to the cytogeneticist and to provide a complete picture. Diseases without a clear-cut genetic basis in which chromosomal instability has been reported, such as scleroderma and systemic lupus erythematosus, are not discussed.

1.1 Safe use of mutagenic chemicals

Some of the assays described in this chapter employ chromosome-breaking agents (clastogens) which are mutagenic and carcinogenic, and it is essential that safety guidelines are followed closely, that appropriate laboratory facilities are available, and that legal requirements and local policies are not countermanded. The following hints may be of value.

(a) **Containment.** Carry out all procedures involving mutagens in an approved exhaust protective cabinet and work in a tray or on polythene-backed absorbent paper, e.g. 'Benchkote' (Whatman). Keep all bottles in racks to prevent spillage. Store reagents in well-labelled sealed containers. Disposable latex or nitrile gloves, and a laboratory coat protected by a plastic apron are essential, plastic oversleeves and a face-mask are recommended.

(b) **Choice of clastogen.** Where possible, use a pre-weighed agent which can be dissolved within its vial. MMC (Sigma) and HN2 (as mustine hydrochloride, supplied by Sovereign Medical), are available in this form. DEB (Sigma) is a volatile liquid, and more difficult to contain safely. Bleomycin (Kyowa) is supplied in an ampoule. Ensure that the manufacturer's hazard data information is available.

(c) **Preparation.** Make a detailed written list of all the steps in the procedure and carry out a dummy run using a safe substitute solution. Have all containers, pipettes, etc., conveniently placed before beginning the treatment, and all solutions ready to make the dilutions.

(d) **Equipment.** Use only disposable bottles and pipettes.

(e) **Dispensing.** When dissolving substances within the vial by syringe and needle always use a second vent needle to avoid build-up of pressure. Make up intermediates in the dilution series in small volumes to minimize the extent of any spillage.

(f) **Cultures.** Keep cultures containing mutagens tightly capped and avoid the use of an open culture system.

(g) **Centrifugation.** Spin in sealed buckets, opening them only under exhaust protection.

(h) **Discards.** Place fluids in suitable decontaminating solutions. Two percentage potassium permanganate is recommended for MMC, 2% sodium thiosulphate for HN2, and 1 N HCl for DEB. MMC is also light-sensitive and HN2 has a half-life in solution of only 8 min. Seal used pipettes and containers securely in plastic bags and send for incineration. Small volumes of decontaminated solutions may be absorbed on vermiculite or Fuller's earth in sealable plastic containers for incineration. If discarding larger volumes of decontaminated solutions through the drains, wear gloves, apron and goggles, and flush with copious volumes of water.

2 Diseases for which chromosome analysis is used diagnostically

2.1 Ataxia telangiectasia

Ataxia telangiectasia has a prevalence of about 1 in 300 000 and has been described in different races. Recently, the gene for A-T, *ATM*, has been identified and localized within chromosome band 11q22.3 (1). Many different mutations occur, both frameshift and missense. The gene appears to have a function in controlling the progression of the cell cycle, and alerting the cell to the presence of DNA damage (2).

2.1.1 Clinical features

The major neurological features include a progressive cerebellar ataxia as the earliest clinical sign, presenting in infancy or early childhood, with diminished or absent deep reflexes, flexor or equivocal plantar responses, choreathetosis, oculomotor dyspraxia, and dysarthria (3). Several other features, for example bulbar telangiectasia, may be variable in presentation or onset may be age dependent. It is now apparent that certain mutations result in a milder phenotype, and in some instances, there is partial expression of the *ATM* gene.

A major feature of A-T is the predisposition to lymphoid tumours, lymphoma or lymphocytic leukaemias. In particular, a much higher proportion of lymphoid tumours affect T cells in A-T patients compared with normal individuals.

Serum AFP levels are elevated, and levels of IgA and IgE may be reduced. Both AFP and immunoglobulin levels can provide additional evidence for a diagnosis of A-T.

2.1.2 Cytogenetic characteristics

2.1.2.1 Spontaneous chromosome abnormalities

The incidence of fragments, chromatid gaps, chromatid breaks, and dicentric chromosomes is often increased, but this may not be observed in all patients. Independent of age, up to 10% of PHA-stimulated lymphocytes display stable translocations and inversions, often involving specific breakpoints on chromosome 7 and 14 (4), and these rearrangements provide a useful aid to diagnosis of A-T. However, it should be emphasized that they do also occur spontaneously in the

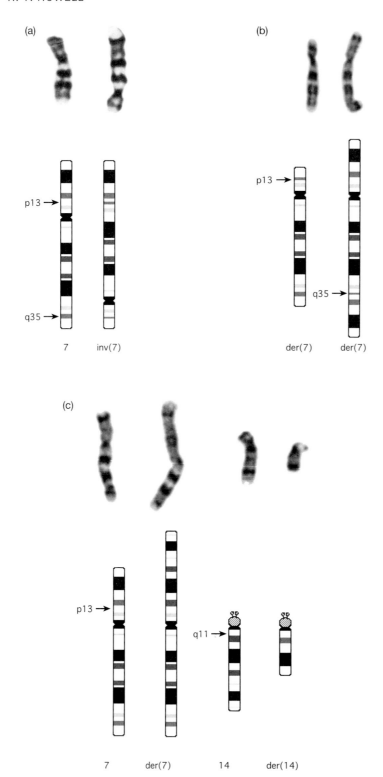

(a)

7   inv(7)

(b)

der(7)   der(7)

(c)

7   der(7)   14   der(14)

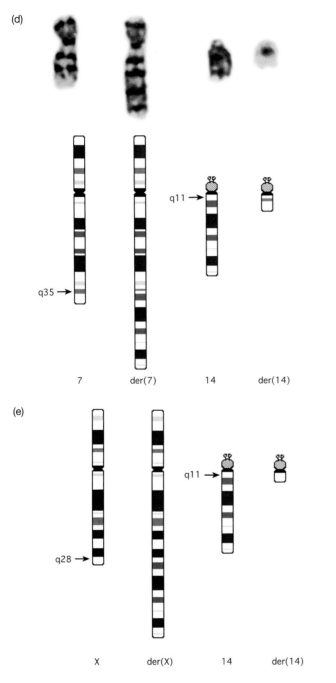

Figure 1 Typical stable rearrangements in ataxia telangiectasia include (a) inv(7)(p13q35); (b) t(7;7)(p13;q35); (c) t(7;14)(p13;q11); (d) t(7;14)(q35;q11); (e) t(X;14)(q28;q11).

normal population, albeit at a frequency 40–50 times lower. Typical rearrangements are inv(7)(p13q35), t(7;7)(p13;q35), t(7;14)(p13;q11), t(7;14)(q35;q11), t(X;14)(q28;q11) (*Figure 1*) t(14;14)(q11;q32) and inv(14)(q11q32) (see *Figure 11* Chapter 4). With the exception of Xq28, these breakpoint sites are the locations of immune system genes and in some instances have been confirmed to occur within T cell receptor genes. Some of these rearrangements may give rise to large clones in A-T patients and cells containing t(14;14), inv(14), or t(7;14)(q35;q32) have been reported to become malignant.

Other non-clonal translocations may be seen and also telomeric dicentrics, formed by the fusion of two chromosomes at the very tips. These dicentrics are observed at a high frequency only in the presence of large translocation clones.

Chromosome abnormalities noted in fibroblasts include telomeric dicentric chromosomes, but no examples of the translocations associated with T lymphocytes have been found. B lymphocytes display high levels of apparently random chromosome rearrangement.

2.1.2.2 Induced chromosome abnormalities

In more than 90% of families, blood cultures irradiated in the G_2 phase of the cell cycle show a much greater increase in chromatid-type damage (*Figure 2*) than normal controls. The differential between A-T and normal in terms of frequency of induced aberrations may be 4–20-fold, so that there is usually no ambiguity

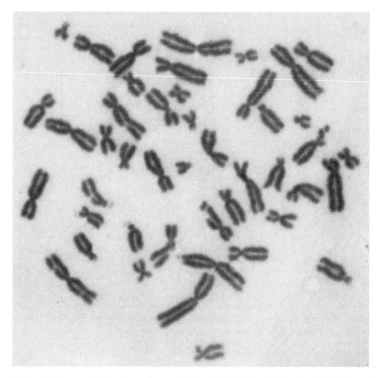

Figure 2 Chromatid breaks and gaps induced by G_2 X-irradiation in ataxia telangiectasia.

about this increased radiosensitivity. However, in about 10% of families without any major difference in clinical features, the level of X-ray induced damage may not be greatly different from that in normal individuals. With irradiation at G_0, the differential in the level of induced chromosome-type aberrations is not as great, but A-T cells show a much higher level of induced chromatid damage, a phenomenon rarely seen in normal cells.

2.1.2.3 Sister chromatid exchanges

Spontaneous SCE levels, and frequencies following exposure to a variety of agents, have all proved to be normal.

2.1.3 Diagnostic techniques

Despite identification of the gene, cytogenetic assays are used routinely as a dependable starting point for laboratory diagnosis. Having confirmed the diagnosis, a specialist laboratory may then undertake molecular analysis (generally by RT-PCR) to characterize the exact gene defects.

2.1.3.1 Blood cultures

The enhanced frequency of chromatid-type damage following G_2 X-irradiation provides the most reliable chromosomal method for diagnosis (*Protocol 1*). Because of the small proportion of patients who may not give a significant positive radiation response, it is important also to look for spontaneous chromosome changes: these are generally high in this group. The response of lymphocytes to PHA is often poor, and a low mitotic index may be expected.

Protocol 1

Induction of chromatid aberrations by G_2 X-irradiation

Equipment and reagents

As for Chapter 1, *Protocols 7* and *9*

- Suitable X-ray source

Method

1 Incubate standard PHA-stimulated blood cultures of the patient and control cultures from a sex-matched normal individual for 65–72 h at 37 °C (see Chapter 1, *Protocol 7*).

2 Expose cultures to 0.5 and 1.0 Gy X-rays. (One can typically use 245 keV, 12 mA, half-value thickness copper filters of 1 mm, a filter object distance of 30 cm and a dose rate of 1 Gy/min.) This operation should be performed as quickly as possible, not allowing the cultures to chill.

3 Incubate cultures for a further 3 h and add colcemid for 1 h before harvesting by conventional methods (see Chapter 1, *Protocol 9*). The period between irradiation and harvest should be 4 h, which is the time taken for most cells in G_2 to proceed to mitosis.

A variety of chromosomally radiomimetic drugs can also be employed, showing a two- to five-fold differential in induced damage between A-T and normal cells after treatment at G_2. Bleomycin (*Protocol 2*), neocarcinostatin, streptonigrin or tallysomycin may be used, but X-ray treatment is preferable since a more reliable and higher differential is generally obtained and the handling of highly toxic drugs can be avoided.

Protocol 2

G_2 bleomycin treatment of blood cultures

Equipment and reagents
As for Chapter 1, *Protocols 7* and *9*

- Bleomycin, vial of 15 000 units (Kyowa)[a]
- Micropipettor
- Sterile distilled water

Method

1 Incubate standard PHA-stimulated blood cultures of the patient and control cultures from a sex-matched normal individual for 65–72 h (see Chapter 1, *Protocol 7*).

2 Add 2.5 ml distilled water to the vial of bleomycin.

3 Add 25 μl of this solution to a 5 ml blood culture, or use 50 μl for a 10 ml culture, to give a final concentration of 30 μg/ml[b].

4 Incubate the cultures for a further 3 h and add colcemid for 1 h before harvesting by conventional methods (see Chapter 1, *Protocol 9*).

[a] Caution: refer to Section 1.1 for information regarding the safe use of this hazardous reagent. May cause heritable genetic damage and birth defects.

[b] The stock solution may be divided into small aliquots and stored frozen for future use provided safe containment facilities are available.

2.1.3.2 Prenatal diagnosis

A few pregnancies at risk for A-T have been screened for spontaneous or induced chromosome breakage by chromosomal radiosensitivity following exposure of amniotic or chorionic cells. In such cases, detailed knowledge of the level of radiosensitivity of the proband is essential (5). However, cytogenetic analysis might not be necessary, if the nature of the gene mutations in the proband has been identified by molecular analysis. The pregnancy at risk may then be screened for the presence of the same mutations.

2.1.4 Analysis and interpretation

A total of 50 banded cells are usually examined to identify the typical translocations and inversions involving chromosomes 7 and 14.

It is usual to examine 50 block-stained cells each, from cultures exposed to 0.5 and 1.0 Gy X-rays at G_2 (*Protocol 1*) and the same number from the matched control cultures. The presence of both translocations and a high level of radiation-induced damage supports a diagnosis of A-T. A high level of translocations with a lower level of induced aberrations would suggest a variant form of the disorder.

2.1.5 Heterozygotes

Although there is some conflicting epidemiological evidence, most studies suggest carriers of the A-T gene to have an increased risk of cancer, particularly breast cancer in women. Most reports indicate normal chromosomal radiosensitivity, although others suggest an increased level of X-ray-induced chromatid-type damage in fibroblasts and lymphocytes overlapping with the normal range. A recent report suggests that it might be possible to identify carriers cytogenetically by G_2 X-irradiation at a dose of 1 Gy (6).

2.2 Nijmegen breakage syndrome

2.2.1 Clinical features

A number of patients have been identified since the original description in 1979, by Hustinx *et al.* (7), who described a boy showing small size, microcephaly, mental retardation, *café-au-lait* spots on the skin, and immunodeficiency. Patients have a high incidence of lymphoid cancers.

2.2.2 Cellular characteristics

Recently, the gene (*NBS1*) for this autosomal recessive syndrome has been cloned and mapped to chromosome band 8q21. All mutations so far analysed have comprised the same 5 base pair deletion, indicating a founder mutation (8). There is evidence that the protein may be involved in response to DNA double-strand breaks, and possibly also meiotic recombination.

2.2.3 Cytogenetic characteristics

2.2.3.1 Spontaneous abnormalities

Studies on the original patient and his mother (7) showed a high level of chromosome rearrangements involving chromosomes 7 and 14, including inv(7)(p13q35), t(7;7)(p13;q35) and t(7;14)(p13;q11), that is, the same rearrangements as in A-T. The frequency of these translocations was 20–25% higher than in the average A-T patient. Spontaneous chromosome breakage in lymphocytes was low, again similar to A-T. SCE frequencies were also normal.

2.2.3.2 Induced aberrations

An increased chromosomal sensitivity to X-rays and bleomycin has been reported. Increased radiosensitivity is seen also as a decrease in colony-forming ability and a failure of inhibition of DNA synthesis.

2.2.4 Diagnosis

A combination of identification of the typical translocations and X-irradiation studies as for A-T should be undertaken. Prenatal diagnosis should be undertaken by a specialist molecular laboratory.

2.3 Bloom syndrome

Only about 100 living persons are known to have this autosomal recessive disease. The disorder is apparently relatively more frequent in Ashkenazic Jews than other ethic groups. The gene has been mapped to chromosome 15q26.1, and the protein product is a DNA helicase involved in unwinding DNA during replication (9). A reduced rate of replication fork progression also implies deficiency of replication rather than repair. Different mutations have been identified.

2.3.1 Clinical features

Growth retardation begins prenatally resulting in low birthweight, and continues postnatally, patients being consistently below the third centile for height and weight. An erythematous rash, prominent over the cheeks and bridge of nose and exacerbated by exposure to sunlight, appears during infancy. Spotty hypo- and hyper-pigmentation of the skin is also found. The facies are distinctively long and thin. Severe immune deficiency, in particular IgA and IgM, is usually found. Clinodactyly is common and polydactyly or syndactyly also occur in some cases. Bloom syndrome patients are susceptible to malignancy, especially acute leukaemia. Cases of Wilms tumour and carcinoma have also been reported. The oldest patient was 48 years, but many do not survive to adulthood.

2.3.2 Cytogenetic characteristics

2.3.2.1 Spontaneous sister chromatid exchange

The most remarkable cytogenetic characteristic of BS cells is the spontaneous frequency of SCE (*Figure 3*). This is consistent with the replication defect, since it has been demonstrated in normal cells that SCE frequencies are elevated when the rate of replication fork progression is retarded. In the original report (10) a mean of 89 SCE per cell was found, in comparison to a mean of seven per cell for the normal controls.

The majority of SCE occur at the second cell cycle in culture where DNA containing BrdU is used as the template for replication, whereas in normal cells the number of SCE occurring at the first and second cycles is the same. A minor population of cells with a normal SCE frequency is noted in some patients with BS, generally compound heterozygotes with two non-identical mutations. The reversion to normal phenotype is attributed to somatic crossing over at a point between the two mutations (9).

2.3.2.2 Spontaneous aberrations

These occur with abnormally high frequency, the original observation (10) identifying isochromatid breaks, commonly with sister chromatid reunion, transverse breakage at the centromere and distinctive symmetrical quadriradial chromatid interchanges in as many as 5% of cells (*Figure 4*). The last appear to be exchanges between identical points on the chromatids of homologous chromosomes, the term symmetrical in this context referring to the fact that the centromeres are opposite rather than adjacent.

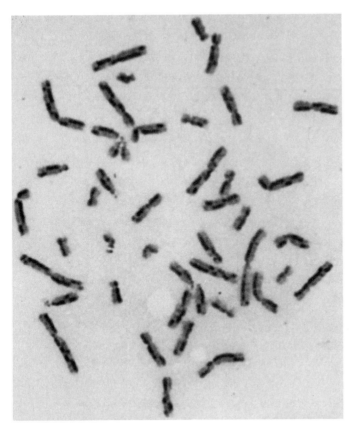

Figure 3 A high spontaneous sister chromatid exchange frequency, characteristic of Bloom syndrome.

2.3.2.3 Induced chromosomal changes

Bloom syndrome cells are known to be hypersensitive to ethylating agents (for example, ethyl methane sulphonate), as measured by SCE response.

2.3.3 Diagnostic techniques

Evaluation of the spontaneous SCE frequency provides the most rapid and reliable means of confirmation or exclusion. Any standard protocol for BrdU incorporation into cultured cells over two complete cycles is suitable (see Chapter 8, *Protocol 1*). The slow growth rate of BS cells means that some adjustment in timing may have to be made in order to recover sufficient harlequin-stained (second) metaphases in the event of the patient being affected. The possibility of poor growth must also be taken into account and duplicate cultures are advisable.

2.3.3.1 Blood

Grow in standard PHA-supplemented medium containing 10 µg/ml BrdU for 3, 4, and 5 days. Prepare slides in the usual way and stain for sister chromatid exchanges (see Chapter 8, *Protocols 1* and *2*).

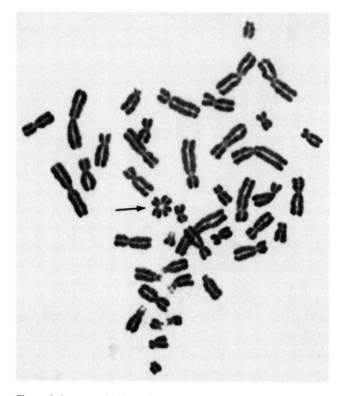

Figure 4 A symmetrical interchange between homologous chromosomes (arrowed), as observed in Bloom syndrome.

2.3.3.2 Amniotic fluid, chorionic villus and solid tissue cultures

Only a single report of prenatal diagnosis of an affected pregnancy has been published (11), where an SCE frequency of about 50 per cell was found in a primary culture of chorionic villus cells. Cells were harvested from a 2 ml tissue culture tube after 12 days' incubation in Chang medium (Irvine Scientific), with 10 µM BrdU added for the final 48 h. Fetal BS cells may grow more slowly than normal cells (which usually traverse one cycle in approximately 24 h), and to maximize the chance of recovering cells that have completed two cycles in the presence of BrdU, back-up or subcultures may be needed, to which BrdU has been added for 3 or 4 days.

2.3.3.3 Semidirect preparations from chorionic villi

Incubation for 48 h in BrdU-supplemented medium will provide a small proportion of second metaphases in normal villi (12). This could be sufficient to provide a rapid exclusion, but it is unlikely to be satisfactory for an affected pregnancy.

2.3.4 Analysis and interpretation

Examination of a small number of harlequin-stained metaphases is sufficient to confirm or exclude Bloom syndrome. The affected patient will have an SCE frequency of 60–100 per cell, compared with a normal baseline of less than 10

SCE per cell. However, note that a minor population of cells with a normal SCE level may be found. In the event of a poor yield of second metaphases, examination of post-second metaphases provides a useful confirmation: the numerous small patches of dark staining on otherwise pale chromatids are very distinctive. Unexpected observation of symmetrical homologous interchanges in the course of routine chromosome analysis indicates that a repeat sample should be requested for SCE studies.

Heterozygotes have normal SCE frequencies.

2.4 Fanconi anaemia

Fanconi anaemia is an autosomal recessive disorder with a heterogeneous genetic basis, the existence of up to eight complementation groups having been suggested. The gene for complementation group A (*FAA*), accounting for about 60% of cases, has been mapped to chromosome 16q, and *FAC* to 9q, but their functions are presently unknown. There is evidence of an impaired capacity to remove DNA interstrand crosslinks induced by alkylating agents, and patients are hypersensitive to the effects of alkylating drugs. The hypersensitivity is manifested as high levels of chromosomal damage in cultures exposed to alkylating agents such as MMC, DEB and HN2. This characteristic is exploited to provide the standard laboratory assay, which is still the method of choice of diagnosis in the majority of cases. Linkage analysis may be possible in certain families and has been employed successfully with the *FAC* gene.

FA cells are known to have an abnormal cell cycle with a G_2 phase transit delay and blockage. Based on this observation a flow cytometric method of diagnosis has also been used (13).

2.4.1 Clinical features

Generalized hypoplasia of the bone marrow results in neutropenia, thrombocytopenia, and reduced numbers of circulating red cells. Other clinical features include hypoplasia or aplasia of the radius associated with a low set or absent thumb, hypogonadism, a variety of cardiac defects, renal hypoplasia, growth retardation and patchy hyperpigmentation. The facial features are said to have a characteristic 'crowded' appearance in some patients. Manifestation of many of these features is variable and therefore a significant proportion of cases may escape confirmation until bone marrow failure occurs.

FA is strongly associated with an increased susceptibility to malignancy, in particular acute myeloid leukaemia, which occurs in approximately 9% of patients (14). Prognosis is poor. Other patients simply succumb to bone marrow failure or aplastic anaemia and survival beyond 20 years was rare in the past. Bone marrow transplantation is increasingly undertaken and improves the prognosis although there is evidence of an elevated risk of non-haematological malignancy. There is recent evidence (15) that up to 25% of patients display a 'somatic mosaicism' with two subpopulations of cells, one responding normally to alkylating agent stress, while the other is hypersensitive. These patients may have relatively mild haematological symptoms and improved survival. There appears to be a high chance of an affected sibling of a somatic mosaic patient also being mosaic (16).

2.4.2 Cytogenetic characteristics

2.4.2.1 Spontaneous aberrations

Cultured cells often contain damage in the form of chromatid breaks and exchanges in a significant proportion of cells. Chromosome type aberrations, such as dicentrics and rings, may also be observed, these being derived from chromatid damage at a previous cell cycle. Spontaneous damage may be detected regardless of time in culture as the inherent chromosomal instability results in the generation of new aberrations at each division. Premature chromosome condensation (PCC) may be noted, resulting from the incomplete disjunction of an unstable aberration at a prior division, and micronuclei may also be seen (See Chapter 8, Section 5)

2.4.2.2 Induced aberrations

Cultures exposed to DNA cross-linking agents including MMC, DEB, and HN2 display multiple aberrations, again as chromatid breaks and exchanges (*Figure 5*), at concentrations of the agent which induce little such damage in normal cells.

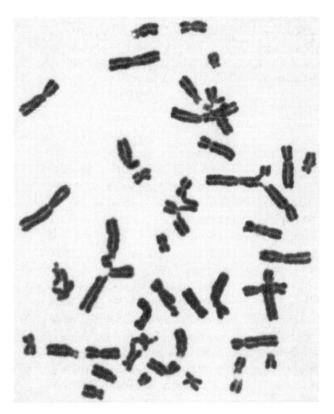

Figure 5 Multiple chromatid interchanges induced by nitrogen mustard in Fanconi anaemia.

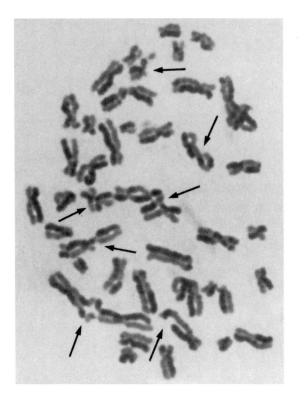

Figure 6 Following alkylating agent treatment of Fanconi anaemia cultures, a high aberration yield in conjunction with only a moderate increase in SCE frequency is typical. This harlequin-stained cell with approximately 30 SCE has four chromatid breaks and three interchanges (arrowed).

2.4.2.3 Sister chromatid exchanges

Spontaneous sister chromatid exchange levels are normal, but there are conflicting reports regarding the response to crosslinking agents. Higher, lower, and normal responses have been reported, possibly a result of cell cycle differences between FA and normal cells. As a general rule, induced SCE frequencies are not grossly abnormal (*Figure 6*).

2.4.2.4 Clonal changes in acute myeloid leukaemia

The most commonly occurring clonal abnormalities in those FA patients who develop AML are monosomy 7, translocations or duplications of the long arm of chromosome 1 (14).

2.4.3 Diagnostic techniques

Clearly, the confirmation of FA is extremely important, and it should be stressed that follow-up of siblings of affected individuals is equally vital. Presymptomatic patients have been identified in this way. A variety of protocols involving MMC, DEB or HN2 treatment at different stages of the culture period are employed to induce damage for the purpose of diagnosis. Pulse or continuous treatments are both effective. In developing these methods, evaluation of SCE response of normal cells exposed to the mutagen provides a good starting point, three to four times the baseline SCE frequency, indicating a satisfactory concentration. It is important to remember that the sensitivity of all cells to alkylating agents varies widely depending on the stage of the cell cycle at which the exposure occurs, and therefore large differences in aberration and SCE response can be demonstrated in cultures treated with the same concentration of mutagen at different times.

2.4.3.1 Blood cultures

Two protocols are given. DEB sensitivity (*Protocol 3*) is widely publicized as a reliable indicator of Fanconi anaemia, and its use is frequently specifically requested by the referring haematologist or paediatrician. There are various protocols for administering DEB, the simplest being to add it for the duration of a 3-day culture.

Treatment of an asynchronously growing culture during approximately the final cell cycle is employed in *Protocol 4*. In a 3-day blood culture, the majority of cells will pass through two or three cycles, although in Fanconi anaemia cells the growth rate may be somewhat retarded. Addition of an alkylating agent over the final 24 h of such a culture mainly results in exposure during the final cycle.

With any agent, treatment after 1 day of a 3-day culture can give variable results because of differences in the time of onset of the first S-phase between slower- and faster-growing cultures.

Protocol 3

DEB treatment of blood, for a 5-ml culture volume, to expose cells to a final concentration of 0.1 µg/ml DEB

Equipment and reagents

- Class 1 or 2 microbiological safety cabinet
- Complete medium (e.g. *Table 3* Chapter 1)
- Sterile distilled water
- BrdU stock solution[b] (see Chapter 8, *Protocol 1*)
- Micropipettor
- DEB[a]. This comes as a 1 ml bottle of liquid (Sigma, Cat. No. D7019)
- Bijou bottles for dilution series, containing 1 ml and 2 ml of distilled water

Method

1 Take four standard blood culture tubes (e.g. Chapter 1, *Protocol 7*) with 5 ml complete medium supplemented with 10 µg/ml BrdU (final concentration).

2 Inoculate two cultures with 0.3 ml of patient's blood, the other two with 0.3 ml blood from a normal control subject.

3 Treat two cultures (one from the patient, one from the control subject) with DEB as detailed in steps 4–6. This can be done at the time of initiation or later the same day. Leave the other pair of cultures untreated for estimation of the baseline SCE frequency.

Protocol 3 continued

4   Using a micropipettor, transfer 10 μl of DEB to 2 ml water and mix well.

5   Change the tip on the micropipettor and transfer 10 μl of this intermediate dilution to 1 ml water and mix well.

6   Change the tip on the micropipettor and transfer 10 μl of the second intermediate dilution to the 5-ml culture.

7   Incubate in the dark for 72 h and harvest by standard methods (see Chapter 1, *Protocol 9*).

[a] Suitable concentrations of other agents: 10^{-6} M MMC or 5×10^{-6} M HN2.

[b] BrdU and DEB may cause heritable genetic damage, and harm to the unborn child. Refer to Section 1.1 for information on safe containment.

Protocol 4

HN2 exposure of blood cultures to a final concentration of 10^{-7} M during the final cell cycle, suitable for a 5-ml culture volume

Equipment and reagents

Culture media and tubes as for *Protocol 3*

- Class 1 or 2 microbiological safety cabinet
- Micropipettor
- BrdU stock solution[b] (see Chapter 8, *Protocol 1*)
- 5 ml syringe and needle, containing 5 ml distilled water

- Spare needle for venting vial
- 10 mg vial of HN2[a,b] (mustine hydrochloride, Sovereign Medical)
- Three bijou bottles, one empty and the others with 0.5 ml and 0.6 ml distilled water, respectively

Method

1   Inoculate four 5 ml cultures with 0.3 ml of blood, two from the patient and two from a sex-matched control in standard medium with 10 μg/ml BrdU added.

2   Incubate in the dark for 48 h at 37 °C.

3   Pierce HN2 vial cap with a vent needle and syringe needle.

4   Add water to the vial and mix well.

5   Take a small amount into the empty bijou bottle.

6   Use a micropipettor to transfer 25 μl to the bottle containing 0.5 ml water.

7   After changing the tip, transfer 25 μl of this intermediate dilution to the bottle containing 0.6 ml water.

8   After changing the tip, transfer 25 μl of the second intermediate dilution to one patient and one control culture. Leave the other two cultures untreated in order to calculate baseline SCE frequencies.

243

Protocol 4 continued

9 Incubate for a further 24 h and harvest by standard methods (see Chapter 1, *Protocol 9*).

[a]Alternative treatments: 10^{-7} M MMC, 10^{-6} M DEB

[b]BrdU and HN2 may cause heritable genetic damage, and harm to the unborn child. Refer to Section 1.1 for information on safe containment.

2.4.3.2 Prenatal diagnosis

Requests for prenatal diagnosis are rare, but becoming more frequent following the diagnosis of upper limb reduction on fetal ultrasound scanning. One specialist laboratory has extensive published experience of a cytogenetic method (17) that involves evaluation of DEB-induced damage in amniotic fluid or chorionic villus cultures and is essentially the same for either type of sample. It may also be applied to postnatal solid tissue cultures (*Protocol 5*). Cell growth from long-term cultures may be impaired and, taking into account that *Protocol 5* involves two successive subcultures, the time required to obtain a result following second trimester amniocentesis may be unacceptably long. Therefore, first-trimester chorionic villus sampling is more appropriate. Alternatively, fetal blood sampling provides a specimen that can be subjected to the more familiar blood treatment methods (*Protocols 3* and *4*). With increasing knowledge of the gene defects there is a greater possibility of the molecular defect being identified in the proband, in which case molecular analysis would be a preferable strategy for prenatal diagnosis.

Protocol 5

DEB exposure to monolayer cultures for prenatal diagnosis of FA

Equipment and reagents

- Class 2 microbiological safety cabinet
- DEB[a]
- BrdU stock solution[a]

- Cultures as in Human cytogenetics: constitutional analysis, Chapter 3, *Protocols 4, 11, 12* or *13*, as appropriate

Method

1 Grow a primary culture in a 25 cm^2 tissue culture flask until it is ready to sub-culture.

2 Make three subcultures (see Human cytogenetics: constitutional analysis, Chapter 3, *Protocol 5*).

3 24 h after subculture add DEB to one flask to a final concentration of 10^{-7} M, keeping one flask as a control and one spare.

4 Incubate for a further 48 h.

5 Subculture the treated and control flasks 1:3 into medium containing 10 μg/ml BrdU (without DEB), seeding the flasks with different densities of cells for sequential harvest.

Protocol 5 continued

6   Harvest using a standard method after 24–96 h, depending on when sufficient cells
    are available, feeding cells as necessary with BrdU supplemented medium (see
    Human cytogenetics: constitutional analysis, Chapter 3, *Protocol 8*).

[a] BrdU and DEB may cause heritable genetic damage, and harm to the unborn child. Refer to
Section 1.1 for information on safe containment.

2.4.4 Analysis and interpretation

There are two approaches to the analysis of the data following mutagen exposure
of cultures. The first is to compare the aberration yield with the induced SCE
frequency in the same culture from the patient (18), the second is to compare the
induced aberration frequency in the patient's culture with that in cultures from a
normal individual matched for sex. Ideally, a combination of these two methods
should be available. Although the aberration yield in the affected patient may be
dramatically abnormal, sufficient cells must be examined to take account of the
possibility of the patient being a somatic mosaic. In the first instance:

(1) Count SCEs in five cells from each of the treated and untreated cultures from
    the patient;

(2) Examine 80 block-stained cells from treated cultures of the patient and re-
    cord the numbers of chromatid-type and chromosome-type gaps, breaks, and
    exchanges and the number of cells sustaining chromosomal damage. The
    number of aberrations per abnormal cell is also a useful statistic, as a somatic
    mosaic may have only a small number of damaged cells, each with multiple
    aberrations.

In untreated cultures from affected and unaffected patients, a baseline frequency
of between 5 and 10 SCE per cell will generally be found. In treated cultures, the
desired mean SCE frequency is between 20 and 50 per cell (*Figure 6*). At extremely
high SCE levels the aberration yield in normal cells will tend to increase and may
lead to ambiguous results.

Given a satisfactory SCE response in treated cultures, unaffected patients and
controls display an overall frequency of chromatid aberrations of between 0 and
0.5 per cell in the same culture. Few cells contain more than one aberration, and
only very occasionally are exchange-type aberrations encountered. Conversely,
the hypersensitive population of cells from the affected patient tend to sustain
heavy chromatid-type damage, often with a high proportion of the damaged cells
having more than one aberration, and many of the aberrations being exchanges
(*Figure 5*). Some chromosome-type aberrations may be encountered, derived
from chromatid damage induced at an earlier cell cycle.

With monolayer cultures, including prenatal diagnosis, the mitotic index of
treated cultures may be low, and it may not be possible to exclude mosaicism. If
necessary, it is possible to score aberrations and SCE in the same cells (*Protocol 6*)
using a simple B-dark harlequin staining method (19).

Protocol 6

Sequential scoring of aberrations and SCE in the same cells

Equipment and reagents

- Chromosome slide preparation from a culture grown in BrdU-supplemented medium (Chapter 8, *Protocol 1*)
- 0.3 M Na_2HPO_4, adjusted to pH 10.4 by the addition of ammonia solution (specific gravity 0.88)

- Sorensen's buffer, pH 6.8
- Giemsa stain
- Leishman stain (optional)
- Methanol in a Coplin Jar
- DPX (Merck)

Method

1   Block-stain the slide in Giemsa or Leishman stain in standard pH 6.8 buffer. Do not coverslip.

2   Score for aberrations, recording the coordinates for all cells.

3   Remove the immersion oil and stain by soaking the slide in a Coplin jar of methanol.

4   Rinse the slide in tap water and place it in a Coplin jar containing 50 ml of the pH 10.4 buffer.

5   Add 2 ml Giemsa stain, mix it well with the buffer and stain for 4 min.

6   Rinse the slide in tap water, blot dry and mount in DPX with a coverslip.

7   Relocate the same metaphases and score SCE in second divisions.

2.4.5 Monitoring bone marrow transplant patients

Bone marrow transplantation is increasingly used for treating FA patients. Confirmation of the disease is vital before preparing the patient for transplant as standard methods for reduction of the marrow must be modified to take account of the hypersensitivity to the drugs employed. Clearly, the exclusion of FA in potential sibling donors is also extremely important.

Sex mismatch transplantation is simply monitored by routine analysis of bone marrow samples, but where the donor is the same sex further stress tests can be performed and the results compared with those obtained prior to the transplant. Circulating lymphocytes of the recipient persist for a considerable time, although the numbers should fall progressively to a low level within a year if the transplant has succeeded. Using the standard blood protocols, a comparison can be made between the pre-transplant results and those obtained in successive samples taken post transplant. The important aspects to take into account when making the comparisons are:

(1) Similar SCE frequencies in cultures exposed to the same treatment regime on different occasions confirms that those cultures received a comparable treatment;

(2) Reduction of the patient's bone marrow by irradiation prior to transplant may result in surviving cells displaying significant levels of chromosome-type damage in the form of dicentrics and rings (see Chapter 8);

(3) An estimate of the ratio of donor to recipient cells can be made by recording in mutagen-treated cultures the numbers of 'significantly damaged cells'; that is, those with more than two breaks, or one interchange, or evidence of radiation-induced damage. Almost all such cells will be recipient in origin, and their frequency may be expected to fall progressively with increasing time following transplant.

2.4.6 Heterozygotes

Parents of children with FA, presumed to be obligate heterozygotes, have been investigated with respect to their chromosomal sensitivity to alkylating agents. As a group, they display a slightly elevated frequency of DEB-induced aberrations, but a considerable overlap with the control population excludes this phenomenon from being of value as a diagnostic test.

2.5 ICF syndrome

ICF syndrome (the acronym stands for immunodeficiency, centromeric heterochromatin instability and facial anomalies) is a recessively inherited disorder involving hypomethylation of DNA. It was recently mapped to chromosome 20, and mutations in the gene *DNMT3B* have been found in some patients. This gene encodes a DNA methyltransferase active in embryonic development and responsible for *de novo* DNA methylation (20). There is evidence that ICF syndrome is a recessively inherited disorder. The molecular defect is unknown but hypomethylation of DNA has been demonstrated (20).

2.5.1 Clinical features

Patients present with facial dysmorphism, developmental delay, mental retardation, recurrent and prolonged infection of the upper respiratory tract, malabsorption and immunodeficiency (21). There is evidence of variability in severity of clinical expression, the cytogenetically affected brother of one patient having only minor clinical signs (22).

2.5.2 Cytogenetic characteristics

The very distinctive chromosomal abnormality associated with this syndrome is observed in PHA-stimulated lymphocyte cultures as uncondensed constitutive heterochromatin in the paracentromeric regions of chromosomes 1, 9 and 16. Stretching or breaking of the centromeric region and association of the centromeres of these chromosomes may be seen, and multibranched chromosomes, particularly involving chromosome 1, occur in up to 40% of lymphocytes (*Figure 7*). Long- or short-arm deletions of 1 and 16, or isochromosome 1q, may also be found. The effect varies between patients, as only in some is there involvement of all three chromosomes. In general, chromosome 1 is the most affected and

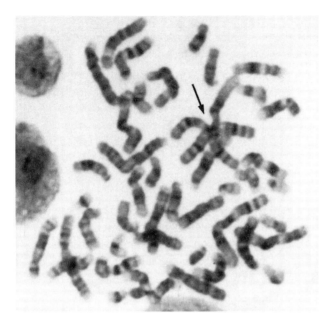

Figure 7 A typical star-shaped configuration in ICF syndrome. One chromosome 1 (arrowed) has four copies of the long arm radiating from the centromeric region.

chromosome 9 the least. Other chromosomes, particularly 2 and 10, are also seen to have abnormal centromeres in some patients.

The instability has been reported to occur in EBV-transformed B lymphocytes but no evidence has been found of multibranched formations in fibroblast cultures. SCE frequencies are normal.

2.5.3 Prenatal diagnosis

There are no reports of attempts at prenatal diagnosis, but amniocytes or chorionic tissue may not be reliable for the detection of the instability, and recourse to fetal blood would probably be necessary.

2.6 Roberts syndrome

This is an autosomal recessive syndrome involving severe deficiencies of the limb long bones associated with cleft palate. The SC–phocomelia syndrome is now considered to represent a variant of Roberts syndrome without cleft palate. Heart and renal defects are also found.

2.6.1 Cytogenetic characteristics

The chromosomes exhibit a characteristic morphology with lack of a defined centromeric constriction, a phenomenon especially clear in C-banded preparations where many of the centromeric C-bands appear as paired dots (*Figure 8*). This apparently results from PCD. Some chromosomes may splay outwards at the centromeres, and particularly distinctive is the 'puffing' of the paracentromeric heterochromatic regions of 1,9, and 16, and the Yq heterochromatin, resulting from despiralization and repulsion between sister chromatids.

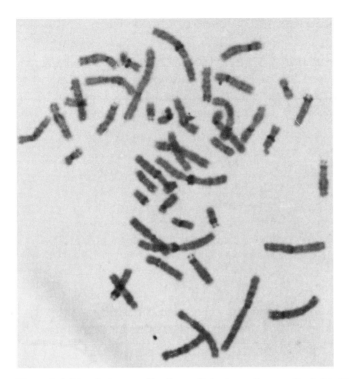

Figure 8 A C-banded preparation from a Roberts syndrome patient showing premature separation of the centromeres, many of the C-bands appearing as double dots. Puffing of the 1 and 9 heterochromatin can be seen. (Photograph supplied by Katie Waters, Kennedy Galton Centre for Clinical Genetics, Harrow, UK.)

The morphological anomaly is apparently related to an authentic abnormality of chromosome behaviour, with random chromosome loss or gain being found in a significant proportion of cells, presumably as the consequence of impaired centromere function. Extra chromosomes may be found in 10–20% of metaphases.

2.6.2 Diagnostic techniques

No specialized culture methods are required, as the centromere puffing phenomenon has been demonstrated in a variety of cultured tissues grown under standard conditions. Examination of C-banded preparations may help.

Prenatal confirmation of Roberts syndrome has been made cytogenetically in amniotic fluid cells following the identification of symmetrical tetra-phocomelia by ultrasound. Benzacken *et al.* (23) reported centromere puffing and chromatid repulsion in more than 10% of amniotic cells, and also noted high frequencies of aneuploid metaphases and micronuclei.

Chromosome analysis may be valuable in detecting mildly affected patients, and there are published examples of the typical chromosome picture occurring in patients with relatively minor reductions of the upper limbs, one such patient being diagnosed as having Baller–Gerold syndrome (24).

2.7 Dominantly inherited premature centromere division

Premature centromere division resulting in metaphase chromosomes without well-defined centromeric constrictions has been reported in association with reduced fertility, and with a possible susceptibility to aneuploid offspring. The PCD manifests in lymphocyte but not long-term monolayer cultures. Dominant inheritance has been suggested, PCD having been demonstrated in parents and offspring (25).

2.8 Werner syndrome

Werner syndrome is a recessively inherited disorder of premature ageing. The main features are growth deficiency and severe degenerative changes affecting different tissues. Premature greying of the hair occurs, cataracts are common, and there are striking skin changes involving thinning and atrophy. A high level of tumours, especially sarcomas, has been noted.

2.8.1 Cellular characteristics

The gene, mapped to the short arm of chromosome 8, encodes a protein with helicase activity, that is, it catalyses DNA unwinding. This gene and the gene for Bloom syndrome belong to a family of RecQ-type helicases.

2.8.2 Cytogenetic characteristics

Chromosome studies to confirm Werner syndrome are rarely requested. However, the observation of multiple different clones containing stable translocations in fibroblast cultures, 'variegated translocation mosaicism' (VTM), is an indicator (26). Fibroblast cultures may be very slow to grow and difficult to passage. Lymphocyte chromosomes do not consistently have the marked increase in spontaneous instability associated with other breakage syndromes, although a somewhat higher level of chromatid breaks, isochromatid breaks and chromatid interchanges may be observed.

Chromosomal sensitivity in lymphocytes to bleomycin has been shown to be normal, but the cells were found to be twice as sensitive to diepoxybutane, and after 4-nitroquinoline oxide exposure the frequency of chromatid gaps and breaks was about four times that of normal cells. SCE frequencies appear to be normal.

3 Other syndromes displaying chromosome instability

3.1 Xeroderma pigmentosum

Xeroderma pigmentosum is an autosomal recessive disorder, with a number of variant forms, resulting from defects in enzymes involved in repair of damage to DNA induced by UV light.

3.1.1 Clinical features

Patients have an extreme sensitivity to UV light and an increased likelihood of developing skin tumours early in life, particularly on sun-exposed areas. The tumours include basal cell and squamous cell carcinomas and malignant melanoma.

3.1.2 Cellular characteristics

In most patients, there is a defect in the initial steps of the nucleotide excision repair pathway. Cells from all patients are hypermutable by UV irradiation and cultured cells from most show an increased sensitivity to the killing effect of UV. At least seven complementation groups are generally accepted, designated XP-A to XP-G, identified by cell fusion studies.

Xeroderma pigmentosum is a multilocus rather than a multi-allelic disorder, and a number of genes and proteins responsible for the disease have been identified.

3.1.3 Diagnostic methods

Classical XP cells can be distinguished from normal cells by detection of the low level of UV-induced unscheduled DNA synthesis (repair synthesis) compared with normals. As well as being a standard method for the postnatal confirmation of XP, this approach has been used in amniocytes to allow prenatal diagnosis and exclusion in a number of cases. Molecular analysis of the gene defect in a proband would now be the logical starting point for prenatal diagnosis.

3.1.4 Cytogenetic characteristics

Unlike A-T, BS or FA, there is no consistent evidence of increased levels of spontaneous chromosome abnormalities in lymphocytes or fibroblasts. Following exposure to UV, however, cells display a higher level of induced SCE and aberrations than normal. The aberrations are mainly chromatid type. Fibroblasts are also unusually sensitive to 4-nitroquinoline oxide and N-acetoxy-aminofluorene. There are no established chromosomal methods for the diagnosis of XP.

3.2 Cockayne syndrome

This is a recessively inherited syndrome involving sensitivity to UV and defective transcription coupled repair, a subpathway of nucleotide excision repair responsible for the preferential removal of DNA lesions from the transcribed strand of an active gene. There are two different genes, *CSA* and *CSB*.

3.2.1 Clinical features

Growth deficiency, mental retardation, weakness with peripheral neuropathy, and deafness are found. The cranium is small and the facies distinctive with a slender nose and sunken eyes. There is no reported increased susceptibility to skin tumours or other malignancy.

3.2.2 Diagnostic methods

Prenatal diagnosis and exclusion has previously been made by the examination of the level of RNA synthesis in cultured amniocytes following exposure to UV light. While in normal exposed cells the level was 50–100% of the unexposed control, in Cockayne syndrome cells the level was reduced to less than 20% of non-irradiated cells (27). Recently, the preferred strategy is molecular analysis, undertaken by a specialist centre.

3.2.3 Cytogenetic characteristics

As with XP, no evidence has been found of increased levels of spontaneous chromosome abnormalities, but UV-induced aberration frequencies have been shown to be about 10 times greater than the normal range, most aberrations being chromatid breaks. UV light also induces a higher than normal level of SCEs.

3.3 Trichothiodystrophy

Hair abnormality associated with defective sulphur metabolism is a feature of a number of different diseases, in some of which photosensitivity is also found. Some of these cases have been shown to have excision repair defects with properties identical to one of the XP complementation groups.

3.4 Rothmund Thomson syndrome

3.4.1 Clinical features

In this autosomal recessive syndrome, there are multiple skin lesions including atrophic and depigmented changes, and telangiectasia; scarring may result from photosensitive dermatitis. Cataracts, sparse hair, skeletal malformations, dystrophic teeth and nails, and hypogonadism are also observed. An elevated incidence of certain malignancies is found, particularly cutaneous epithelioma and osteosarcoma.

3.4.2 Cellular characteristics

There is evidence for a diminished DNA repair capacity in fibroblasts, for enhanced *in vitro* radiosensitivity of lymphocytes and for undue *in vivo* sensitivity to cancer chemotherapy, indicating the possibility of a DNA repair defect

3.4.3 Cytogenetic characteristics

An elevated level of chromosome damage following G_2 irradiation has been reported (28).

Acknowledgement

The contribution of Professor AMR Taylor to the previous version of this chapter that appeared in the second edition of this Volume (1992) is gratefully acknowledged.

References

1. Savitsky, K., Sfez, S., Tagle, D. A., Ziv, Y., Sartiel, A., Collins, F. S. *et al.* (1995). *Hum. Mol. Genet.* **4**, 2025.

2. Lehmann, A. R. and Carr, A. M. (1995). *Trends Genet.* **11**, 375.

3. Boder, E. (1985). In *Ataxia telangiectasia: genetics, neuropathology and immunology of a degenerative disease of childhood* (ed. Gatti R. A. and Swift M.), pp. 1–63. Alan R. Liss, New York.

4. Taylor, A. M. R. (1982). In *Ataxia telangiectasia. A cellular and molecular link between cancer, neuropathology and immune deficiency* (ed. B. A. Bridges and D. G. Harnden), pp. 53–82. John Wiley, Chichester.

5. McConville, C. M., Woods, C. G., Farrall, M., Metcalfe, J. A., and Taylor A. M. R. (1990). *Hum. Genet.* **85**, 215.

6. Tchirkov, A., Bay, J-O., Pernin, D., Bignon, Y-J., Pascale, R., Grancho, M. *et al.* (1997). *Hum. Genet.* **101**, 312.

7. Hustinx, T. W. J., Scheres, J. M. J C., Weenmaes, C. R., ter Haar, B. G. A., and Janssen, A. H. (1979). *Hum. Genet.* **49**, 199.

8. Matsuura, S., Tauchi, H., Nakamura, A., Kondo, N., Sakamoto, S., Endo, S. *et al.* (1998). *Nat Genet.* **19**, 179.

9. Ellis, N. A., and German, J. (1996). *Hum. Mol. Genet.* **5**, 1457.

10. Chaganti, R. S. K., Schonberg, S., and German, J. (1974). *Proc. Natl. Acad. Sci. USA* **71**, 4508.

11. Howell, R.T., and Davies, T. (1994). *Prenat. Diagn.* **14**, 1071.

12. Zahed, L., Murer-Orlando, M., and Bobrow, M. (1988). *Hum. Genet.* **80**, 127.

13. Schindler, D., Kubbies, M., Hoehn, H., Schinzel, A., and Rabinovitch, P. S. (1985). *Lancet* **i**, 937.

14. Auerbach, A. D. and Allen, R. G. (1991). *Cancer Genet. Cytogenet.* **51**, 1.

15. Lo Ten Foe, J.R., Kwee, M. L., Rooimans, M. A., Oostra, A. B., Veerman, A. J. P., van Weel, M. *et al.* (1997). *Eur. J. Hum. Genet.*, **5**, 137.

16. Nobbs, M. and Howell, R.T. (1998). *J. Med. Genet.* **35**(Suppl. 1), S48.

17. Auerbach, A. D., Ghosh, R., Pollio, P. C., and Zhang, M. (1989). In *Fanconi anemia; clinical, cytogenetic and experimental aspects* (ed. Schroeder-Kurth, T. M., Auerbach, A. D. and Obe, G.), pp. 71–82. Springer-Verlag, Berlin.

18. Howell, R. T. (1991). *J. Med. Genet.* **28**, 468.

19. Aghamohammadi, S. Z., and Savage, J. R. K. (1990). *Chromosoma* **99**, 76.

20. Hansen, R. S., Wijmenga, C., Luo, P., Stanek, A. M., Canfield, T. K., Weemaes, C. M., Gartler, S. M. (1999). *Proc. Natl. Acad. Sci. USA.* **96**, 14412.

21. Maraschio, P., Zuffardi, O., Dalla Fiovi, T., and Tiepolo, L. (1988). *J. Med. Genet.* **25**, 173.

22. Gimelli, G., Varone, P., Pezzolo, A., Lerone, M., and Pistoia, V. (1993). *J. Med. Genet.* **30**, 429.

23. Benzacken, B., Savary, J. B., Manouvrier, S., Bucourt, M., and Gonzales, J. (1996). *Prenat. Diagn.* **16**, 125.

24. Huson, S. M., Rodgers, C. S., Hall, C. M., and Winter, R. M. (1990). *J. Med. Genet.* **27**, 371.

25. Madan, K., Lindhout, D., and Palan, A. (1987). *Hum. Genet.* **77**, 193.

26. Salk, D. J. (1982). *Hum. Genet.* **62**, 1.

27. Lehmann, A. R., Francis, A. J., and Gianelli, F. (1985). *Lancet* **i**, 486.

28. Kerr, B., Ashcroft, G. S., Scott, D., Horan, M. A., Ferguson, M. W. J., and Donnai, D. (1996). *J. Med. Genet.* **33**, 928.

Further reading

Auerbach, A. D., and Verlander, P.C. (1997). *Curr. Opin. Pediatr.* **9**, 600.

Cohen, M. M., and Levy, H. P (1989). In *Advances in human genetics* (ed. Harris H. and Hirschhorn K.), Vol. 18, pp. 43–149. Plenum Press, New York.

Sandberg, A. A. (1990). *The Chromosomes in human cancer and leukemia*, 2nd edn, pp. 174–215. Elsevier, New York and Amsterdam.

Woods, C.G. (1998). *Arch. Dis. Child.* **78**, 178.

Appendix 1
List of suppliers

Abbott Diagnostics Division, Abbott House, Norden Road, Maidenhead, Berkshire SL6 4XF, UK.
Tel: 01628 644203

Advanced Protein Products Ltd, UK, Unit 18H Premier Partnership Estate, Leys Road, Brockmoor, Brierly Hill, West Midlands DY5 3UP, UK.

Agar Scientific Ltd, 66a Cambridge Road, Stansted, Essex CM24 8DA, UK.

Amersham
Amersham International plc, Lincoln Place, Green End, Aylesbury, Buckinghamshire HP20 2TP, UK.
Amersham Corporation, 2636 South Clearbrook Drive, Arlington Heights, IL 60005, USA.

Amersham Pharmacia BioTech
Pharmacia Biotech (Biochrom) Ltd, Unit 22, Cambridge Science Park, Milton Road, Cambridge CB4 0FJ, UK.
Tel: 01223 423723
Fax: 01223 420164
URL: http://www.biochrom.co.uk
Pharmacia and Upjohn Ltd, Davy Avenue, Knowlhill, Milton Keynes, Buckinghamshire MK5 8PH, UK.
Tel: 01908 661101
Fax: 01908 690091
URL: http://www.eu.pnu.com

Anachem, 20 Charles Street, Luton, Bedfordshire LU2 0EB, UK.

Anderman and Co. Ltd, 145 London Road, Kingston-upon-Thames, Surrey KT2 6NH, UK.
Tel: 0181 541 0035
Fax: 0181 541 0623

Antec International Ltd, Winham Road, Sudbury, Suffolk, UK.
Tel: 01787 377305

Applied Biosystems
Applied Biosystems, Kelvin Close, Birchwood Science Park North, Warrington, Cheshire WA3 7PB, UK.
Applied Biosystems, 850 Lincoln Center Drive, Foster City, CA 94404-1128, USA.
Applied Biosystems GmbH, Brunnenweg 13, Weiterstadt D–64331, Germany

Applied Imaging
Applied Imaging, 2380 Walsh Avenue, Building B, Santa Clara, CA 95051, USA.
Applied Imaging International Ltd, Bioscience Centre, Times Square, Scotswood Road, Newcastle upon Tyne NE1 4EP, UK.

Appligene Oncor, Pinetree Centre, Durham Road, Birtley, Chester-le-Street, Co Durham DH3 2TD, UK.

Appligene Oncor Molecular Cytogenetics Division, Qbiogene, Salamander Quay West, Park Lane, Harefield, Middlesex UB9 6NZ.
Tel: 01895 453 7605   Fax: 01895 453705

Baxter Diagnostics Inc., Deerfield, IL 60015-4633, USA.

Beckman Coulter Inc.
Beckman Coulter Inc., 4300 N Harbor Boulevard, PO Box 3100, Fullerton, CA 92834-3100, USA.
Tel: 001 714 871 4848
Fax: 001 714 773 8283
URL: http://www.beckman.com

Beckman Coulter (UK) Ltd, Oakley Court, Kingsmead Business Park, London Road, High Wycombe, Buckinghamshire HP11 1JU, UK.
Tel: 01494 441181   Fax: 01494 447558
URL: http://www.beckman.com
Beckman Instruments UK Ltd, Progress Road, Sands Industrial Estate, High Wycombe, Buckinghamshire HP12 4JL, UK.

Becton Dickinson and Co.
Becton Dickinson and Co., 21 Between Towns Road, Cowley, Oxford OX4 3LY, UK.
Tel: 01865 748844   Fax: 01865 781627
URL: http://www.bd.com
Becton Dickinson and Co., 1 Becton Drive, Franklin Lakes, NJ 07417-1883, USA.
Tel: 001 201 847 6800
RL: http://www.bd.com
Becton Dickinson Europe, 5 Chemin des Sources, 38241 Meylan, France.

BDH Laboratory Supplies, Broom Road, Poole, Dorset, UK.

Bibby Sterilin Ltd, Tilling Drive, Stone, Staffordshire ST15 0SA, UK.

Bio 101 Inc.
Bio 101 Inc., c/o Anachem Ltd, Anachem House, 20 Charles Street, Luton, Bedfordshire LU2 0EB, UK.
Tel: 01582 456666   Fax: 01582 391768
URL: http://www.anachem.co.uk

Bio 101 Inc., PO Box 2284, La Jolla, CA 92038-2284, USA.
Tel: 001 760 598 7299
Fax: 001 760 598 0116
RL: http://www.bio101.com

Biomedical Specialties, Box 1687, Santa Monica, CA 90406, USA.

Bio-Rad Laboratories Ltd
Bio-Rad Laboratories Ltd, Bio-Rad House, Maylands Avenue, Hemel Hempstead, Hertfordshire HP2 7TD, UK.
Tel: 0181 328 2000   Fax: 0181 328 2550
URL: http://www.bio-rad.com
Bio-Rad Laboratories Ltd, Division Headquarters, 1000 Alfred Noble Drive, Hercules, CA 94547, USA.
Tel: 001 510 724 7000
Fax: 001 510 741 5817
URL: http://www.bio-rad.com
Bio-Rad Micromeasurements Ltd, Haxby Road York, North Yorkshire YO3 7SD, UK.
URL: http://www.bio-rad.com/index1.html

Biological Industries Ltd, Media House, Dunnsrood Road, Ward Park South, Cumbernauld, Glasgow G67 3ET, UK.

BioWhittaker UK Ltd, BioWhittaker House, 1 Ashville Way, Wokingham, Berkshire RG41 2PL, UK.

Boehringer Mannheim
Boehringer Mannheim Corp., 9115 Hague Road, PO Box 50414, Indianapolis, IN 46250-0414, USA.
URL:http://biochem.boehringer-mannheim.com/
Boehringer Mannheim UK (Diagnostics and Biochemicals) Ltd, Bell Lane, Lewes, E Sussex BN7 1LG, UK.

Boro Labs Ltd, Paices Hill, Aldermaston, Berkshire RG7 4QU, UK.

BRSL (Brian Reece Scientific Ltd), 12 West Mills, Newbury, Berkshire RG14 5HG, UK.

Calbiochem–Novabiochem Corp., P.O. Box 12087, La Jolla, CA 92039-2087, USA. URL: http://www.calbiochem.com/

Cambio Ltd, 34 Millington Road, Cambridge CB3 9HP, UK.

Camlab Ltd, Trinity Hall farm Industrial Estate, Nuffield Road, Cambridge CB4 1TH, UK.

Chiron Diagnostics (formerly Ciba Corning Diagnostics) Ltd, Colchester Road, Halstead, Essex CO9 2DX, UK.

Citifluor Ltd, University of Kent, Canterbury, UK.
Tel: 01227 827733

Collaborative Biomedical Products, Two Oak Park, Bedford, MA 01730, USA.

Collagen Biomaterials, Palo Alto, CA 94303, USA.

Corning
Corning Inc., PO Box 5000, Corning, NY 14831, USA.
Corning Costar UK, One The Valley Centre, Gordon Road, High Wycombe, Buckinghamshire HP13 6EQ, UK.

Costar, 1 Alewife Center, Cambridge, MA 02140, USA.

CP Instrument Co. Ltd, PO Box 22, Bishop Stortford, Hertfordshire CM23 3DX, UK.
Tel: 01279 757711   Fax: 01279 755785
URL: http://www.cpinstrument.co.uk

Cytocell Ltd, Somerville Court, Banbury Business Park, Adderbury, Banbury, Oxfordshire OX17 3SN, UK.

DAKO Ltd, Denmark House, Angel Drove, Ely, Cambridge CB7 4ET.
Tel: 01353 669911   Fax: 01353 668989

Difco Laboratories (see Becton Dickinson).

Dupont
Dupont (UK) Ltd, Industrial Products Division, Wedgwood Way, Stevenage, Hertfordshire SG1 4QN, UK.
Tel: 01438 734000   Fax: 01438 734382
URL: http://www.dupont.com
Dupont Co. (Biotechnology Systems Division), PO Box 80024, Wilmington, DE 19880-002, USA.
Tel: 001 302 774 1000
Fax: 001 302 774 7321
URL: http://www.dupont.com

Eastman Chemical Co., 100 North Eastman Road, PO Box 511, Kingsport, TN 37662-5075, USA.
Tel: 001 423 229 2000
URL: http://www.eastman.com

Eastman Kodak
Eastman Kodak Ltd, P.O. Box 66, Station Road, Hemel Hempstead, Hertforshire HP1 1UJ, UK.
Eastman Kodak, 25 Science Park, New Haven, CT 06511, USA.
European Collection of Animal Cell Culture, Division of Biologics, PHLS Centre for Applied Microbiology and Research, Porton Down, Salisbury, Wiltshire SP4 0JG, UK.

Falcon (Falcon is a registered trademark of Becton Dickinson and Co.)

Fisher Scientific
Fisher Scientific, Fisher Research, 2761 Walnut Avenue, Tustin, CA 92780, USA.
Tel: 001 714 669 4600
Fax: 001 714 669 1613
URL: http://www.fishersci.com
Fisher Scientific Co., 711 Forbest Avenue, Pittsburgh, PA 15219-4785, USA.
Fisher Scientific UK Ltd, Bishop Meadow Road, Loughborough, Leicestershire LE11 5RG, UK.
Tel: 01509 231166   Fax: 01509 231893
URL: http://www.fisher.co.uk

Flow Laboratories, Woodcock Hill, Harefield Road, Rickmansworth, Hertfordshire WD3 1PQ, UK.

Flowgen Instruments Ltd, Broadoak Enterprise Village, Broadoak Road, Sittingbourne, Kent ME9 8AQ, UK.

Fluka

Fluka, PO Box 2060, Milwaukee, WI 53201, USA.   Tel: 001 414 273 5013
Fax: 001 414 2734979
URL: http://www.sigma-aldrich.com
Fluka-Chemie AG, CH–9470, Buchs, Switzerland.
Fluka Chemical Co. Ltd, PO Box 260, CH–9471, Buchs, Switzerland.
Fluka Chemicals Ltd, The Old Brickyard, New Road, Gillingham, Dorset SP8 4JL, UK.
Tel: 0041 81 745 2828
Fax: 0041 81 756 5449
URL: http://www.sigma-aldrich.com

Gibco BRL

Gibco BRL (Life Technologies Inc.), 3175 Staler Road, Grand island, NY 14072-0068, USA.
Gibco BRL (Life Technologies Ltd), Trident House, Renfrew Road, Paisley PA3 4EF, UK.

Grant Instruments (Cambridge) Ltd, Barrington, Cambridge CB2 5QZ, UK.

Greiner

Greiner Labortek Ltd, Station Road, Cam, Dursley, Gloucestershire GL11 5NS, UK.
Greiner Labortke GmbH, Maybachstrasse 2, D–7443 Frickenhausen, Germany.

Hamilton

Hamilton (GB) Ltd, Lyne Riggs Estate, Lancaster Road, Carnforth, Lancashire LA5 9EA, UK.
Hamilton Company, PO Box 10 030, Reno, Nevada 89520, USA.
Hamilton Bonaduz AG, PO Box 26, CH-7402, Bonaduz, Switzerland.
Hamilton Deutschland GmbH, P.O. Box 110 565, D-64220 Darmstadt, Germany.

Philip Harris Scientific, 618 Western Avenue, Park Royal, London W3 0TE, UK.

Heraeus

Heraeus Instruments GmbH, PO Box 1563, Hanau, D–63405, Germany.
Heraeus Instruments Inc., 11A Corporate Boulevard, South Plainfield, NJ 07080, USA.
Heraeus Instruments Ltd, Unit 9, Wates Way, Brentwood, Essex CM15 9TB, UK.

Hewlett-Packard Company, 2850 Centreville Road, Wilmington, Delaware, USA 19808
URL: http://www.zorbax.com/

Histolab Products, Hulda Lindgrens Gata6 SE 42131, Gothenburg, Sweden.

Hoslab, PO Box 25, Baxter Road, Ilford, Essex IG1 2HQ, UK.

Hybaid

Hybaid National Labnet Corp., PO Box 841, Woodbridge, NJ 07095, USA.
Hybaid Ltd, Action Court, Ashford Road, Ashford, Middlesex TW15 1XB, UK.
Hybaid Ltd, 111-113 Waldegrave Road, Teddington, Middlesex TW11 8LL, UK.
Tel: 01784 425000   Fax: 01784 248085
URL: http://www.hybaid.com
Hybaid US, 8 East Forge Parkway, Franklin, MA 02038, USA.   Tel: 001 508 541 6918
Fax: 001 508 541 3041
URL: http://www.hybaid.com

Hyclone

Hyclone Europe Ltd (formerly Northumbria Biologicals Ltd), Unit 9, Atley Way, North Nelson Industrial Estate, Cramlington, Northumberland NE23 9WA, UK
HyClone Laboratories, 1725 South HyClone Road, Logan, UT 84321, USA.
Tel: 001 435 753 4584
Fax: 001 435 753 4589
URL: http://www.hyclone.com

IBF Biotechnics, 35 Avenue Jean Jaures, 92390 Villeneuve La Garenne, France.

ICN

ICN, Unit 18, Thames Business Park,Wenman Road, Thame, Oxfordshire OX9 3XA, UK.
ICN Pharmaceuticals Inc., Biomedicals Products Division, 3300 Hyland Avenue, Costa Mesa, CA 92626, USA.

IEC

IEC, Unit 7, Lawrence Way, Brewers Hill Road, Dunstable, Bedfordshire LU6 1BD, UK.
IEC, 300 Second Avenue, Needham Heights, MA 02194, USA.

Imperial Laboratories (Europe) Ltd, West Portway, Andover, Hampshire SP10 3LF, UK.

International Biotechnologies Inc., 25 Science Park, New Haven, Connecticut 06535, USA.

Invitrogen

Invitrogen BV, PO Box 2312, 9704 CH Groningen, The Netherlands.
Tel: 00800 5345 5345
Fax: 00800 7890 7890
URL: http://www.invitrogen.com
Invitrogen Corp., 3985 B Sorrenton Valley Building, San Diego, CA 92121, USA.
Invitrogen Corp., 1600 Faraday Avenue, Carlsbad, CA 92008, USA.
Tel: 001 760 603 7200
Fax: 001 760 603 7201
URL: http://www.invitrogen.com
Invitrogen Cor., c/o British Biotechnology Products Ltd, 4-20 The Quadrant, Barton Lane, Abingdon, Oxfordshire OX14 3YS, UK.

Irvine Scientific, Santa Ana, CA 92705, USA.

Jencons Scientific Ltd, Cherrycourt Way Industrial Estate, Stanbridge Road, Leighton Buzzard, Bedfordshire LU7 8UA, UK.

Jouan

Jouan, rue Bobby Sands CP 3203, 44805 Saint-Herblain Cedex, France.
Jouan Inc., 110-B Industrial Drive, Winchester, VA 22602, USA.
Jouan Ltd, Merlin Way, Quarry Hill Road, Ilkeston, Derby DE7 4RA, UK.

Kyowa Hakko UK Ltd, 258 Bath Road, Slough SL1 4DX, UK.

Leec Ltd, Private Road No 7, Colwick Industrial Estate, Nottingham NG4 2AJ, UK.

Leica

Leica Microsystems Imaging Solutions Ltd, Clifton Road, Cambridge CB1 3QH, UK.
Leica UK Ltd, Davy Avenue, Knowlhill, Milton Keynes MK5 8LB, UK.

Leo Laboratories Ltd, Longwick Road, Princes Risborough, Buckinghamshire, HP27 9RR, UK.

Life Technologies

Life Technologies Inc., 8451 Helgerman Court, Gaithersburg, MN 20877, USA.
Life Technologies Inc., 9800 Medical Center Drive, Rockville, MD 20850, USA.
Tel: 001 301 610 8000
URL: http://www.lifetech.com
Life Technologies Ltd, PO Box 35, Free Fountain Drive, Incsinnan Business Park, Paisley PA4 9RF, UK.
Tel: 0800 269210   Fax: 0800 838380
URL: http://www.lifetech.com

LIP Equipment and Services Ltd, Dockfield Road, Shipley, W Yorkshire BD17 7SJ, UK.

LKB

LKB Instruments Ltd, LKB House, 232 Addington Road, Selsdon, South Croydon, Surrey CR2 8YD, UK.
LKB Instruments, 9319 Gaither Road, Gaithersburgh, MD 20877, USA.

MDH Ltd. (Microflow), Walworth Road, Andover, Hampshire SP10 5AA, UK.

Medical Air Technology Ltd, Wilton Street, Denton, Manchester M 34 3LZ, UK.

Merck
Merck, Frankfurter Strasse, 250, Postfach 4119, D–64293, Germany.
Merck Industries Inc., 5 Skyline Drive, Nawthorne, NY 10532, USA.
Merck Ltd (BDH), Hunter Boulevard, Magna Park, Lutterworth, Leicestershire LE17 9XN, UK.
Merck UK Ltd, Customer Service Centre, Magna Park, Lutterworth LE17 4XN, UK.
Tel: 0800 223344

Merck Sharp & Dohme
Merck Sharp & Dohme Research Laboratories, Neuroscience Research Centre, Terlings Park, Harlow, Essex CM20 2QR, UK.
URL: http://www.msd-nrc.co.uk
MSD Sharp and Dohme GmbH, Lindenplatz 1, D–85540, Haar, Germany.
URL: http://www.msd-deutschland.com

Metachem Diagnostics Ltd, 29 Forest Road, Piddington, Northampton NN7 2DA, UK.

MetaSystems GmbH, Robert Bosch Str. 6, D-68804 Altlussheim, Germany.
Tel: 00 49 6205 39610
Fax: 00 49 6205 32270

Michrom BioResources, Inc., 5673 W. Las Positas Boulevard, Suite 291, Pleasanton, CA 94566, USA.

Millipore
Millipore Corp., 80 Ashby Road, Bedford, MA 01730, USA.
Tel: 001 800 645 5476
Fax: 001 800 645 5439
URL: http://www.millipore.com
Millipore (UK) Ltd, The Boulevard, Blackmoor Lane, Watford, Hertfordshire WD1 8YW, UK.
Tel: 01923 816375   Fax: 01923 818297
URL: http://www.millipore.com/local/UK.htm

Molecular Probes
URL: http://www.probes.com/
Molecular Probes, Inc., 4849 Pitchford Avenue, Eugene, OR, 97402-9165, USA

Murex Biotech Ltd, Central Road, Temple Hill, Dartford, Kent DA1 5LR, UK.

New England Biolabs (NBL)
New England Biolabs (NBL), 32 Tozer Road, Beverley, MA 01915-5510, USA.
Tel: 001 978 927 5054
New England Biolabs (NBL), c/o CP Labs Ltd, P.O. Box 22, Bishops Stortford, Hertfordshire CM23 3DH, UK.

Nikon
Nikon Corp., Fuji Building, 2-3, 3-chome, Marunouchi, Chiyoda-ku, Tokyo 100, Japan.
Tel: 00813 3214 5311
Fax: 00813 3201 5856
URL: http://www.nikon.co.jp/main/index_e.htm
Nikon Inc., 1300 Walt Whitman Road, Melville, NY 11747-3064, USA.
Tel: 001 516 547 4200
Fax: 001 516 547 0299
URL: http://www.nikonusa.com
Nikon UK Ltd, Instruments Division, Nikon House, 380 Richmond Road, Kingston Upon Thames, Surrey KT2 5PR, UK.

North East Laboratory Supplies, 7 Cumbie Way, Aycliffe Industrial Estate, Newton Aycliffe, Co. Durham DL5 6YA, UK
Tel: 01325 301320

Novex, 11040 Roselle Street, San Diego, California, 92121 USA.
URL: http://www.novex.com/

Nunc A/S, Kamstruprej 90, Postbox 280, DK–4000, Denmark.

Nycomed
Nycomed Amersham, 101 Carnegie Center, Princeton, NJ 08540, USA.
Tel: 001 609 514 6000
URL: http://www.amersham.co.uk

Nycomed Amersham plc, Amersham Place, Little Chalfont, Buckinghamshire HP7 9NA, UK.
Tel: 01494 544000   Fax: 01494 542266
URL: http://www.amersham.co.uk

Oncor
Oncor Inc., 209 Perry Parkway, Gaithersburgh, MD 20877, USA.
Oncor Instrument Systems, 9581 Ridgehaven Court, San Diego, CA 92123, USA.

Optivision (Yorkshire) Ltd, Ahed House, Dewsbury Road, Ossett, W. Yorkshire WF5 9ND, UK.

Perkin-Elmer
Perkin-Elmer Ltd, Maxwell Road. Beaconsfield, Buckinghamshire HP9 1QA, UK.
Perkin Elmer Ltd, Post Office Lane, Beaconsfield, Buckinghamshire HP9 1QA, UK.
Tel: 01494 676161
URL: http://www.perkin-elmer.com
Perkin Elmer-Cetus (The Perkin-Elmer Corporation), 761 Main Avenue, Norwalk, CT 0689, USA.

Perseptive Biosystems, Inc., 500 Old Connecticut Path, Framingham, MA 01701, USA.
URL: http://www.pbio.com/

Pharmacia (please see also Amersham Pharmacia Bio Tech)
Pharmacia Biosystems Ltd, (Biotechnology Division), Davy Avenue, Knowlhill, Milton Keynes MK5 8PH, UK.
Pharmacia Biotech Europe, Procordia EuroCentre, Rue de la Fuse-e 62, B–1130 Brussells, Belgium.
Pharmacia LKB Biotechnology AB, Bjorngatan 30, S–75182 Uppsala, Sweden.

Phenomenex, 2320 W. 205th Street, Torrance, CA 90501-1456, USA.

Pierce, PO Box 117, Rockford, IL 61105, USA.
URL: http://www.piercenet.com/

Polysciences Inc., Warrington, PA 18976-2590, USA.

PolyLC Inc., 9151 Rumsey Road, Suite 180, Columbia, MD 21045, USA.
E-mail: polylc@aol.com

Promega
Promega Corp., 2800 Woods Hollow Road, Madison, WI 53711-5399, USA.
Tel: 001 608 274 4330
Fax: 001 608 277 2516
URL: http://www.promega.com
Promega UK Ltd, Delta House, Chilworth Research Centre, Southampton SO16 7NS, UK.
Tel: 0800 378994   Fax: 0800 181037
URL: http://www.promega.com

Protana A/S, Staermosegaardsvej 16, DK–5230 Odense M, Denmark

PSI (Perceptive Scientific International Ltd)
PSI, Halladale, Lakeside, Chester Business Park, Wrexham Road, Chester, Cheshire CH4 9QT, UK.
PSI, 2525 South Shore Boulevard, Ste 100, League City, TX 77573, USA.

Qiagen
Qiagen Inc., 28159 Avenue Stanford, Valencia, CA 91355, USA.
Tel: 001 800 426 8157
Fax: 001 800 718 2056
URL: http://www.qiagen.com
Qiagen Inc., c/o Hybaid, 111–113 Waldegrave Road, Teddington, Middlesex, TW11 8LL, UK.
Qiagen Inc., 9259 Eton Avenue, Chatsworth, CA 91311, USA.
Qiagen UK Ltd, Boundary Court, Gatwick Road, Crawley, West Sussex RH10 2AX, UK.
Tel: 01293 422911   Fax: 01293 422922
URL: http://www.qiagen.com

Raymond A. Lamb Ltd, Units 4 and 5, Parkview Industrial Estate, Alder Close, Lottbridge Drove, Eastbourne, East Sussex BN23 6QE.
Tel: 01323 737000   Fax: 01323 733000

Roche Diagnostics

Roche Diagnostics Corp., 9115 Hague Road, PO Box 50457, Indianapolis, IN 46256, USA.
Tel: 001 317 845 2358
Fax: 001 317 576 2126
URL: http://www.roche.com
Roche Diagnostics GmbH, Sandhoferstrasse 116, D–68305 Mannheim, Germany.
Tel: 0049 621 759 4747
Fax: 0049 621 759 4002
URL: http://www.roche.com
Roche Diagnostics Ltd, Bell Lane, Lewes, East Sussex BN7 1LG, UK.
Tel: 01273 484644   Fax: 01273 480266
URL: http://www.roche.com

Schleicher and Schuell

Schleicher and Schuell Inc., Keene, NH 03431A, USA.
Tel: 001 603 357 2398
Schleicher and Schuell Inc., D–3354 Dassel, Germany.

Scotlab Ltd, Kirkshaws Road, Coatbridge, Lanarkshire ML 8AD, UK.

Shandon Scientific Ltd, 93-96 Chadwick Road, Astmoor, Runcorn, Cheshire WA7 1PR, UK.
Tel: 01928 566611
URL: http://www.shandon.com

Sigma-Aldrich

Sigma-Aldrich Chemie GmbH, Reidstrasse 2, D-89555 Steinheim, Germany
Sigma-Aldrich Co. Ltd, The Old Brickyard, New Road, Gillingham, Dorset XP8 4XT, UK.
Tel: 01747 822211   Fax: 01747 823779
URL: http://www.sigma-aldrich.com
Sigma-Aldrich Co. Ltd, Fancy Road, Poole, Dorset BH12 4QH, UK.
Tel: 01202 722114   Fax: 01202 715460
URL: http://www.sigma-aldrich.com

Sigma Chemical Co., PO Box 14508, St Louis, MO 63178, USA.
Tel: 001 314 771 5765
Fax: 001 314 771 5757
URL: http://www.sigma-aldrich.com

Stratagene

Stratagene Europe, Gebouw California, Hogehilweg 15, 1101 CB Amsterdam Zuidoost, The Netherlands.
Tel: 00800 9100 9100
URL: http://www.stratagene.com
Stratagene Inc., 11011 North Torrey Pines Road, La Jolla, CA 92037, USA.
Tel: 001 858 535 5400
URL: http://www.stratagene.com
Stratagene Ltd, Unit 140, Cambridge Innovation Centre, Milton Road, Cambridge CB4 4FG, UK.

Techne (Cambridge) Ltd, Duxford, Cambridge CB2 4PZ.
Tel: 01223 832401
Fax: 01223 836838

Technicon Instruments Ltd, Evans House, Hamilton Close, Basingstoke, Hampshire RG21 2YE, UK.

Thermoquest Scientific Equipment Group Ltd, Unit 5, The Ringway Centre, Edison Road, Basingstoke, Hampshire RG21 6YH.
Tel: 01256 817282
Fax: 01256 817292

Ultraviolet Products, Unit 1, Trinity Hall Farm Estate, Nuffield Road, Cambridge CB4 1TG
Tel: 01223 420022
Fax:01223 420561

Unipath Ltd, Basingstoke, Hampshire, UK.

United States Biochemical, PO Box 22400, Cleveland, OH 44122, USA.
Tel: 001 216 464 9277

Vector Laboratories

Vector Laboratories, 16 Wulfric Square, Bretton, Peterborough PE3 8RF, UK.
Vector Laboratories Inc., 30 Ingold Road, Burlingame, CA 91010, USA.

Vydac/The Separations Group, Inc., 17434 Mojave Street, Hesperia, CA 92345 USA.
URL: http://www.vydac.com/

Vysis

Vysis Inc., 3100 Woodcreek Drive, Downers Grove, IL 60515-5400, USA.

Vysis GmbH, Vor dem Lauch 25, D–70567 Stuttgart-Fasanenhof, Germany.

Vysis (UK) Ltd, Rosedale House, Rosedale Road, Richmond, Surrey TW9 2SZ, UK.

Wako Chemicals USA Inc., BioProducts Division, 1600 Bellwood Road., Richmond, VA 23237, USA.
URL: http://www.wako-chem.co.jp

Wellcome Reagents, Langley Court, Beckenham, Kent BR3 3BS, UK.

Whatman

Whatman International Ltd, Springfield Mill, James Whatman Way, Maidstone, Kent ME14 2LE, UK.

Whatman International Inc., 9 Bridewell Place, Clifton, NJ 07014, UK.

Don Whitley Scientific Ltd, 14 Otley Road, Shipley, West Yorkshire BD17 7SE, UK.

Carl Zeiss

Carl Zeiss Inc., Microscope Division, 1 Zeiss Drive, Thornwood, NY 10594, USA.

Carl Zeiss Ltd, PO Box 78, Woodfield Road, Welwyn Garden City, Hertfordshire AL7 1LU, UK.

Appendix 2
Safety considerations

Introduction

It is essential that the cytogeneticist be fully trained in all aspects of safety in the laboratory. This must include a basic awareness and understanding of potential hazards, namely pathological (samples), chemical (reagents) and physical (equipment), as well as safety procedures to minimize both the occurrence and the consequences of accidents. Written procedures for storage, safe handling, disposal, spillage and correct use of equipment must be available in the laboratory, as well as copies of appropriate local health and safety regulations for reference. *Croner's Laboratory Manager* (1) is a useful source of information.

It is beyond the scope of this book to deal with this topic in any great detail, but the following information gives a brief overview of basic safety considerations for the cytogeneticist. It is assumed that general safety regulations, such as forbiddance of eating, drinking and smoking in the laboratory, as well as accident procedure and record-keeping, are already in place.

Personal protective equipment

All cytogenetic procedures involve the use of unfixed human tissues and/or hazardous reagents, therefore, a fully fastened protective laboratory coat must be worn at all times. Likewise, disposable latex or nitrile gloves (as appropriate for the substance being handled) must be worn for all handling procedures. Facemasks, goggles, plastic aprons and oversleeves must be available for the handling of those reagents which are of particularly high risk (e.g. clastogens).

Safety cabinets

Two types of safety cabinet are essential for cytogenetic work: the fume hood (for hazardous reagents) and the microbiological safety cabinet (for containment of potentially infective pathogenic material).

Reagents

Throughout this book, attention is drawn to hazardous reagents in protocols, with a brief cautionary footnote as to the nature of the hazard. These footnotes are by no means a comprehensive summary of all known hazards associated with that reagent, nor does the absence of a cautionary note imply that a reagent is of no hazard whatsoever. Rather, the cautions are for guidance only and the reader is urged to check material safety data sheets issued by suppliers as well as any other available information (companies such as Sigma provide this information via their website). Most reagents are now designated with 'Risk phrases' (R numbers) to indicate hazards, and Safety phrases (S numbers) to indicate precautions. Disposal of chemicals and reagents must be in accordance with local regulations (see ref. 2 for more information).

Equipment

All equipment must be used in accordance with the manufacturers instructions, and regularly serviced where appropriate. Care must be taken when siting some equipment, e.g. placement of safety cabinets to avoid cross-interference, spacing of centrifuges.

Specimens and live cultures

Unfixed human tissues may harbour potentially infective pathogens, and must therefore be handled in a microbiological safety cabinet which provides some protection to the operator. A Class 1 cabinet will provide adequate protection from samples of moderate risk to the operator, but is not designed to ensure sterility of the culture (these may be used for short-term cultures such as blood and bone marrow). Class 2 cabinets provide adequate protection from samples of moderate risk to the operator as well as a sterile environment for the culture, and are therefore favoured for long-term culturing (such as from tumours). Samples of known high-risk may require a Class 3 cabinet, which provides full protection to the operator. Local safety regulations must apply according to the pathogen involved; ref. 3 is a useful source of information.

It must be remembered that patients suffering from malignant disorders are often immunocompromised, and thus particularly susceptible to pathological infection which is potentially hazardous to staff handling samples.

Disposal of unfixed material such as surplus sample, supernatants, cultures, etc., must be into a disinfectant approved by local regulation. In most cases, overnight disinfection in a 5% sodium hypochlorite solution is suitable, although some laboratories use proprietary disinfectants such as Virkon. It is vital that disposal, and spillage containment procedures are properly approved by the hospital or company housing the cytogenetic laboratory, and that incineration facilities are available where appropriate.

General considerations

Avoidance of glass and needles

A primary route of infection with pathogens is through an open wound. For this reason, it is essential in the cytogenetics laboratory to minimize the use of glass and needles. Disposable plastic culture vessels, pipettes and 'quills' are widely available and are adequate substitutes for glass and needles in most cases. Where 'sharps' have to be used, such as blades for mincing tissue, these must be disposed of in an appropriate container prior to incineration.

Pregnant women

A number of reagents used in the cytogenetics laboratory are of particular risk to pregnant women. It is essential that all procedures are evaluated for such risk so that they are rendered safe for the unknowingly pregnant, by means of adequate precautionary technique and full compliance on the part of staff.

References

1. Croner (1997). *Croner's Laboratory Manager* Croner Publications Ltd., Kingson-upon-Thames.
2. HMSO (1988). *Control of substances hazardous to health regulations (COSHH).* HMSO, London.
3. HMSO (1987). *Code of practice for the prevention of infection in clinical laboratories and post-mortem rooms.* HMSO, London.

Appendix 3
Ideograms of G-banded chromosomes at three levels of resolution

Ideograms of G-banded chromosomes adapted from ISCN (1995) An International System for Human Cytogenetic Nomenclature, ed: Mitelman, F. S. Karger, Basel, by B. Czepulkowski, Cytogenetics Department, Leukaemia Science Laboratories, The Rayne Institute, London. Each chromosome is depicted at the 400, 500 and 550–850 band per haploid set level (from left to right).

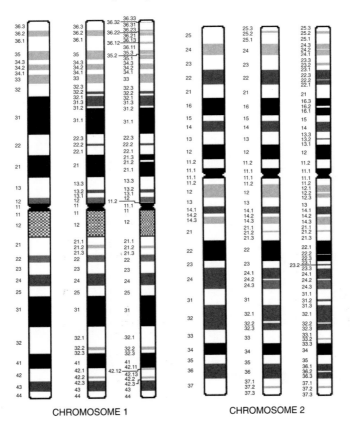

CHROMOSOME 1   CHROMOSOME 2

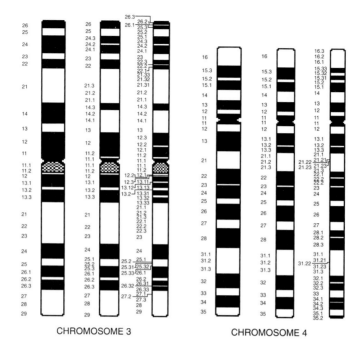

CHROMOSOME 3

CHROMOSOME 4

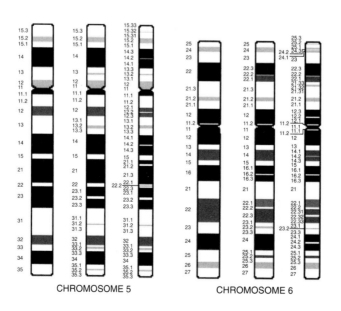

CHROMOSOME 5

CHROMOSOME 6

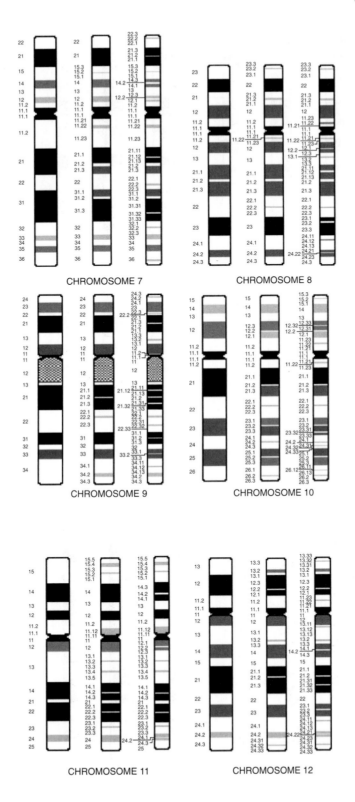

CHROMOSOME 7

CHROMOSOME 8

CHROMOSOME 9

CHROMOSOME 10

CHROMOSOME 11

CHROMOSOME 12

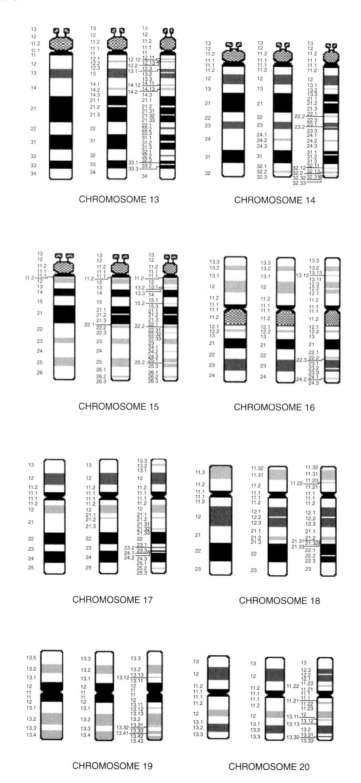

CHROMOSOME 13

CHROMOSOME 14

CHROMOSOME 15

CHROMOSOME 16

CHROMOSOME 17

CHROMOSOME 18

CHROMOSOME 19

CHROMOSOME 20

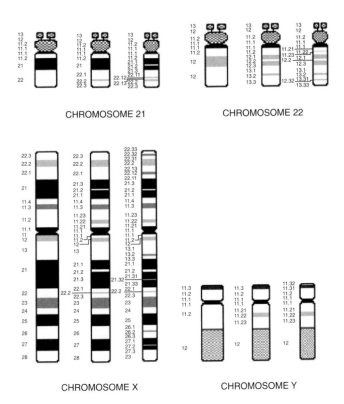

CHROMOSOME 21

CHROMOSOME 22

CHROMOSOME X

CHROMOSOME Y

Appendix 4
Glossary

This glossary was compiled by B. Czepulkowski, Cytogenetics Department, Leukaemia Science Laboratories, The Rayne Institute, London.

acute lymphoblastic leukaemia (ALL)—A progressive malignant disease characterized by large numbers of immature cells of the lymphoid series in bone marrow, peripheral blood and lymph node, spleen, and other organs

acute myeloid leukaemia (AML)—A malignant neoplasm of blood-forming tissues characterized by uncontrolled proliferation of immature cells of myeloid lineage

acute non-lymphoblastic leukaemia (ANNL)—Any leukaemia that is not of lymphoid origin; synonymous with acute myeloid leukaemia.

acute promyelocytic leukaemia (APML)—Malignancy of blood forming tissues, characterized by bleeding, scattered bruises, and proliferation of promyelocytes in bone marrow.

adenocarcinoma—Any of a large group of malignant epithelial cell tumours of the glands.

anaemia—A decrease in haemoglobin concentration in blood below the normal range. It reflects either a decrease in haemoglobin or red cell production, an increase in red cell destruction or blood loss.

aplasia—A lack of development of organ or tissue, or the cellular products of the organ or tissue.

aplastic anaemia—A deficiency of all formed elements of the blood representing a failure of the cell generating capacity of the bone marrow.

ascites—An abnormal intraperitoneal accumulation of a fluid containing large amounts of protein and electrolytes. It is a complication of cirrhosis, congestive heart failure, nephrosis, malignant diseases, peritonitis, or various fungal and parasitic diseases.

Auer rod—Abnormal, needle shaped, pink-staining inclusion in the cytoplasm of myeloblasts and promyelocytes, which contain enzymes and represent abnormal derivatives of cytoplasmic granules.

basophil—A granulocyte characterized by a segmented nucleus and cytoplasmic granules, which stain purple when exposed to a basic dye. Represents 1% or less of the total white blood cell count. Basophil numbers increase in MPD.

B cell (or B lymphocyte)—A type of lymphocyte that expresses monoclonal immunoglobulin on its surface and differentiates into plasma cells upon suitable antigenic stimulation.

benign—A tumour or condition which is not malignant.

B-lineage—B lymphocytes and their precursors.

blast cell—An immature cell which is a leukocyte precursor, e.g. lymphoblast, myeloblast.

Budd-Chiari syndrome—A disorder of hepatic circulation marked by venous obstruction, leading to liver enlargement and severe portal hypertension.

Burkitt's lymphoma—A malignant neoplasm common in African children, composed of mature B cells with distinct cytological features. The Epstein–Barr virus is one of the aetiological factors in the development of this lymphoma.

carcinoma—A malignant epithelial neoplasm that tends to invade the surrounding tissues and metastasize to distant regions of the body.

chronic granulocytic leukaemia (CGL)—A malignant neoplasm of the blood-forming tissues characterized by proliferation of cells of granulocytic lineage (e.g. neutrophils, basophils and usually eosinophils) and also megakaryocytes. More frequent in older patients.

chronic lymphocytic leukaemia (CLL)—A neoplasm of the blood-forming tissues characterized by the proliferation of small, long-lived lymphocytes of B lineage. Neoplastic cells are present in the bone marrow, blood, liver, spleen, and lymph nodes. It is rare under the age of 55 years and is more common in men than women.

chronic myeloid leukaemia (CML)—A malignant neoplasm of the blood forming tissues characterized by proliferation of cells of the granulocytic lineage with or without monocyte or megakaryocyte proliferation. The term is sometimes used as a synonym for CGL (see above) and sometimes more broadly.

differentiation—The process whereby a cell becomes committed to a certain lineage, also used more loosely to imply maturation.

di Guglielmo's disease—see erythroleukaemia.

disseminated intravascular coagulation (DIC)—A grave coagulopathy caused by over-stimulation of the body's clotting and fibrinolytic processes in response to disease or injury. Observed in APML.

eosinophil—A granulocyte, larger than a neutrophil, with a bilobed nucleus and coarse cytoplasmic granules that stain intensely with the acid dye eosin. They constitute 1–3% of the white blood cells.

eosinophilia—An increase in the number of eosinophils in the blood, accompanying many inflammatory and some malignant conditions.

Epstein-Barr virus (EBV)—The herpes virus that causes infectious mononucleosis.

erythrocyte—Major cellular element of the circulating blood; the red blood cell, which transports oxygen.

erythrocyte sedimentation rate (ESR)—The rate at which red cells settle out in a tube of anti coagulated blood. A high ESR indicates usually inflammation, but this test can also be used to indicate the presence of a tumour.

erythrocytosis—An abnormal increase in the number of circulating red blood cells.

erythroleukaemia—A malignant blood disorder characterized by proliferation of erythropoietic elements in the bone marrow The disease can have an acute or chronic course.

erythropoiesis—The process of erythrocyte production.

essential thrombocythaemia (ET)—Thrombocytosis consequent on neoplastic proliferation of megakaryocyte precursors.

Ewing's sarcoma—A malignant tumour developing from the bone marrow, usually arising in the long bones or pelvis. Most frequent in adolescent boys.

Fanconi anaemia—The commonest inherited form of aplastic anaemia.

follicular lymphoma—A nodular well differentiated lymphocytic malignant lymphoma, where neoplastic cells form follicles and distort the structure of the lymph node.

grade—An expression of the degree of malignancy of a tumour, high grade being more aggressive than low grade.

graft-versus-host-disease (GVHD)—An immune response directed at host tissues occurring when incompatible immunocompetent cells (for example, lymphocytes in bone marrow) are engrafted.

granulocyte—One of the leukocyte types, characterized by the presence of cytoplasmic granules, e.g. basophil, eosinophil, neutrophil.

granulocytopenia—A decrease in the total number of granulocytes.

hairy cell leukaemia (HCL)—A rare neoplasm of the blood-forming tissues characterized by pancytopenia, large spleen, and the presence in the blood and bone marrow of abnormal B-lineage lymphocytes with many fine projections on their surface, giving rise to the name of the disease. It is much more frequent in men, usually at about age 50 years or older.

haemopoiesis—The production of all types of blood cells.

haemostasis—The termination of bleeding by mechanical or chemical means or by the coagulation process of the body.

hepatomegaly—Enlargement of the liver, which can be caused by hepatitis or other infections, biliary obstruction or malignancy.

hepatosplenomegaly—Enlargement of both the liver and spleen.

histiocyte—See macrophage.

Hodgkin's disease—A malignant disorder characterized by progressive enlargement of lymphoid tissue, plenomegaly, and the presence of Reed–Sternberg cells (atypical cells, usually of B lineage, with multiple or hyperlobulated nuclei containing prominent nucleoli.

idiopathic thrombocytopenic purpura (ITP)—Bleeding into the skin and other organs owing to platelet deficiency consequent on increased destruction of platelets; although often designated 'ideopathic' it is actually autoimmune in nature.

leukaemia—A malignant neoplasm of the blood-forming organs characterized by diffuse replacement of bone marrow with leukocyte precursors; immature and abnormal white cells may also be present in the circulation and other tissues.

leukaemoid reaction—Clinical syndrome resembling leukaemia in which the white cell count is raised in response to allergy, inflammation, infection or haemorrhage.

leukocyte—White blood cell. There are five types classified according to cytological features: (a) mononuclear cells (lymphocytes and monocytes), (b) granulocytes (neutrophils, basophils and eosinophils).

leukocytosis—Increase in the number of circulating white blood cells.

leukopenia—Decrease in the number of circulating white blood cells.

lymph node—Small oval structures in the lymphatic system composed mainly of T and B lymphocytes. Lymph nodes filter lymph and mount an immune response to antigenic stimuli.

lymphocyte—A leukocyte with predominantly agranular cytoplasm originating in the bone marrow or thymus, B, T, and NK cells. They normally comprise 25% of the total white cell count, but increase in response to infection.

lymphocytopenia—Decreased number of circulating lymphocytes.

lymphocytosis—Increased number of circulating lymphocytes.

lymphoma—A neoplasm of lymphoid tissue. Various lymphomas differ in the degree of cellular differentiation and content.

macrocytic anaemia—Blood disorder characterized by impaired erythropoiesis and presence of red blood cells that are larger than normal.

macrophage—Phagocytic cell of the reticulo-endothelial system derived from a peripheral blood monocyte, synonymous with histiocyte.

malignant—Tending to become worse, causing death. Describes a cancer that is metastatic and tending to recur even upon removal of the tumour tissue.

maturation—The process by which a cell acquires characteristics of a more mature, or end stage in any given lineage.

mean corpuscular volume (MCV)—Evaluation of volume of red cells, derived from the ratio of volume of packed red cells to total number.

megakaryocyte—Bone marrow cell which produces platelets and releases them into the circulating blood.

megaloblast—Abnormally large nucleated immature erythroid precursor showing nuclear maturation that is retarded in relation to cytoplasmic maturation.

megaloblastic anaemia—Blood disorder characterized by anaemia and megaloblastic erythropoiesis.

melanoma—A group of malignant neoplasms, primarily of skin, that are composed of melanocytes.

metastasis—The process by which tumour cells are spread to other parts of the body.

monoclonal antibody—An antibody produced by a single clone of cells, usually a hybridoma.

monocyte—Large mononuclear leukocytes with an ovoid or kidney-shaped nucleus.

monocytic leukaemia—Malignancy of blood-forming tissues where the predominant cells are monocytes and their precursors.

monocytosis—Increase in the number of circulating monocytes.

mononucleosis—Abnormal increase of mononuclear leukocytes in the blood; usually refers to infectious mononucleosis in which the abnormal cells are highly abnormal lymphocytes mainly of T cell lineage.

multiple myeloma—Plasma cell neoplasm which characteristically causes osteolytic bone lesions

mycosis fungoides—Rare chronic cutaneous lymphoma resembling eczema or a cutaneous tumour.

myeloblast—The earlier morphologically recognizable precursor of granulocytes.

myelocyte—Immature white blood cell, more mature than a promyelocyte, which can be identified as belonging to the basophil, neutrophil of eosinophil lineage. Normally found in the bone marrow.

myelodyplastic syndromes (MDS)—A group of bone marrow diseases characterized by dysplastic (morphologically abnormal) and ineffective haemopoiesis, consequent on replacement of normal polyclonal haemopoietic cells by a neoplastic clone of cells showing abnormalities of proliferation and maturation.

myeloproliferative disorders (MPD)—A group of conditions characterized by increased effective proliferation of one or more haemopoietic components of the bone marrow, and in some cases the liver and the spleen.

necrosis—Localized tissue death that occurs in groups of cells in response to disease or injury.

neoplasia—The process in which a genetically altered precursor cell gives rise to an abnormal clone of cells which show abnormality in proliferation and maturation. Neoplasms vary in their degree of abnormality leading to clinical features, which allow them to be classified as benign or malignant.

neuroblastoma—Highly malignant tumour composed of primitive neuro-ectodermal cells derived from the neural plate. May originate in any part of the sympathetic nervous system but most common in the adrenal medulla of young children.

neutropenia—Decrease in the number of circulating neutrophils. Associated with acute leukaemia or any condition where normally functioning bone marrow is replaced by abnormal cells.

neutrophil—A polymorphonuclear granular leukocyte, the granules of which stain easily with a mixture of basic and acidic dyes. They are essential for phagocytosis and proteolysis.

normoblast—Nucleated precursor cell of the circulating erythrocyte. After extrusion of the nucleus from the normoblast, the young erythrocyte becomes known as a reticulocyte.

oncogene—A gene which is important in initiating or sustaining the process of neoplasia.

pancytopenia—Abnormal condition characterized by marked reduction in all major cellular elements of the blood, red cells, white cells and platelets.

petechiae—Tiny purple or red spots that appear on the skin owing to minute haemorrhages within the dermis.

plasma cell—The most mature cell in the B-lymphocyte lineage capable of secreting antibody.

platelet—Smallest cells of the blood; they are anuclear and essential for normal haemostasis.

polycythaemia—Abnormal increase in the number of erythrocytes in the blood.

polycythemia rubra vera (PRV)—Polycythemia consequent on neoplastic proliferation of red cell precursors.

prevalence—The number of cases of a given condition present in a defined population at a point in time, e.g. 1 per 1 000.

prognosis—The expected outcome of a disease.

promyelocyte—Granulocytic precursor, more mature than a myeloblast but less mature than a myelocyte.

purpura—haemorrhage into the skin or mucous membranes, often consequent on thrombocytopenia.

Reed-Sternberg cells—Neoplastic cell, usually of B lineage, occurring in Hodgkin's disease. Number and proportion of the cells are a basis for the histological classification of Hodgkin's disease.

remission—A state in which all detectable evidence of neoplasm has disappeared.

reticulocyte—Immature erythrocyte with mesh like pattern of threads and particles composed of RNA, apparent on staining with certain dyes. Usually make up only 1–2% of circulating erythrocytes.

retinoblastoma—Neoplasm developing from the retinal germ cells which is often congenital and hereditary. It is the most common malignancy of the eye in childhood.

rhabdomyosarcoma—Malignant tumour of muscle cells.

secondary leukaemia—Leukaemia attributable at least in part to prior radiotherapy, chemotherapy or exposure to other identifiable mutagens.

sideroblastic anaemia—Anaemia characterized by the presence of abnormal ring sideroblasts in the bone marrow; these are erythroblasts with an abnormal ring of iron-containing granules around the nucleus. May be secondary (e.g. to certain drugs) and reversible, or a manifestation of MDS.

splenomegaly—Enlargement of the spleen.

Stage—An expression of the extent of anatomical spread of a tumour. Tumours are often staged from Stage I (localized) to Stage IV (widely disseminated).

systemic lupus erythematosus (SLE)—Chronic inflammatory disease affecting many systems of the body. Symptoms and signs include arthritis, erythematous rash, weakness, fatigue, and weight loss.

T cell (or T lymphocyte)—A lymphocyte involved in cell-mediated immunity, the maturation of which is influenced in the thymus. Mature T cells express antigenic structures on their surface which are detected by certain monoclonal antibodies and enable them to form rosettes with sheep red blood cells.

thrombocytopenia—Reduction in the number of circulating platelets, usually due either to reduced production in the bone marrow or to increased destruction in the blood.

thrombocytopenic purpura—A bleeding disorder characterized by a decrease in the number of platelets resulting in multiple bruises, petechiae, and haemorrhage into the tissues.

thrombocytosis—Increase in the number of circulating platelets in blood (see also essential thrombocythaemia, ET).

T-lineage—T cells and their precursors.

tumour—A neoplasm growing as a discrete mass of neoplastic tissue.

Wilm's tumour—A malignant neoplasm of the kidney, in most cases occurring in young children under 5 years old.

Index